The Perennial Quest for a Psychology with a Soul

The Perennial Quest for a Psychology with a Soul

Dr. Joseph Vrinte

MLBD PUBLICATIONS

Motilal Banarsidass Publications

MOTILAL BANARSIDASS
PUBLICATIONS
4741/23, Ansari Road, Daryaganj, New Delhi - 110002 (India)
Email: mlbd@mlbd.com | sales@mlbd.com | exports@mlbd.com
Website: www.mlbd.com

The Perennial Quest for a Psychology with a Soul
by
Dr. Joseph Vrinte

First Edition Published in 2023

Published in India by Motilal Banarsidass Publications

ISBN : 978-93-91759-40-7 (HB)

Printed and bound in India

To all those Aurobindonians and
Wilberians who agree that the integral
systems of Sri Aurobindo and
Ken Wilber are not complete.

Preface

This book is offered as an explorer's source book in the mapping of various psychological problems inherent in Sri Aurobindo's integral sadhana and Ken Wilber's integral psychology. The purpose of this book is not to extol or decry one of the two integral thinkers at the cost of the other. This comparative study, therefore, does not aim at setting one approach against the other, but at showing how the two could be complementary in spiritual psychology and human nature.

There are possible dangers in working with spiritual and psychological domains simultaneously and the various pitfalls are extensively elaborated in this book, because knowing about them can lessen the dangers. However, in this attempt at clarification of the different problems related to Sri Aurobindo's and Ken Wilber's visions, the clarification itself does not constitute a solution to the problems involved in their models.

A few preliminary questions may be helpful in order to avoid certain confusions. Are Ken Wilber's and Sri Aurobindo's integral views simply two parallel approaches aiming at the same end but are they using a different language, or do they have the same ideas about developmental areas, but differ in their concept of growth? Are there many pitfalls in prematurely trying to juxtapose the two approaches and are they two separate directions in which human life is moving? If Yes, are the divergences essentially a matter of terminology, or do the differences affect a genuine plurality of problems?

This comparison does not magnify differences without

acknowledging the overlap in issues, as both theories share considerable common ground. Nevertheless, it is not the author's intention to adapt Sri Aurobindo's metaphysical Yoga psychology to Ken Wilber's integral psychology, even though it seems that there are some important insights that are similar. Sri Aurobindo's *The Life Divine* and *The Synthesis of Yoga* are mainly works on Yoga and only indirectly on psychology.

The author has tried to use a language that is comprehensible for everyone without falling into generalities. In spite of this, the contents of this book may not always be easily digestible.

This study is comprised of three parts, which are subdivided into twelve chapters.

Part One gives the background which is needed for parts two and three.

The first chapter commences with a brief overview of some of the fundamentals of the aim and nature of psychotherapy as well as some of its limitations. Psychotherapy aims at helping clients to grow and promoting insight and inner freedom. It can be seen as an initiating process for the development of an integrated ego, and its constructive application can be used as a bridge or adjunctive aid to help seekers to a turning point on the spiritual journey.

However, it seems that most brands of psychotherapy focus only on one or some aspects of human functioning and are therefore severely limited in the degree to which they are capable of enlarging the client's awareness and modifying man's behaviour.

Chapter two elaborates on the relation between conventional psychotherapy and traditional spiritual discipline. Both approaches are concerned with human suffering and self-analysis through a change of automatic patterns of awareness and thinking from which much human suffering originates, yet they differ regarding the fundamental nature of reality and the concept of the self. Nevertheless, in their partially overlapping areas of interest the two approaches can be complementary aspects of the process of self-realisation. Each approach has its own importance; each may be regarded as a different stage in the course of the seeker's development.

Chapter three discusses the metaphysical nature of spiritual discipline and the metaphysical nature of the self. A spiritual discipline is not based on an uncritical acceptance of certain doctrinal interpretations; it demands an initial acceptance of the prescribed methods, but at a later stage, with knowledge and insight, the researcher maybe able to debate certain issues which are related to a specific spiritual discipline. In looking at the metaphysical nature of the Self, as distinguished from the psychological nature of the self, the author describes the concept of the Self as explored in the Upanishads, Advait Vedanta, Patanjali's Yoga, Sri Aurobindo's metaphysical system, and conventional Western psychotherapy.

The fourth chapter deals with the transpersonal movement and gives a general overview of transpersonal psychology, transpersonal psychotherapy and transpersonal psychiatry.

The transpersonal movement, as a subject for scientific investigation, affirms that the transpersonal realm is not the exclusive domain of priests, yogis or mystics but also of scientists; it is an open system undergoing continuous development. In this development it brings together the ancient wisdom of all the great spiritual traditions of the world and the pragmatism of modem Western science.

Transpersonal psychotherapy is an approach to healing through the integration of the physical, vital, mental and spiritual aspects of the person. The spiritual dimensions and potentials of the seeker are explored from a psychological perspective. In transpersonal psychiatry the mystical experience can be transformative and healing, and the transpersonal psychiatrist, who treats individuals with a spiritual orientation, acknowledges the link between the biological and spiritual aspects of man.

Part Two elaborates extensively on Ken Wilber's integral psychology and Sri Aurobindo's metaphysical Yoga psychology.

Chapter five describes the main works of Ken Wilber, from his first book, *The Spectrum of Consciousness,* to his latest work, *A Theory of Everything,* so that the reader gets a better understanding of Ken Wilber's multidisciplinary approach.

In the sixth chapter the author examines briefly some of the main works of Sri Aurobindo *(The Life Divine, The Synthesis of Yoga, The Human Cycle* and *Letters on Yoga),* the aim of his integral Yoga and the concept of integral transformation. The aim of the practitioner of integral Yoga must be the possession of God, to be as perfect as God in His being, and to live a divine life on earth so that all mankind may attain the same divine perfection. Sri Aurobindo's integral transformation enables the spiritual seeker to live in the Divine not only in the absorbed ecstasy of trance, but also to live the Life Divine on earth at all times, in all parts and elements of the being— physically, vitally, mentally and spiritually.

The seventh chapter describes and attempts to analyse Sri Aurobindo's concept of the psycho-spiritual nature of man, in terms of the various layers of consciousness and in terms of the different parts of the being. This classification is helpful for psychological self-knowledge, discipline and practice, but should not be erected into too rigid a formula. As these things run very much into each other, a synthetic sense of these powers is as necessary as the analytical.

In the eighth chapter insight is gained into sadhana in integral Yoga and its difficulties. Sadhana as a science of spiritual discipline is a conscious effort to find God or the divine within and to transform one's whole nature. Sri Aurobindo's integral sadhana, as an intensive preparative process for a divine life or Gnostic kingdom of heaven on earth, is not an easy sadhana. The path of integral sadhana is steep and does not avoid regions of darkness. Its difficult, complex course is not a path for any ordinary seeker to follow, but only for those who accept to seek its aim and for those whose inner strength is supplemented by the true aid of the Guru. However, Sri Aurobindo maintains that those who are sincere, faithful in heart and rely on the Divine will arrive at the kingdom in spite of all difficulties.

Part Three attempts to render a critical and constructive dialogue between Ken Wilber and Sri Aurobindo regarding their integral views and their metaphysical vision respectively.

Chapter nine opens with a comparison of conventional psychotherapy and integral sadhana. Systems of psychotherapy and Sri Aurobindo's sadhana include the development of insight and increasing awareness pertaining to aspects of behaviour of which the seeker has been more or less unaware. But for Sri Aurobindo psychological difficulties do not disappear by the mind's brooding on them; he wants the seeker to put one's whole sress on faith, aspiration and surrender to the Divine, as it is from something outside and above the difficulties that the solution must come. After discussing the role of the ego and the place of God in transpersonal psychotherapy and in integral sadhana, the author concludes this chapter with a comparison of transpersonal psychotherapy and integral sadhana. Both approaches take consciousness as the true subject matter of psychology but, unlike transpersonal psychotherapy, Sri Aurobindo's yoga of integral perfection regards man as a divine spiritual being, involved in mind, life and body, and his Yoga aims not only at the realisation but also at the perfection of the seeker's divine nature. Integral sadhana and transpersonal psychotherapy can be viewed as complementary, however, each representing different levels of health and growth, and each simply dealing with different ranges of human development.

Chapter ten offers a critical evaluation of Ken Wilber's commentary on the shortcomings of Sri Aurobindo's integral Yoga. Does Sri Aurobindo make a sufficiently strong link between his spiritual objectives and social, economic, cultural and scientific goals that can be tested by established social or scientific criteria?

The eleventh chapter examines Ken Wilber's critical interpretations of various aspects of Sri Aurobindo's metaphysical vision, and concludes with a critical estimate of Ken Wilber. It may be useful to compare various aspects of Sri Aurobindo's vision with his own 'all quadrant, all level' model but, when they are applied to life, are the similarities used in the same way in both systems?

The concluding chapter presents a critical summary of Sri Aurobindo's metaphysical Yoga psychology and the place of psychopathology in it. Sri Aurobindo is not an academic psychologist, but a Yogi who takes psychology in his stride. Are the psychological aspects of Sri Aurobindo's metaphysical vision, which are based on the practice of his integral Yoga, applicable to the discoveries of clinical psychology or contemporary applied psychology? In a critical estimate of Sri Aurobindo's integralism, the author asks himself if Sri Aurobindo's metaphysical vision is able to withstand the rise of Western psychology's scientific development, and if the followers of Sri Aurobindo's vision are able to use certain contemporary ideas in a constructive manner without deconstructing the major contents of his vision. It takes a brief look at the Ashramites of the Sri Aurobindo Ashram, seen through the eyes of a long-time ashramite and at Auroville, the city of human unity, founded in 1968.

The reflections and critical comments at the end of the last three chapters are not meant as criticism on their vision, but as an elucidation of their agreements and disagreements and a genuine appreciation of their integral approach.

—DR. JOSEPH VRINTE

Acknowledgement

This research work started taking shape during a period of extensive reading and exposure to the works of Sri Aurobindo, Ken Wilber and other transpersonal psychologists. At this time I was living in Auroville, an inspiring place which generated many ideas and processes discussed in this book. Many of its inhabitants were extremely helpful in ways known and unknown. They were a source of encouragement and inspiration. They offered me critical challenges, but also illuminating and confronting encounters, which enabled me to write about and explore some of the views in this work. I offer my special thanks to Annemarie, Alain Grandcolas, Doris, and Dhanya for their support and encouragement in difficult times, and my personal appreciation to Auralee, who has made this a much better written book, after devoting many hours of editorial labour to make the English flow.

This work is not merely an intellectual academic study, but is also one of observation and analysis of my personal perceptions and inner experiences while living in Auroville. Some of the contents of these subjective introspective experiences are therefore debatable, and naturally, open for discussion.

This second edition of the "The Perennial Quest" is offered as a tribute to Sri Aurobindo on his 150th birth anniversary

August 2023

Acceptance community
Auroville, Tamil Nadu-605 101
(India)
josephvrinte@yahoo.co.in

Contents

Part I:

Aspects of the Transpersonal Psychology Movement and Sri Aurobindo's Integral Yoga

Chapter One

Psychotherapy

INTRODUCTION

In this chapter references to some systems of psychotherapy will be made to clarify and expand upon their contributions to transpersonal psychotherapy. The various kinds of psychotherapy will not be specifically summarised, however, as that is not in the scope of this book.

It is to be understood that before entering therapy, the individual is not content with his or her present living; there is an inability to cope with life situations or a defective integration of personality. A sense of insecurity, social failure, frustration, fear, anxiety, despair or other mental strains pave the way to seeking the guidance of a therapist or a counsellor. When the distress or the emotional conflict seriously affects the individual's life, then psychotherapy becomes a possibility; when the misery is accompanied by intense confusion regarding one's conduct in everyday life or when the client does not respond positively to the crisis, he or she will most likely consult a psychotherapist.

At present, life is influenced by unprecedented scientific and technological development. A different lifestyle from that to which the individual is accustomed and other rapid changes may become a source of intensive stress. To find relief from these stressful situations one often looks at material solutions, sometimes in the form of neuropsychological treatment. However, such means offer only temporary relief, and the individual still does not feel in tune with life. In wider perspective, what is lacking or missing is related to the meaning of life, and this in turn often relates to the quest for spiritual knowledge. This introspective quest is reflected in the development of new forms of psychotherapy.

Traditional psychotherapy is highly influenced by the medical model where all kinds of emotional, psychosomatic and interpersonal problems are considered as symptoms of disease. Often the decrease of symptoms is labelled as progress, while the intensity of the symptom is viewed as an indication of the severity of the pathological process. However, it seems that this symptomatic orientation is often an artificial and superficial compromise as it touches only the surface of the problem and leaves aside the underlying cause which is much more difficult to come to grips with. Psychotherapy also pays attention to basic maintenance and survival needs, such as security, self-esteem, love and social needs and the obstacles to the gratification of these needs.

The term 'psychotherapy' originated from the nurturing or care of the breath or spirit, but later on it became associated with medical practice. As an ideology and set of practices, psychotherapy thus passed from the spiritual domain into the secular, scientific realm and form of explanation, and today's psychotherapists are the heirs of *shamans* and priests. As the science and art of relieving human suffering by psychological methods, psychotherapy aims at healing the disturbed client. In general, psychotherapy is a process of treatment which endeavours to restore "normal" psychological functioning, to relieve emotional distress; to restore the meaning and significance in the client's life as also to release hidden human potentials.

This process brings to the client's awareness the underlying deep-rooted origins of one's psychological disturbances. But psychotherapy also attempts to help the client in understanding oneself as a whole, through increased self- knowledge and through the discovery of the various unknown aspects of his of her personality. Psychotherapy is not only used as a means of curing psychopathological symptoms or modifying character structure; it is also the art of helping the client encounter one's life situation, and of alleviating interpersonal problems. The client's negative self assumptions as well as one's distorted views about one's interpersonal relationships are gradually modified in order to provide him or her with a new base of confidence.

The therapist, with the help of methodical interactions, tries to return to the client something that has been lost, and help him or her to remove obstacles to maintain a healthy life. In the process of self-improvement, the therapist functions as a guarantor by penetrating deep into the client's world and making these inner contents accessible to the client. While guiding the client's "troubled soul" on his or her way to recovery, the therapist does not function merely as a magician who juggles away the client's psychological problems.

Theories and techniques of psychotherapy are not only based upon certain ethical and evaluative presuppositions, but are also based upon the *Zeitgeist* in which the therapist and his adherents live. Each system of psychotherapy explicitly or implicitly explores the image of man, the nature of one's conflicts and methods for resolving these conflicts. Out of these theories each system formulates a model of psychotherapy, which guides the therapist in one's therapeutic advice.

At present there is no universally recognised way to classify various different therapies, but Abraham Maslow meaningfully divided major theoretical trends into four types, often called 'forces'. These four fundamental forces are:

1. the classical psychoanalytic,
2. the cognitive-behavioural,
3. the existential-humanistic, and
4. the transpersonal approaches.

Although the first three, "forces" often, have different and conflicting views regarding human nature and development and their specific goals, and also differ regarding the content of psychotherapy and the mechanisms of change, they nevertheless agree on the process or theory of therapeutic change and offer important perspectives for securing this change within the individual. They also share some common general goals such as development of self-acceptance, increased awareness and insight, uprooting of neurotic defences, achievement of human freedom and a meaningful life. They all aim at human maturity, which does not consist merely of social adjustment but also attainment of autonomy and free will.

Excessive unsubstantiated claims regarding the applicability and importance of psychotherapy has caused some severe criticism about its negative effects. While examining various psychotherapeutic theories and procedures, one is confronted with a perplexing set of ideas and techniques.

Present-day psychotherapeutic systems differ a great deal from each other in their descriptions of the fundamental dynamics involved with the human personality, in their approach to the nature and dynamics of psychopathological problems and in their interpretation of therapeutic techniques. Each of the newly evolved psychotherapeutic models claims new knowledge and healing methods that are supposed to be more effective and comprehensive than the existing ones. Some of the new therapies have survived, others have been in existence for only one or two decades.

However, the influence of various kinds of psychotherapy in curing mental disturbances still seems extremely uncertain. It seems that any psychotherapy, while appropriate for one area of human psychological disturbance may be invalid or even harmful for other areas. There continues to be exploitation of clients by therapists or by incompetent practitioners, using ineffective or inappropriate methods of therapy resulting in negative side effects, etc. Often therapists translate the reality of the client's life to the constructs of their own model. They may impose their worldview upon clients to help them through caring, controlling, manipulation, interpretation and insight.

But genuine change in the client has to be accompanied by the development of a strong desire and determination to change. Insight into deep-rooted issues by itself is not sufficient, it must be followed up by the ability to see across and behind. The client may deal with one's crisis and yet not be able to integrate insight into his or her inner 'processes'. The release of repressed affects brought about under the influence of the psychotherapist may be purifying, but it may also impair the individual's self-worth. Other motives may spring up later, which will subsequently cause the accumulation of the same feelings again. In such cases, emotional and rational insight can be used to produce relief and gradual necessary changes. This is what the client has to learn.

Therapeutic techniques facilitate the disclosure and resolution, of the client's major conflicts within a certain time limit. These techniques are powerful instruments that cause decrease and disappearance of the client's troubles and conflicts and reduction of symptoms which does not necessarily constitute a cure. Successful elimination of symptoms helps the client to learn to behave more adaptively even if at the cost of one's creativity and contentment. When clients who are not sufficiently well-integrated shed repressive aspects of their life, they may only be overwhelmed by anxiety, accompanied by a loss of impulse control. In such cases clients may become dependent upon the therapist's techniques to move step by step. There may be a tendency to continue exploring problem areas, and the continuous preoccupation with examining unresolved situations. This, of course is different from a more aware client reaching a basic openness to the transpersonal realm of being.

With the existence of more than 250 different kinds of therapies it should be apparent that in its therapeutic efficiency no single approach has found the only one true path. Most brands of psychotherapy rely for their credibility on focusing on one aspect of human functioning and making it central to their system. *All psychotherapies are therefore limited in the degree to which they are capable of modifying man's behaviour or enlarging the client's awareness.* For many people, therapy may become an end in itself, in which the therapeutic experience— the verbalizing insight—fails to change the client's basic life commitments. In other words, psychotherapy as an end becomes a way of life rather than a means for change and autonomy.

CONCLUSION

What used to be called the "cure of souls" is now called psychotherapy and man is witnessing an increasing medicalisation of psychotherapy due to increasing economic, cultural and political controls. The number of specific problems seems to have multiplied in the last quarter century. There is a pressing need for specialised psychotherapeutic techniques to meet the changing character structure and symptomatology. Present-day culture is saturated with beliefs about human nature and society, which provides sufficient ground on which psychotherapy can develop itself. Consumerism and the largely materialistic aims of our society do not accept anxiety, confusion, fear, panic and depression for a happy life and where they do arise they have to be removed as quickly as possible from the psychological field. These problems are most frequently treated with the help of tranquillising and anti-depressive drugs. This kind of treatment is, of course, largely physical in nature; i.e., it effects an alteration of behaviour via the body's chemistry.

In recent years, conventional psychotherapy has been 'refined' with explorations in neurophysiology, which have generated a gigantic medical and pharmacological industry. These pharmacological discoveries do not solve the problems of interpersonal dynamics and the meaning of life in general. Psychotherapy could offer an alternative approach for facing and understanding these problems by giving them their proper place in a new way of life, rather than making the client' insensible to these conflicts by provision of anaesthesia or other escape routes. Nevertheless, even an alternative psychotherapeutic approach for relief of such problems is often restricted to the more socially privileged sections of society, i.e., a relatively small proportion of the population.

Differences between systems of psychotherapy render certain therapies more effective for certain clients, but each system cannot claim to be complete. Each system, therefore, can be considered as a contribution to a specific area of insight and to the construction of a more comprehensive system. Psychotherapy neither claims a dramatic instant cure nor does it pretend to create perfectly balanced superhumans who are well-integrated with themselves and with the universe. It does not promise salvation through magical therapeutic techniques and it cannot guarantee the individual a kind of enjoyable end-state in which all life's obstacles are surmounted. A modestly held therapeutic goal moves on the ground of everyday life, i.e., the goal is not remote from the present psychological reality and, as such, psychotherapy helps the client to grow and promotes insight and inner freedom, rather than enslavement and mechanization due to one's unconscious tendencies. This increased self-awareness and extended awareness of life's possibilities enable the client to venture into new and unknown paths. Psychotherapy can be seen as an initiating process for the development of an integrated ego and the accompanying alleviation and removal of severe psychological problems. However, studies in recent years regarding the beneficial aspects of psychotherapy do not always clearly indicate lasting benefits.

It seems to this author that any form of therapy without a spiritual dimension, i.e., the absence of a mainstream spiritual principle of faith often offers only superficial positive solutions which ultimately turns out to be fallible and unreliable. Psychotherapy may offer some relief but, at a more complex level the seeker does not want merely to recover from mental disturbances but aims simultaneously at transcendence into a higher realm of being. Many clients who visit a therapist view their difficulties not so much as medical problems but more as symptoms of "a troubled soul". Such clients do not suffer from serious personal anguish, but seek self-actualisation of their potential; they do not seek a therapist for guidance in eliminating their conflicts, but to discover' themselves and. find self-enlightenment. Traditional methods of psychotherapy have very often added new approaches to their therapeutic process, such as teachings of Eastern disciplines, meditation, self-awareness, self-actualisation, etc., and the boundaries between treatment and growth have become more obscure. By bringing about reconciliation between the ego and various repressed experiences, psychotherapy also endeavours to integrate the split between the individual and the world. This is not merely a matter of adjusting the client to society; therapy is more than just adjustment.

Various schools of traditional psychotherapy (Freudian, humanistic and behavioural) offer complementary views regarding human behaviour in relation to intrapsychic forces, inter-subjective processes, family circumstances and environmental influences. However, they all leave out the spiritual realm, and then their solutions appear to be only partial. As long as psychotherapy remains preoccupied with the limited surface structures of the self, it may not be able to eliminate human suffering completely nor to transform the structure of psychic life. As long as a psychotherapist maintains "the continued acceptance of the dualistic view of man [the traditional split between spirit and nature] he leaves the client upon one horn of the dualistic dilemma, which is at best the achievement of courageous despair."[1] As long as consciousness cannot be conceived without the duality of subject and object one will never be deemed capable of transcending ego conditions. In psychotherapy, there is always a danger of the fortified ego being called up for questioning. But ego transcendence need not always lead to an invasion of consciousness by the primordial contents of the unconscious; it may also lead to an insight-perception of the whole. When the psychotherapist teaches the client to stop identifying him or herself with the ego, then the development of a new actualisation of the self takes place, where opposites are no longer compromised but meet. As such psychotherapy can function as a stepping-stone to self-transcendence, which enables people to realise the ultimate need of the Divine within.

Constructive application of psychotherapy can be used as a bridge or adjunctive aid to help seekers to a turning point on the spiritual journey. Without paying attention to the unconscious and defensive processes', of the ego, people may get lost in neurotic behaviour; in such cases psychotherapy helps to sort this problem out. Thereafter, the client can continue his or her onward journey of self-discovery and embark consciously on his or her spiritual quest. In this way, psychotherapy can serve as a valuable preparation before entering onto the path of Sri Aurobindo's integral sadhana, where the ego is sacrificed for the universal and transcendental Seif. This does not, however, make psychotherapy a necessary approach to the transcendence of the ego or any other spiritual goals.

NOTES

1. A. Watts; *Psychotherapy East and West*, p. 92

Chapter Two

Conventional Psychotherapy and Traditional Spiritual Disciplines

INTRODUCTION

It is not easy to take up the relation between conventional psychotherapy and traditional spiritual disciplines as both subjects are rather complicated and comprehensive and their respective adherents do not always support each other. Though this brief overview and comparison contains broad generalizations it nevertheless tries to create a fuller understanding of the two approaches and the impact they have on each other.

In expanding the underdeveloped ego-structure, conventional psychotherapy frequently lays stress on an analysis of conflicts made by uncovering the roots of psychopathological processes. With the accent on psychopathology its attention is focused on the negative and maladaptive aspects of human nature. It does not encourage spiritual awakening, which is fostered by an emphasis on synthesis, an integrative healing or growth-oriented process. Psychotherapy accentuates the development and strengthening of the personality; the therapist guides the client to a better understanding of his or her personality structure and attempts to remove the obstacles that prevent such development. Moreover, psychotherapy is concerned with the psychological well-being of the client, i.e., the relief of discomfort through the justification of unfulfilled desires, anxieties, frustrations and maladaptive behaviours for the sake of living a 'normal' fulfilled life.

As a treatment of psychological distress or as a way of self-reflection and self-improvement, psychotherapy aims at a breakthrough of insight, which heals conflicts and reconciles the individual with oneself and one's surroundings. It tries to create a sense of well-being despite common human malady; alienation from oneself, one's fellow creatures and nature. Well-being is related to human potentiality, man's inherent capacity for growth and fulfilment, to become what one potentially is.

Traditional psycho-spiritual practices or spiritual disciplines such as Buddhism, Vedanta or Christian mysticism aim at the realisation of one's own true Self, and do not place much importance on the development of an outer personality. They speak about an essence or soul behind the relatively surface personality; beneath the mask of personality, beneath the flow of the 'I and me', there exists a Self that is pure, timeless and not conditioned by nature or society. This deeper Self is responsible for man's inner spiritual growth. In the course of spiritual development, instinctual and social motivations are gradually transcended and, going beyond ego motivations, the liberated seeker finds one's true self. The self-realised person now joyfully participates in the social process, without the conventional moral distinctions of right and wrong, with a selfless dedication to the growth of human welfare. Those who undertake the struggle to overcome the obstacles to spiritual realisation are yearning for the Divine, beyond recognisable psychological motivations such as duty or satisfaction of religious, intellectual, moral or social life.

In conquering the unknown, traditional spiritual disciplines increase the seeker's vision and accommodate him or her to the world rather than give the individual a sense of possession. All traditional spiritual disciplines aim at clarifying the contents of consciousness. Aided by one's restraint of the natural greed of the outer self and a growing indifference toward inappropriate habits or excessive desires, one creates an opening to the more spiritual contents of consciousness. Through the practice of spiritual discipline, the seeker learns to tap inner resources, which include the exploration of healing capacities that may be latent or undeveloped within the suffering individual. The discipline brings into awareness the obstacles to spiritual development, such as greed, attachment, desire, rejection, anger, etc. Renunciation of these obstacles is often practised in order to foster a growing freedom from them. It is not much concerned with the psychopathological aspects of extreme fear and depression and although it does not pathologically deny the gratification of A. Maslow's 'basic needs', it emphasizes more spiritual needs. All other needs are subordinated to these primarily spiritual 'metaneeds', and when they are not fulfilled, a pathological condition may arise.

Emotional inclinations are an inherent part of any being and often act as veils. Spiritual discipline tries to analyse the workings of these veils, to elevate them and to so transform all sorts of limitations. It is this idea that forms the core of traditional spiritual practices.

Both approaches, conventional psychotherapy and traditional spiritual discipline, are concerned with changing automatic patterns of awareness and thinking, from which much of human suffering originates, though they differ in their perception of the fundamental nature of reality and the concept of self. The reality that underlies the world of appearances is accessible to spiritual or mystical intuition but not always to sense-organs. The experience of this underlying reality clarifies the true nature of the self and gives meaning to the aim of life.

In conventional psychotherapy, self is considered as a kind of object (an ego) which is separated from all other objects. This, limits the self to a particular aspect of human life and does not take into consideration the universal and transcendental aspects of the self, beyond space, time and causality. The self as object is functional: self-preservation and the satisfaction of basic needs are its most important motives. They strengthen the object-self and enable the organism to influence its environment.

Spiritual discipline does not consider the self as separate; it synthesises what the object-self separates and allows the self to be united with its surroundings. This pure, subjective consciousness is a unifying principle. In its therapeutic aims, psychotherapy could use this mode of subjective self-experience to supplement its object-self mode, in order to gain a change in the perception of self. Spiritual growth requires a harmony between the object-self and true Self in order to achieve further development.

The beginner practitioner on the path of spiritual discipline is not totally free from egocentricity all at once and disturbing tendencies like desire, attachment, etc., need to be gradually controlled so that they do not hinder the process. After all, fulfilment of desires does not clarify the underlying essence of suffering, i.e., egocentricity and ignorance. A full elaboration of the concept of the self in Western psychotherapy, in Eastern spiritual disciplines and in Sri Aurobindo's metaphysical system will be made in the following chapter.

The psychotherapeutic treatment aims at developing a strong and well-adjusted ego and imparting an autonomous self-esteem to the client who can then have meaningful relationships in social life. Psychotherapy seeks to improve the outer self so that it is more productive, more enjoyable and less complicated: The seeker of spiritual growth, on the other hand, uses detachment from the external physical world in order to get what he or she needs at a certain stage: to be reunited with the universal Spirit. Thus seekers sacrifice their egos to serve other purposes. Spiritual discipline aims at purification, detachment and liberation from desires of the material world, and the attachment to Spirit through the dynamic interaction of energy fields.

Conventional psychotherapies value theoretical discussions, speculative analyses and intellectual understanding as important factors in the process of self-knowledge; spiritual discipline is more concerned with the immediate actual experience, often muted, of the seeker's own awareness' in the exploration of consciousness. As an art of transcendence, spiritual discipline enables the seeker to experience the depth of one's being and one's interconnectedness with the world.

Psychotherapy has the tendency to 'psychologize' these processes, which are reduced in experiential meaning when they are merely understood through preconceived ideas and thoughts. According to J. Deikman, "In psychotherapy, you [the psychotherapist] are basically working to help the client clarify the motivations that underlie behaviour that is frustrating or restricting him or her at the level of interpersonal relationships and also with regards to their work efficiency and creativity ... Now all kinds of behaviours might be improved in the course of spiritual development, but only as a secondary by-product of something that really has a different focus. Indeed, spiritual development may require a certain degree of health to have things go well. Thus, I could see psychotherapy as providing a very important foundation from which someone might gain access to larger dimensions of reality... psychotherapy might be a basis for more effective spiritual development, but it is not the same thing... Psychotherapy and spiritual development are two different levels of the same continuum, but they do not substitute for each other. They work synergistically with each other."[1] In other words, ways of attaining liberation and thereby reunion with the universal Spirit should not be identified as psychotherapy.

Actually, the most important difference between the two approaches lies in the usage of the prefix 'psyche'; the therapeutic attitude regards the psyche or mind, more or less, as a clinical entity which is inherently intelligent by nature and is limited to the body. Eastern spiritual discipline regards the mind as a psychic apparatus or internal instrument, as something far more extensive and holistic than the individual's mental functioning. The mind in Eastern psychology is only an instrument of knowledge and experience and is in itself non-intelligent. This inner instrument connects *Atman* (Spirit) with the external environment and functions as a mediating link between the two. The various schools of Indian philosophy interpret this inner instrument differently, but almost all of them agree that it performs a psychological as well as a metaphysical function. In its psychological function it constitutes reason, ego, mind and memory, and from its metaphysical function evolves the world.

Western psychotherapy approaches the psyche as a balanced system of mental and emotional functions, archetypal structures and libidinous dynamisms. The mental field in psychotherapy is often studied indirectly, by making inferences about mental operations through observing outward behaviour. In spiritual discipline the mind is studied directly through introspection or meditation; the trained mind is able to observe itself without being overwhelmed by thoughts.

Do all these differences lie only in approach and not in principle? In their pursuit of relief from human suffering, could these apparently different approaches be viewed as interdependent on each other in the process of healing? Conventional Western psychotherapy, as well as traditional spiritual discipline, aims to bring about changes in consciousness and both explore the essence and nature of man, his well-being and the meaning of existence.

Human suffering and pain are often the product of ignorance and both approaches endeavour to reintegrate the personality through increased self-knowledge and insight; the self is expanded by making the unconscious conscious and, by the removal of ignorance, the seeker is able to discover and reunite itself. For A. Watts the two resemblances between Eastern ways of life [the Eastern ways of liberation] and Western psychotherapy are: "first the transformation of consciousness, of the inner feeling of one's own existence; and second the release of the individual from forms of conditioning imposed upon him by social institutions ... If, then, there are in other cultures [spiritual] disciplines having something in common with psychotherapy, a theoretical knowledge of their methods, objectives, and principles may enable the psychotherapist to get a better perspective upon what he himself is doing."[2]

Psychotherapy as a science need not be in conflict with spiritual discipline when it includes an intuitive approach to a different definition of reality in which there is a place for the rational as well as the non-rational dimensions of human experience. By adding a contemplative awareness to their psychological concepts and techniques, psychotherapists are more able to help those people who are alienated from their roots.

There are partially overlapping areas of interest and the two approaches could be complementary aspects in the process of self-realisation. Each has its own importance; each may be regarded as a different stage in the course of the development of the spiritual seeker. According to B. Boorstein, "Spiritual approaches have specific psychotherapeutic value when seen as being used to resolve our fear systems; they help us cultivate compassion, forgiveness and acceptance, and help us learn to temper our anger ... I see myself at the same time as working with patients on the problems they have with internal conflicts, such as guilt and fear and conflicts with family and friends and in work relationships."[3] Clients who need psychotherapy suffer from painful psychological problems that interfere with their daily life and they want direct relief from their symptoms as well as the satisfaction of their frustrated desires. Relief from suffering in spiritual discipline requires a different orientation—the transcendence of egocentricity, the discovery of one's real Self and the determining ultimate goal of life. What is most urgent needs to be tackled first. If psychopathology is predominant, then it is best to tackle it first, as spiritual discipline cannot replace psychotherapy in such cases.

Psychotherapy is primarily concerned with the art of healing psychological disturbances through behaviour modification, resolution of psychodynamic conflicts and personal growth. It can be effective in resolving stubborn psychological blockages and could be considered as a fruitful preparation for the client's long road of spiritual awakening. To break down habitual resistances and explore underlying vulnerabilities takes resilience and patience. Some seekers may lack sufficient grounding to enter the path of spiritual discipline, especially when defensive structures gradually collapse and various ego structures are dissolved or changed.

Breaking down old structures and allowing new ones to unfold at an inappropriate time may block spiritual development, i.e., the seeker may not have developed the awareness to cope with the powerful spiritual process. Only at the point when the therapeutic interaction is directed toward the spiritual aim of life, then and only then is the seeker ready to realise that "all life is Yoga", a journey in which one's whole life is seen in the light of this motive. On the other hand, in its positive understanding of human nature, spiritual discipline has sometimes the tendency of underestimating the psychopathological aspects of man. By interpreting man exclusively in the light of the Divine within, it often ignores the seeker's hereditary factors and past history. Spiritual discipline can easily be misused as a way of avoiding uncomfortable life situations and cannot usually be substituted for psychotherapy and its process of removing various obscurities and clearing out defences.

Thus neither of these approaches is self-sufficient; each one is deficient and incomplete on its own. By making the two approaches complementary, the excesses and shortcomings of each are checked and refined by the other. One approach need not exclude the other. When both are used simultaneously and in the proper context, each enhances the value of the other. Psychological techniques alone cannot fundamentally remedy the present complicated human situation; metaphysical explanations often need to be added for a complete experience of human life. In the absence of a metaphysical background and spiritual instruction, the basic wholeness of the individual cannot be realised because man is not merely a psychophysical organism but is in essence Spirit; the soul is essentially divine. A deeper understanding of the psyche and the spiritual quest for inner growth cannot be satisfied by psychotherapy alone; it needs to be supplemented by spiritual practice.

Spiritual discipline can be used constructively as an addition to psychotherapy. However, in a strict sense, in facilitating the process of healing, spiritual issues are not the same as psychological problems. Even though psychological and spiritual issues are perplexedly interwoven and even though it is possible, in some cases, to eliminate psychological conflicts with the help of spiritual insight, this does not mean that the approach of psychological insight through 'working it out' is more direct and amenable than spiritual insight. Then, many individuals get involved in various spiritual traditions in order to heal themselves of early unresolved psychological conflicts and traumas, but this does not mean that spiritual needs always indicate unfulfilled childhood needs. More often, spiritual longings are derived from the seeker's most developed level of psychological maturity.

The domains of both approaches remain distinct to the extent of the difference in the client's or seeker's goals. Psychotherapy, on the one hand, is able to reduce neurotic egocentricity and unassimilated childhood experiences and create new and effective ways to meet one's needs. It aims at a strong identification and integration of one's personality, and the client works out various kinds of psychological blockages, as these obstructions may continue to attract one's attention and as a consequence may impede spiritual development. Spiritual discipline, on the other hand, aims at the disidentification with or release of one's surface personality i.e., identification with one's body, thoughts and feelings, imprisons the seeker. This experiential process cannot always be comprehended by our thoughts and feelings.

The initial stages of spiritual discipline are often characterised by a relentless self-analysis, and it requires patience and will-power to overcome stubborn impulses, mechanical automatisms and acquired habits. As long as the seeker has not found his or her 'soul' or centre of spiritual consciousness, psychological difficulties could be the source of setbacks in one's spiritual progress. Spiritual discipline does not usually offer the seeker a well-developed theoretical map for working out specific psychological problems. With the guidance of a psychotherapist one may be in a better position to work out intrapsychic conflicts and interpersonal misunderstandings. When these obstacles are elaborated, spiritual practice may become more subtle as these psychological difficulties come to have less effect on the practitioners. By then the seeker may be able to get more in contact with God's Grace and the Divine within.

In the final analysis it seems clear that the seeker who embarks on the journey to spiritual realisation experiences him or herself, initially, as a psychological being; and then as a spiritual being. By going within, the seeker first encounters the unconscious psychological structures of his ego (defences, anxieties, frustrations, desires, etc.), and in dealing with these mental dilemmas he or she removes these difficulties.

On the journey of the discovery of the true Self, psychotherapy may be able to help the seeker to explore psychological hindrances at a deeper level and thus help spiritual practices immensely. Spiritual practice alone may not be able to penetrate deeper into these hidden psychological layers; psychotherapy could be helpful as a valuable preparation for the spiritual unfolding of the seeker, though it is certainly not a prerequisite for it. Spiritual practice may enable the individual to resolve psychological conflicts without undergoing psychotherapeutic guidance. At the same time, it seems clear that psychological insight is often more accessible to resolve emotional conflicts and traumas than spiritual insight. Could it be that the psychotherapeutic approach deals more directly with the elimination of psychological problems, as compared to the insight of spiritual disciplines? The transpersonal psychotherapist seeks a balance between spiritual discipline and various forms of psychotherapy.

POSSIBLE OBSTACLES ON THE WAY TO DIVINE AWAKENING WITHIN

The process of spiritual development has its challenges and difficulties. There are many dangers besetting the spiritual journey and the spiritual path is sometimes sharp, like a razor's edge. The various difficulties are meaningfully described by E. Deutsch as follows: "There is no royal road to Spirit. Transformation is perhaps the most difficult task which man can impose upon himself. It is filled with the most bitter disappointments, the most trying demands; one makes progress and falls back from it to a point lower than from where one began; one conquers one aspect of one's diverted nature only to find another one taking its place; one is discouraged by others, even forcibly discouraged by demands made upon one by society; and there is no resting place along the way. Every time one stops, one is retreating; every time one thinks one has arrived, one discovers a chasm still to be bridged. But there is within us this power for self-transformation; man does possess the strength to conquer his distorted, diverted self. The power for self-transformation is not a magical or occult power; it is the power of the Divine urging us on to the completion of our destiny."[4]

Any form of spiritual discipline carries with it the potential to aggravate the seeker's difficulties; the spiritual path is often unpredictable and difficult to navigate. It may expose conflicts that have been previously denied or fended of in a variety of ways. An inevitable component of spiritual discipline may create unavoidable struggle and stress due to a growing awareness of painful traumas that are difficult to face. Even self-awareness in itself can, at times, be painful and these difficulties need to be placed in a proper perspective by the seeker. Being overwhelmed by spiritual impressions or experiences may cause a conflict between conscious and unconscious processes which ends in a spiritual crisis. S. Grof defines *spiritual crisis* or spiritual emergency as "critical and experientially difficult stages of a profound psychological transformation that involves one's entire being. They take the form of non-ordinary states of consciousness and involve intense emotions, visions and other sensory changes, and unusual thoughts, as well as various physical manifestations. These episodes often revolve around spiritual themes ... People who are in such a crisis suddenly feel uncomfortable in the formerly familiar world and may find it difficult to meet the demands of everyday life. They can have great problems distinguishing their inner visionary world from the external world of daily reality."[5]

As the stage of spiritual awakening approaches, which is often accompanied by an increased awareness of a higher power, the seeker, in the process of change, may become aware of one's own impurities and may experience a temporary incapacity to cope with daily life.

It also happens that, in their spiritual enthusiasm, seekers suppress useful and noble aspirations and even deny legitimate and healthy needs such as human love and compassion along with higher intellectual joys, etc. But for the beginner spiritual practitioner, who is still not able to draw power from direct spiritual experiences, study, service to humanity and fulfilment of duties are more essential than the withdrawal from them.

Suppression of the elements of the so-called 'lower' nature—ego, rationality, sexuality—may result in pathological conditions; these elements can be turned into unique potentials in the constructive development of one's personality. Spiritual growth need not imply suppression; on the contrary, during a stage of occasional fulfilment, higher spiritual dimensions may gradually be comprehended.

Spiritual practice can also be used to compensate for some major forms of psychopathology such as narcissistic withdrawal from the world and other such self-defeating behaviours.

For most seekers, in fact, transcendental bliss is not the ultimate goal of life. Though the transcendental Self has been described as essentially self-sufficient and eternally perfect, this does not mean the rejection and renouncement of the world. The seeker needs a certain maturity without which he or she might be tempted to withdraw from society. Seekers who are complaining of experiencing maladaptive symptoms or interpersonal disorders and whose spiritual discipline advocates a detachment from the material world to meet the seeker's psychic need may, in effect, be creating new pathological symptoms. The same seeker may realise his or her interconnectedness with the world and the responsibility for one's own reality. He or she should be encouraged to use any situation as a self-created opportunity for growth in this world rather than escaping into asceticism and avoiding painful confrontations with the reality of life, or running away from constructive creation in this world. Using spiritual techniques without a prior clear-cut understanding of the ultimate goal of dynamic self-integration with the sacred realm might easily provide a naive attempt at an escape from the hardships of life into an assumed Utopia.

One of the causes of negative side effects for the beginner practitioner is related to the lack of sufficient mental preparation, patience and will-power. Often seekers will try to control the mind in the midst of all kinds of latent and unmanifest disturbances and neglect these disturbances. But sooner or later these hindrances will return, sometimes even more strongly and forcefully. It needs a certain maturity to overcome one's ego attachment and unless the seeker has some conscious control of one's lower physical, vital and mental nature he or she may break down or become exhausted.

Others with personality disorders or with suppressed or uncontrollable emotions may hand over their responsibility to the Divine in the hope that these will be taken over. By denying their own human potential to help themselves—not an ill-fated attempt to overreach their capabilities—and becoming fully dependent on a higher power, the seeker may escape into another illusion.

Walking the spiritual path is, therefore, not something to be jumped into naively. Seekers can deceive themselves into thinking that they are developing spiritually when in fact they are strengthening their egocentricity through misplaced spiritual discipline. An intense process of change is often accompanied by an intense crisis. On the one hand, there is a relief because certain restrictive mental processes are losing their grip but, on the other hand, the old ego habits are not given up without paying the price. Seekers with ego defects or low ego strength who are not sufficiently integrated may not be able to handle upcoming repressed material which could be very threatening. With an excessive strain on their psychological resources they become incapable of assimilating such material. According to S. Kakar, "The past, hidden in the darkness of the long forgotten, found form and awakened ... In my own work with gurus and disciples, I found that many of the latter shared a common pattern in their lives that had led them to a search for the guru and to initiation in his cult. Almost invariably the individual had gone through one or more experiences that had severely mauled his sense of self-worth... Unable to rid themselves of the feelings of 'I have lost everything and the world is empty'... they had been on the lookout for someone, somewhere, to restore the lost sense of self-worth and to counteract their hidden image of a failing depleted self—a search nonetheless desperate for its being mostly unconscious."[6]

These difficulties are sometimes caused by a greater sensitivity to or emergence of previously repressed psychological conflicts. When these old unconscious tendencies come up, they can drag the seeker downwards into a mental crisis. It seems that a certain minimal amount of ego strength is essential for undertaking spiritual practices.

Just as difficulties can be involved in developing the strength and control of the ego level, there can also be difficulties encountered by some seekers when they move beyond their ego level. On the one hand, there is the possibility that the spiritual experience is mistaken for a regression to a pre-egoic condition (the ego of the newborn infant has no basis for conflicts), i.e., a failure to realise the ego. On the other hand, there is the confusion of ego inflation, which is mistaken for spiritual experience, i.e., a failure to realise the limits of the ego when it identifies itself with God. In the false identification of the subjective ego consciousness with the spiritual Self, the seeker is under the delusion of being all-powerful. As Grof puts it, "Instead of emerging from the experience [encounter with the divine] with the understanding that they are divine and so is everyone and everything else, they feel that they are God and have a message for the world."[7]

When the discovery of the seeker's divinity remains attached to the ego, it may end up in a psychotic delusion of grandeur instead of a genuine spiritual insight. Along with the practice of discipline goes that of non-attachment; the two should go together because if non-attachment is not observed and the seeker remains attached to the things of the world, he or she may well use his or her newly acquired powers for selfish ends.

The dramatic and disorganised unconscious material which comes up to the surface from deep levels of the psyche, whenever it is hurried, can be overwhelming and the seeker may have difficulty functioning in everyday reality. Other problems may arise during the practice of spiritual discipline, when the seeker is unable to assimilate the inflow of spiritual forces due to an unbalanced mental-emotional excitement or inadequate ego development. In such situations, the individual is not likely to be liberated from unconscious deep-rooted fears, habitual resistances, repressed unconscious processes or any other psychopathological obstacles in general, through spiritual discipline alone. Psychological obstructions of a serious nature are impediments in spiritual growth and therefore remain demanding the seeker's psychological attention:

Even though these problems are temporary reactions, they do not always disappear by themselves.

The quest for the inner man does not always progress without difficulties. On the road to inner growth the seeker is bound to be confronted with his or her own limits, such as fear, insecurity, anxiety, isolation, resistance, etc. Some problems may be genetically determined; others may originate from childhood traumas and, later in life, other blockades may come into existence due to loneliness, fear of aggression or terror through physical or emotional violence. The spiritual quest is not the mere absence of these anxieties, fears, anguish, etc., but a frame of mind in which these processes do not irritate the seeker any more: one is free in the midst of these obstacles. Exploring the inner world with serious emotional problems and simultaneously aiming to move beyond the limitations of the ego to a deeper, higher Self appears counter-productive. Before recognising the Divine within, seekers could be aided first of all to regain some of their human potentials before moving toward superhuman potentials.

However, it should be clear that the various psychological problems which can arise during an encounter with the higher realms are often the result of spontaneous efforts of the organism to heal itself. All these obstacles are not only related to problems in interpersonal relationships but can also be used as opportunities for healing emotional and psychodynamic disorders. By converting these obstacles into stepping-stones the seeker can continue his or her spiritual journey to 'inner' continents and Self-discovery.

NOTES

J. Deikman, 'Mindfulness, spiritual seeking and psychotherapy', *Journal of Transp. Psychology,* Vol.23, No.9, 1991, p.39-43.

2. A. Watts, *Psychotherapy East and West,* p.21.

3. B. Boorstein, *Clinical studies in Transpersonal psychotherapy,* pp.25-26.
4. E. Deutsch, *Humanity and Divinity,* p.105.
5. C. Grof and S. Grof, *The Stormy Search of Self,* pp.31-35.
6. S. Kakar, *The Analyst and the Mystic,* p.47-48.
7. C. Grof and S. Grof, *The Stormy Search of Self,* p.71

Chapter Three

Metaphysical Psychology

THE METAPHYSICAL NATURE OF SPIRITUAL DISCIPLINE

Metaphysics is an inquiry into the general meaning and character of reality as opposed to appearances, the distinction between the real and the apparent.

Traditional Western metaphysics claims to have achieved some understanding of the immanent nature and the structure of existence or reality and partly of the essence of the supreme or transcendent Reality, God, soul and the world. A metaphysical worldview implies human power and divinity; life is part of a spiritual journey and within each individual resides the mystic who knows that the ego is just a limited aspect of an infinite Self. The individual creates his or her own reality, rather than its being determined by God's chance or luck and one is, therefore, himself responsible for one's acts using any situation or circumstance as a self created opportunity for growth and wholeness.

In psychological language, the soul, which is identical with the divine Reality, moves beyond the limitations of the senses, the rational mind, space and time and explores regions beyond ordinary human potentials towards inner and higher realms, i.e., the spiritual realm.

An absolute truth is not merely known but also lived; it is appreciated as true by a certain kind of life. As such, metaphysics can be described as a reflection of the nature of the innermost reality in man and its relation to external existence. Reflection is seen as a way of life, lifting man to higher levels of being in order to experience them, rather than forming a hypothetical model of thought and the application of this model to a human level.

The truth of transcendental dimensions of reality cannot always be adequately understood and expressed in conventional language. The communication of the contents of these intuitive experiences takes place mostly through figurative, metaphorical and symbolic statements, suggestions or mythical images, even though our capacity to interpret these messages is limited as they are partly obscure in what they seek to reveal.

Metaphysics implies a coordinated ordering of the structure of being and the reality that is so disclosed in experience. Concepts such as supramental or transcendental consciousness, liberation, etc., which lie beyond all known categories and relations are difficult concepts for the more mundane. Objective research, on the other hand, may preclude or undermine a true understanding of these experiences and processes. All such data of reality consists of pure experience. The human experience itself falls short of the 'pure' experience as it is incomplete in respect of its data: many aspects of reality do not enter directly into the structure of one's experience. Metaphysics tries to discover the general characteristics of the complete pure experience, which is inclusive, systematic and direct. While the perceptive capacity of our senses is restricted, our intelligence too is limited in penetrating to the bottom of the principles that govern science. Science *per se* is not concerned with the unity of experience; it can reach probable and practical truth, but never an eternal, metaphysical truth. Can the limitations of science be removed through contemplative introspection on the deeper aspects of the problem, i.e., the absolute truth within the soul? Through focusing on this divine principle, the seeker can experience something of it, even without directly understanding it with the intellect.

Though the student of metaphysics aspires for deliverance from the physical or material framework, he or she interprets and identifies the beyond within the framework of known entities. This 'beyond' as a product of reason, as a mental abstraction, cannot be itself confirmed. It must remain in the realm of speculation.

Western metaphysical thought does not always go beyond intellect in its methods and, therefore, often remains restricted in mind-constructs, pointing vaguely to a fragmentary representation of the supreme Truth. This speculation about truth has its utility in helping the mind to seek the idea of the beyond.

Metaphysical principles in the East, on the other hand, go a step further by uplifting man to the level of spiritual understanding rather than their embodiment in concrete life. The history of Eastern metaphysics has been the history of endlessly diverse explorations with spiritual truth, an attempt at unravelling the different aspects of ultimate Reality.

Logical reasoning is indispensable as it gives the mind a certain clarity and subtlety of ideas and removes confusions. Logical reasoning, as a partially enlightened guide, is therefore part of the preparation for the method of metaphysical dialectics. Man's intellect needs to know the nature of spiritual reality. In this way, it helps to create a mental formulation of the spiritual truth which can be applied later on, in the more advanced stages of the spiritual journey. Reason does liberate man from narrow dogmas and superstitions and enables one to control and order the environment. It unites individuals and is very useful when applied to the control of one's impulsive nature. However, reason also separates man from the rest of nature and prevents the individual from affirming the totality of his being. The non-rational, non-personal transcendent levels of reality, the infinite, cannot be identified with finite reason, as the Absolute transcends logical thought.

Intellect and reason restrain man from coming into intimate unity with the Divine; the former functions in the presence of time, forms and relations, whereas the latter is unformed, timeless and beyond qualities. Intellect can describe the nature of the transcendental self in terms of limited psychological and philosophical concepts, but it cannot explain the beyond.

Reason cannot establish certitudes regarding the mystery of nature, the purpose of human life and other ultimate questions. It cannot create an emotive relatedness to the mystery of the universe, and it is not able to connect the individual with his or her transcendent realm of being or existence. Often these questions cannot be proved or demonstrated, but through introspection one can understand them.

There are rational explanations for spiritual experiences, but reason is not the best way to study them. Positivistic methodology exposes the meaninglessness of many metaphysical speculations. But a rational spiritual psychology, based on a rational foundation, insists on the experiential and existential nature of man.

A spiritual experience is not mere sense-experience or reason, but the direct experience of the innermost reality. Scientific materialism denies any affirmation regarding spiritual transcendence, i.e., the central spiritual dimension of man. It interprets life purely intellectually, as if the only distinctive character of man's nature is reason. Empirical science observes only the periphery of existence and the motivating factors remain outside its scope. It is not concerned with the ultimate questions of life; it does not offer an answer to why the universe is as it is and it still has to discover a theory about the origin of life from lifeless material; it may therefore need the help of metaphysical explorations.

Even though it is clear to the common man that modern empirical science does not have all the answers to the fundamental questions of existence, for a large number of scientists the exploration of such questions does not lead to any final solutions. For them, in fact, these questions have no answer at all. Each field of science has its own inner contradictions; there are still more than enough mysteries and science represents, at the most, the best available insights. As a human activity science is always subject to change. There are still details in science that are not understood and that might, one day, upturn all basis of science as we have known so far. It may be questioned if the role of science in contemporary human experience has given us a real sense of unity with nature. Scientific theories are often based on a confusing succession of intellectual outpourings of those who try to make a coherent sense of what they deduce.

The methods of objective, reductionistic and mechanistic science are not wrong in themselves but they are only applicable on the basis of rational logic, whereas self-knowledge or self-realisation is an open system rather than a situation to be observed and quantified. Unless science extends to involve awareness, subjectivity, openness and 'awe' in the exploration of complex spiritual phenomena it will hardly be able to understand the mystery of human psyche or the material world. Through its scientific methods, science enables the researcher to manipulate, calculate and exploit their understanding of objects but the scientist does not penetrate into the essential meaning of these objects. It does not explore their origin and the destiny of future man. Science does not share a common 'existential' ground with the spirit and does not validate underlying forces and hidden causes. The real nature and essence of human reality and the world around us does not come merely by intellectual know-how. It comes to the seeker by direct experience during spiritual practice.

At present, metaphysics has a confusing multiplicity of contradictory meanings, ranging from clear thinking about the deeper levels of reality up to hypothetical propositions and irrational formulations. Due to these contradictory meanings, scientists do not consider metaphysics as a science and tend not to give it any importance. But does art in general—poetry, painting, music, theatre, etc ,—has no meaning because it is not a science? Has metaphysics, therefore, no meaning because it is not covered under the title science? Science and metaphysics, as different orders of reality, each have their own range and their own method of inquiry. The truths of the physical universe can throw some light on the nature of the Force that is active in the universe. Nevertheless, science cannot dictate its conclusions on metaphysics any more than metaphysics can impose its conclusions on science. The scientist experiences the world through specialisation of a rational analysis whereas the student of metaphysics does it through his or her mystical intuition. Can there be a synthesis in which the scientist supplants the scientific method for the introspective, contemplative method? Both actually supplement one another for a complete worldview.

A similar idea has been expressed by A. Watts: "Something that has constantly worried me about almost all schools of psychotherapy is what I am going to call a lack of metaphysical depth, a certain shallowness which results from having a philosophical unconscious which has not been examined."[1]

The transpersonal psychologist criticises the focus on objectivity of scientific psychology. Only by going beyond the ordinary waking state of consciousness can the researcher become aware and open to new and more inclusive models of the psychological constitution of man. Nevertheless, the transpersonal psychologist also expects from each seeker the use of one's reason rather than the simple following of the teaching of any spiritual discipline in blind obedience or devotion.

A spiritual discipline is not based on an uncritical acceptance of certain doctrinal interpretations, however, it demands an initial receptivity and acceptance of the prescribed methods before the seeker can critically examine them. Initially, there should be no doubts and no critical judgements but at a later stage, with knowledge and insight, the researcher may be able to debate certain issues which are related to a specific spiritual discipline. F. Staal affirms that psychology gets deepened and enlarged when it includes special aspects of mysticism in its research. He observes, however, that "some contemporary psychologists are attempting to place psychology in a larger framework. But in doing so they choose for irrationalism and get entangled in problems ... a rational investigation needs to be done towards this second stream of knowledge [intuitive knowledge]. It should not be surprising when we discover that our insight increases enormously by researching this stream. But it would be a *petitio principi* when we take for granted from the beginning that we are dealing here with a complement of rational knowledge; this is just one of the problems we are investigating."[2]

It seems that in order to understand the human personality as an integrated part of a holographic universe, some of the transpersonal psychologists are still limited by the very concepts of the scientific paradigm itself. These transpersonal psychologists are willing to accept spirituality but they still operate and struggle out of a postmodern mechanistic scientific worldview with a limited understanding of the universe. They use the methods of reductionistic science to prove the validity of spiritual phenomena, which cannot be studied by empirical methodology only. It seems odd that many transpersonal psychologists do challenge parts of the mechanistic worldview but still remain involved in the same worldview in order to gain acceptance as scientists. As the reader will see later on, Sri Aurobindo—in order to avoid this contradiction of the scientific and theoretical assumptions which underlie transpersonal psychology—wants the seeker to get in touch with the deeper inner being, which offers each of us every possible opportunity to heal.

The concept of *Jnana* as knowledge or insight is not merely an expression of anti-intellectualism; knowledge is something which is objective and true, whether intellectual or anti intellectual. In transpersonal psychology, a critical evaluation combined with an experimental as well as a rational and experiential approach to spirituality is essential if spirituality is ever to become a part of psychological research.

In creating such a scientific approach, the transpersonal psychologist should attempt to bridge the gulf between the spiritual nature of man and the essence of science. The scientific and questioning mindset is an asset in the quest of spirituality and one's intellect and common sense need therefore never be abandoned in the spiritual quest. But as long as science remains restricted to external observation and excludes meaning, it can never know the meaninglessness of metaphysical speculation.

From a metaphysical point of view, the Self recognises the Divine reality which is immanent in life, mind and nature. By reducing the contents of spiritual knowledge and experiences to the subject of comprehensive observations and making them understandable in intellectual terms, many of the transpersonal psychologists seem to leave out the deep-rooted metaphysical dimensions of spirituality which underlie each spiritual tradition. To make the spiritual experience amenable to research by science and make it 'naturalistic' involves some form of reductionism. This naturalistic theory of spiritual experience considers that the 'higher', pre-existent in the 'lower', emerges from the lower through some means. In its attempt to naturalise spirituality, some transpersonal psychologists try to bring down the Eternal and Infinite experience to the level of the finite and the temporal. Such psychologists are unable to go beyond the transpersonal. Other transpersonal psychologists emphasise the transcendental experience but in their naturalistic approach they split off the transcendental experience from God and each and every experience becomes more or less natural rather than supernatural. Such an approach denies the source of spiritual experience: in spiritual traditions the divine origin refers to God.

Although the transpersonal approach is experiential at its core—by moving toward the depth of one's inner being the seeker is able to discover the realm of his or her spiritual being—many transpersonal psychologists still have not sufficiently developed a well-integrated metaphysical worldview. As concluded by B. Cortright, "the transpersonal field has not yet come to the point of trying to establish a consensual view of reality."[3]

Transpersonal psychologists are not students of metaphysics, however, as empirical scientists of the Spirit they take the inner life of the seeker seriously and, therefore, they enrich one's understanding of the human psyche.

THE CONCEPT OF 'SELF' IN METAPHYSICS

The Psychological Nature of the Self

Spiritual activity such as the search for self-realisation has different meanings in the East and the West. There is a confusion regarding the exact meaning of the concept of the self, I, and the person, which becomes more complicated when the terms psyche, soul and Spirit are added. The self in Western psychotherapy is often related to the physical body and such operations of the psyche as emotions (urges and feelings), cognition (images and the observing centre) and reason (thinking and imagination and will or functional capacities). The self is often equated with the personality, ego or I; these expressions, however, need careful definition and analysis.

The psychological self as a conceptual centre of being is a collection of attributes and attitudes that identifies the person as a particular human being, i.e., the body, the personality, the character, the memories, attitudes, roles and skills and all the things that constitute 'who I am'. This psychological self consists of the sum-total of capacities to reflect on the information that the various sense organs register and to direct and control these experiences. The self functions as a means of organising information and as a source of reflection. The individual experiences the mass of information in consciousness as the self; this self, however, has its own features that cannot be predicted or directed.

The will, cognition and emotion need the self for activating them, i.e., the I appears to be one with the act of willing, seeing and feeling. The self is thus something the person creates to account for the multiplicity of impressions, emotions, thoughts and feelings that the brain records. Without this centralising faculty all the sensory inputs will jostle one another in what may be termed senseless chaos. Ken Wilber credits the self on the mental level with the following basic functions:

(1) the locus of identification, the I/me experience;
(2) the organizing principle of unity;
(3) the navigator between progression and regression;
(4) the centre of free will and of the defence mechanisms;
(5) the centre of assimilation of past and present experiences.

At present, the concept of self is often identified with external objects and relationships, and the development of the self is mostly dependent on external accomplishments. This self as a concept, however, cannot be localised and has no actual reality of its own.

The term self is used interchangeably with the term personality or 'I' in everyday usage. Personality is related to an enduring set of traits, beliefs, attitudes, motivations and response patterns that characterise an individual and which distinguishes one person from another. Being the core of personality, the 'I' organises and integrates all the factors of individuality into a unity.

As the object of self-consciousness, the self or I is also often referred to as the ego. There is a distinction between the self as I and the self as 'ego' but this distinction is relative and not absolute. The I as a concrete self is inescapably emotional and cognitive as well as moral; it is this 'I' and its subjectivity— the ego—which thinks, feels and makes man aware of his or her body. The ego as a self-centred consciousness refers to that aspect of the mind which establishes a duality between I and not-I but, it also enables consciousness to reflect upon itself and create self-responsibility within the individual. As such, the ego is treated as a product of psychological forces generated by the interactions of the individual and one's socio-physical environment.

The ego or I as an organising force acts in the specific locus of the individual's organism ('I' want) but the I is also identical with awareness, the 'I' as a witness to all events (I am). But this 'I' as awareness is limited by beliefs and assumptions of the individual and is, therefore, cut off from a wider awareness, i.e., man confuses this I awareness (mental function) with the universal awareness and is caught in illusions of separateness. To know the real nature of the 'I' requires the freedom and transcendence of the I from its ego involvement; in its transcendence, the ego becomes noumenon, i.e., its independent existence can be reasoned but never perceived by the mind.

In spiritual discipline the ego-self is often seen as an obstacle during the process of growth, as it consumes all the seeker's vital energy, which interferes with the discovery and manifestation of one's deeper self. Traditions of spiritual discipline affirm that beneath the I and me there exists an unchanging Self beyond the personal empirical self, beyond duality and distinction, and one which can be known by immediate intuitive experience. This Self lies at the deepest recesses of our being and can be realised within the depth of stillness.

In transpersonal psychology the self is related to pure consciousness or pure Ground of being. One of the central subject matters in transpersonal psychology is the movement and growth of this consciousness, which is not conditioned or modified by the physical, vital and mental structures of the self but transcends the self. However, consciousness as 'Pure Ground of Being' is mostly obscured by the contents of the self and the seeker wrongly identifies this pure consciousness with contents of consciousness such as sensations, affects and cognition. In combination with spiritual practice transpersonal psychotherapy is able to remove this misplaced identification and to explore and develop the divine nature of consciousness which illuminates and sustains the outer contents of consciousness. The exploration of a growing awareness need not always be accompanied by the transpersonal psychotherapist but may also come in silence with the help of the Divine Grace.

The Metaphysical Nature of the Self

The terms psyche, soul and Spirit are often used indiscriminately and interchangeably. Eastern spiritual disciplines do not categorize self, soul and spirit as in the West. By confusing soul with psyche there is a tendency to confuse psychotherapy with sadhana.

The psyche in psychotherapy has its own logic; it allows the individual to experience him or herself and the world empirically and is closely linked with pathology, mortality and limitations.

The term psyche often refers to the ground of psychological self-awareness at any level of consciousness. As the principle of mental and emotional life this psychological psyche has spiritual needs. When these needs (Maslow's metaneeds) are not fulfilled or don't get sufficient attention from the soul, the psyche often turns beyond psychotherapy to sadhana.

The soul as a psychological concept is commonly used as a simple subject of awareness, and refers to the subtle separate self-sense, but in Indian philosophy the soul is immortal and is free from mental, vital and physical imperfections. The soul is the indestructible essence of the individual; it transcends birth and death, and is the priciple of ultimate individual growth. The soul when disunited from the body becomes Spirit, the ultimate Reality, i.e., the soul relates the seeker to the Divine, whereas Spirit is identical with the Divine. Spirit is beyond subject-object reality, beyond reason, and a spiritual life is in its essence not the realisation of an ethical life but the realisation of the ultimate Reality.

For Sri Aurobindo, psyche and Spirit are two different concepts and should not be confounded. The psyche is related to psychological principles, whereas Spirit is identified with metaphysical principles. Each realm has its own rules and perspectives.

Spirit as Brahman is always in Oneness with the Divine. The Self as the highest centre of pure consciousness, also called Atman, is free, eternal and transcendent. This

Self is more than the universal or individual mind, life and body; they are only its forms and not the true Self. By detaching oneself from all identifications with these forms, the individual can get back to the consciousness of the true Individual, the eternal Being and pure Existence. The Self is immanent in all things. It is something self-existent, pure and eternal.

Sri Aurobindo makes no distinction between the Self and Spirit; the Self is the divine element within the individual that is not affected by evolution. Spirit is always one with the Divine and in its nature it is either transcendent or universal. When it individualises it is called *Jivatman,* which remains aware of its oneness with the universal and transcendent but at the same time feels its central identity/ individuality as a portion of the Divine.

In the embodied individual the Spirit develops as a psychic being, a pure power of light, love and refined essence of being, "the inner voice of the mystic." The word psychic is ordinarily used in psychology as anything phenomenal (such as the ego) but Sri Aurobindo uses the word psychic for the soul, differentiating it from the mental-vital consciousness. As he explains, "the word psychic is used in English to indicate anything that is other or deeper than the external mind, life and body or it indicates sometimes anything occult or supraphysical; but that is a use which brings confusion and error and we have almost entirely to discard it."[4] He uses the term psychic as "a spark come from the Divine which is there in all things and as the individual evolves it grows in him and manifests as the psychic being, the soul, seeking always for the Divine and the Truth."[5]

The soul, as a representative of the *Jivatman,* is not a compound but a thing in itself: it is a Power of the Divine Consciousness which does not disintegrate and is always turned towards Truth, Good and Beauty. This psychic part within the individual has in its origin divine possibilities, but this divine element is at first hidden behind the ordinary consciousness; once it grows by the accumulation of deeper and higher movements of consciousness it develops into a psychic individuality, the *Psychic Being,* which is the secret cause of man's turning to the spiritual life.

The psychic being stands behind the mental, vital and physical nature, transforming it until all is ready for union with the Divine. The *Psychic entity,* the soul in its essence, and the *psychic being,* the soul in its individual form are, therefore, not the same. The soul as the eternal essence is the divine spark that dwells at the centre of each being, whereas the psychic being is shaped progressively around the soul during terrestrial evolution. According to Sri Aurobindo, "It is the psychic personality in us that flowers as the saint, the sage, the seer; when it reaches its full strength, it turns the being towards the knowledge of Self and the Divine, towards the supreme Truth, the supreme Good, the supreme Beauty, Love and Bliss, the divine heights and largeness, and opens us to the touch of spiritual sympathy, universality, oneness."[6]

The psychic being can be located in the transpersonal realm as it forms the depth-dimension of the inner reality and opens the individual towards universality as it has a permanent relation with it.

The Self in the Upanishads

In *Mandukya Upanishad* a description is given of different types of the 'Self' that occur in the various states of consciousness. The Upanishads acknowledge a meta-psychological model in which there exists a relationship between the Self and underlying states of consciousness. The Self is the inmost centre of diverse waking, dreaming and deep sleep states and the state of pure spiritual consciousness. Consciousness does not belong to the body or the mind but resides in the Self or Atman; it is the power of consciousness that illuminates all gross physical and mental bodies at the individual level, and the external universe at the cosmic level. The nature of each state that the Atman passes through may be summarized as follows:

1. In *the waking state* of the self, the self has a gross body and makes use of the sense-organs and the intellect; its consciousness is directed toward the external world and the sensual enjoyment of gross objects. In this waking state the Atman identifies itself with the physical body and its consciousness is involved in the operation of the senses together with the mind. The mind is busily engaged in receiving and registering the sense impressions of gross external objects through the external sense organs.
2. In *the dream state* of the self, the self uses psychic force and its consciousness is directed toward internal unconscious forces such as desires, instincts and drives. The sense-organs are quiescent, i.e., perception without sensation. The mind is still active, though independently of the sense-organs, and works on the impressions left behind from waking experiences. Consciousness is partly awake and partly asleep; its experiences are conditioned by past impressions rather than by present external objects.
3. In *the deep-sleep state* the self attains to a state of complete rest and its consciousness is directed toward integrated self-awareness or the undifferentiated blissful state of consciousness. In this state all experiences become unified with the inner and universal self. All distinctions between body, mind and senses are lost and the Self perceives through its own light. This state appears to man's surface consciousness as a state without any consciousness, because the wakening consciousness is rooted in duality and

it cannot long sustain this experience of unity. Nevertheless, limitations still exist in this state though in latent form. The Atman is still stupefied by the unmanifest, i.e., the root of ignorance persists and therefore the Atman does not realise its true nature.

4. The *pure-consciousness state,* the *Turiya state,* is not really a condition of the mind but a complete and unchanging experience. The original nature of Atman can be discovered only when the seeker disentangles oneself from the other three states and goes beyond them—beyond the senses, thought and speech because its nature is the source and not the object of consciousness. It is tranquil and without a second and it transcends yet includes consciousness and unconsciousness. By its intrinsic nature it possesses no activities, qualities or form and, therefore, it cannot be fully described as it lies outside the limits of empirical investigation; however, it can be realised directly and intuitively. This Self is the unconditioned substratum and the common ground of all the other.

The Upanishads give a detailed description of these four experiences of the soul and the various phenomena with which these are associated. The first two states fall under psychology, for in these states the mind functions fully but the other two states are over-mental or super-mental (above and beyond the realms of the mental) and reveal the real nature of the soul.

The Upanishadic concept of the Self is not merely a metaphysical system fit for intellectual analysis. It is really an experience related to the exploration of the deeper levels of the Self. This experiential valuation of the various states of consciousness confronts the Western psychologist who regards the waking state as more real than the dream state, in contrast to the Upanishadic view, which regards dream and deep-sleep states as closer to the Self''s true nature than the waking state.

Contrary to the concept of an inert state, waking or sleeping, Sri Aurobindo's view is of an 'inclusive' evolutionary model of interpenetrating planes or levels of consciousness. He makes a meaningful distinction between the surface consciousness of the self as the ordinary waking consciousness, the subconscient below, the subliminal behind and the superconscient above the surface consciousness. Sri Aurobindo emphasises the subliminal consciousness, which is similar to the deep-sleep state beyond the surface consciousness and which "gives access to new mental and vital and subtle physical planes of universal consciousness."[7]

Sri Aurobindo also refers to the deep-sleep state as the Supramental Spirit where the seeker enters the Superconscient. He agrees with the Upanishadic view that the fourth state of the Self is the true Self and the first three states are three different orders of one Reality. But he refuses Sankara's Advait Vedanta's illusionist view of the "unreal" psychological states of the waking, dream and deep-sleep states. These three planes are a harmonised and unified experience and the interpenetrating planes of consciousness are, therefore, not unreal. For Sri Aurobindo all four phases of human experience are real aspects of man's individuality.

The Self in Advait Vedanta and Yoga

The psychological self that is cognised is not 'the true self, as the latter cannot be cognised as an object of knowledge. Consciousness may stand for the ultimate unchanging metaphysical self or for the changing psychological self; the former cannot be objectified as it is the objectless subject and the latter is only conscious of its contents. The Eastern spiritual traditions affirm the reality of the psychological self, but this is relegated to a lower or practical realm. The individual has self-consciousness in the practical realm but this is not the true Self as it is conditioned by the internal instrument, i.e., the mind, sense-organs and ego. Deep within all individuals resides the true Self, which may be termed Atman, but often it dwells so deep within that the individual remains aware only of his or her body, mind and senses, and as a consequence erroneously identifies the Atman with the internal instrument, and the body. Spiritual growth is related to the process of realising the Atman. According to Yoga and Vedanta, consciousness is not a quality or attribute of the Self or Atman but its very essence, i.e., a self-existing entity, not caused or produced but real and timeless. Not being an attribute of anything it is eternal, infinite and without complexity.

Atman aims at the disclosure to the individual of one's true essence, whereas Brahman, as the cosmic principle, aims at the discovery and realisation of the universe as a whole. The two concepts are often correlated and identified, i.e., 'I am Brahman/ and this ultimate Reality once apprehended dons the spiritual character.

The real Self is devoid of attributes and cannot be perceived by the mind, but this Atman is not unknown, and like the Atman in the *Mandukya Upanishad,* it can be realised through immediate intuitive knowledge.

The Advait Vedanta of Sankara

For Sankara the essential nature of the Self is pure subject when it is detached from the objective elements that are superimposed on it. He maintains that the Self, Atman, is completely identical with Brahman and the individual's Self is just like the supreme Self. Sankara classifies the Self, pure consciousness, as a transcendental and empirical reality; the former is one, inactive and unchanging; whereas the latter is many, active and changing. The transcendental reality of the absolute consciousness, 'Atman', is self-luminous, eternal and unmodified by qualities. As such there is no selfconsciousness in the sense of ego-consciousness. The true self-consciousness is not the consciousness of the self as an object used in introspection. Sankara's central conception is related to the reflective inwardness of the Brahman to man and this Brahman has to be realised by every seeker as the Atman. In Advaita's ontology and epistemology, one's true underlying Self is the individual aspect of Brahman. Besides this absolute Self, Sankara also accepts the existence of an individual empirical self as '*Jiva*', which is constituted of self and not self (ignorance). The individual Self, as pure consciousness, is unlike the empirical self with its unconscious life activities and conscious psychological activities that form the empirical attributes of the soul. The Jiva is composed of a finite ethical personality and its conscious aspects are due to the Atman, as the latter is the onlooker of the experiences of the former. As the eternal consciousness, the Jiva is the Self as Atman seen under the conditions of space and time and limited by the internal instrument; the latter functions as an awareness-mechanism which acts through other senses but which is ultimately a delusive adjunct of the Self. To the Jiva belongs change, activity and dynamism, the unconscious creative energy of *Prakriti* [nature] in Yoga and ignorance in Vedanta. This Jiva, as an agent of action and enjoyer of the results of these actions, is subject to transmigration. However, Sankara does not deny the reality of 'Jiva' *in its spiritual aspects;* when ignorance is destroyed the Jiva remains in its essential nature of the Atman.

For Sri Aurobindo the Atman is only one aspect of the Divine, as the Divine contains everything, including Nature. This is unlike Sankara's view, which regards the Atman or universal Self as identical with Brahman; for Sankara nature is ultimately unreal, an illusory manifestation of Brahman. Sri Aurobindo also differs with Sankara regarding the postulate of Jiva. The Jiva in Sri Aurobindo's Yoga is seen as a portion of the Divine, manifested as the individual self to preside over the individual's evolution without getting itself involved in it. For Sankara the Jiva is a mixture of the self and not self (ignorant and unreal), whereas for Sri Aurobindo there is no unreality in the Jiva; it is the Divine itself though not in its wholeness.

Patanjali's Yoga

In Yoga, the *Purusha* or true Self is the independent unifying principle of the total psyche, including self-consciousness, the unconscious and the superconscious. This Self is pure consciousness and not a substance endowed with consciousness as an attribute.

The *Prakriti* in the form of a psychological self consists of mind, intellect, memory and ego and is designed as a practical tool for participation in the world. These psychic functions, however, impose limitations upon the Spirit in the form of an alienation from one's own spiritual essence. Spiritual growth aims at the realisation of the individual's spiritual essence and the removal of the false identification of the different psychic functions with the true Self.

In Patanjali's Yoga the psychological self is also referred to as the internal instrument which is made up of *manas,* (recording faculty) *ahamkara,* (ego-sense or I-ness), *buddhi,* (discriminative faculty) and *chitta* (faculty of memory). Through the senses *chitta* comes into contact with the external world. In its initial contact *chitta* gets in touch with *buddhi,* the organ that recognises, discriminates and determines. In the next stage ahamkarah, or the individuation principle as the subject of all psychological experience, tests reality according to its individual interest. Finally, manas, as the organiser of sensations, is responsible for all kinds of conscious actions.

This internal instrument, as the sum-total of mental functioning, corresponds to the Western concept of mind, but Yoga adds a metaphysical significance to it. Liberation is the isolation of the pure transcendental Self from the internal instrument. This transcendental Self cannot come into its own unless it leaves behind the discursive rational mind and its activities.

Status of the Self in Sri Aurobindo's Metaphysical System

Sri Aurobindo regards Self as an entity in itself and the ultimate source of consciousness with illuminative and transformative capabilities; it is considered as a portion of the Divine involving itself in Matter. The Self is not a substance endowed with consciousness as an attribute; the Self is pure consciousness itself, intrinsically luminous and eternally perfect. Sri Aurobindo harmonises the values of nature (cosmic action) and Spirit (transcendence), the imperfect world and the supreme Good, "the real self is the eternal who is obviously capable of both the mobility in Time and the immobility basing Time—simultaneously, otherwise they could not both exist; nor, even, could one exist and the other create seemings."[8] This statement affirms the experience of both the mobile multiple world and the immobile self absorbed state as poles of the individual's experience.

The Self is the principle of all existence; though one, it reveals itself in three ways—as (1) transcendent, (2) universal and (3) individual.

(1) The transcendental Self is beyond the individual and the cosmos; it is existence identical with the essential Divine Being. Brahman is the Self of the selves, i.e., the transcendent Self as supracosmic Existence. The essential oneness of this Self is due to its infiniteness but Brahman is also one in the many, the synthetic unity of the manifold. Participating in becoming involves Brahman's own being, and creation of the universe is part of the complete self-manifestation of all that is Brahman. This transcendental consciousness is described by Sri Aurobindo as "a Transcendent

who is beyond all world and all Nature and yet possesses the world and its nature ... it is the Source of our being, the Source of our works and their Master. But the seat of the Transcendent Consciousness is above in an absoluteness of divine Existence."[9] This Superconscient Transcendence is not only an Existence but also a Power.

(2) The real Self as universal consciousness is Brahman the cosmic Spirit or Self who uses the cosmos for the working out of the being as Brahman. This eternal Brahman manifested in time or the Spirit manifested in infinite self-extension is the indwelling Spirit inherent in all creation. In the world process, Brahman creates out of a joyous expression of being, "out of delight", and is present in the world rather than separate from it. The creation of the world is part of the complete self-manifestation of all that Brahman is; without this manifestation Brahman would not be All. Spirit cannot do without creation, as it forms the very basis of its existence. Both Spirit and the world are necessary for perfect life. For Sri Aurobindo a cosmic Self or Spirit not only supports but also originates and contains the whole cosmic action. Although he admits the primacy of Spirit, this does not mean that the world is an illusion. The universal Self is above the individual's personality and bodily existence and exceeds it altogether, yet it contains everything in the Cosmos.

(3) The true Individual Self is the vehicle in which Brahman seeks to emerge most completely. The existence of man, as a vehicle in which Brahman seeks to reveal itself, includes the capability of man to become God without ceasing to be man. Because the individual directs all one's energy

and knowledge to externals, one is not able to find one's real Self or the real Self of the world in which one lives. Man wrongly identifies the Self with body, life and mind or with the limitations of the ego and, unless man turns his or her vision inward, he will remain separated from other selves and God. The ego is only a knot in the lower nature and has no separate existence; our apparent separate individuality is only a surface movement serving as a practical nucleus for the pragmatic aspects of life. This ego or immediate self is the basis or raw material for growth toward the Universal and Transcendental self. Behind the individual ego is Purusha, the real individual. The true Individual Self, the Jivatman, the immanent Divine and the central being of each living entity is immutable and free, unaffected by desire, ego and ignorance.

The existence of individuality is real because "his heart, his will, the strongest and intensest parts of his being remain without a meaning, void of purpose or justification, or become merely a random foolishness agitating itself like a vain and restless shadow against the eternal repose of the pure Existence or amidst the eternal inconscience of the universe."[10]

The first step in sadhana is to affirm and possess powerfully and completely one's own individuality. For Sri Aurobindo "this primary egoistic development with all its sins and violences and crudities is by no means to be regarded, in its proper place, as an evil or an error of Nature; it is necessary for man's first work, the finding of his own individuality."[11] Without a strong individuality the seeker cannot attain oneness with all; the development of individuality is, therefore, an essential precondition for spiritual realisation. Although a fortified individuality is necessary for effective action in practical life, Sri Aurobindo maintains that such individuality is not the highest state of being, as it does not provide a means for the fulfilment of the progressing soul. As such the development of the egoistic individuality is only a stage which was essential for the practical life in the world; but it has to be passed for the fulfilment of the goal of one's life— the finding of one's true Self.

The individual can never get rid of the ego completely and even in self-extinction the ego is not abolished altogether but transcended. What is dissolved is not the seeker's individuality but the ignorance which separates the person from the Divine. Once this ignorance is removed he or she will "find either his transcendent Self or his true Person", the true individual. Sri Aurobindo does not deny the reality of the individual self. Individuality has a persistent reality of itself which is veiled from Brahman and which must be realised, i.e., God must be revealed to Himself in man and with this self discovery the realisation of God in life becomes possible.

In describing the importance of the individual Self, Sri Aurobindo writes, "The Self as individual is no less real than the Self as cosmic Being or Spirit and both are powers of the Eternal." This explains "the necessity for the growth of the individual and his discovery of himself as a condition for the discovery of the cosmic Self. ... For it is no longer sufficient to suppose an illusory or temporary individual ... if the individual is a persistent reality, an eternal portion or power of the Eternal, if his growth of consciousness is the means by which the Spirit in things discloses its being ... then, secure behind all the changings of our personality, upholding the stream of its mutations, there must be a true Person, a real spiritual Individual, a true Purusha."[12]

Sri Aurobindo regards the Self as a portion and power of the Divine embodied in the individual. This Self must in its intrinsic nature be pure, transcendent and eternally perfect. The experience of the individual only finds its own truth when it is known in terms of the universal and transcendental.

According to Sri Aurobindo, "the Transcendent, the Universal, the Individual are three powers overarching, underlying and penetrating the whole manifestation ... Out of the individual we wake into a vaster freer cosmic consciousness; but out of the universal too with its complex of forms and powers we must emerge by a still greater self exceeding into a consciousness without limits that is founded on the Absolute. And yet in this ascension we do not really abolish but take up and transfigure what we seem to leave; for there is a height where the three live eternally in each other, on that height they are blissfully joined in a nodus of their harmonised oneness."[13] For Sri Aurobindo, there is the need of realising all the states of the Self—the individual, universal and transcendent—because of the unity of ultimate Reality which manifests itself in trinity. This unity is not an organic unity but a spiritual relation in which the individual is closely related with the universal and the universal is closely related with the transcendent, while the transcendent expresses itself through the individual and universal. It is one, the All and One. When the individual and the universal are combined within it, the Self is regarded as transcendent. Sri Aurobindo's Self is a concept which can be understood only by insight, which requires not only human effort but also an unfolding granted by the Divine Grace.

The Self in Conventional Western Psychotherapy and Traditional Eastern Spiritual Disciplines

In spiritual discipline the realisation of the Self is the remedy against all human suffering. But Western psychotherapy lacks a sufficient theory of the observing self and remains more or less lost in the object-self (made up of thoughts, sensory perception and the will to act) as the centre of all experiences. According to A. Deikman, who explains the phenomenological basis of the self, "Psychotherapy is imperfect because it misses the centre; it does not see the observing self as the centre of all experience, but places it at the periphery."[14]

In spiritual discipline the observing self, unlike the psychological observing ego, is that which is consciousness itself. It transcends thinking, feeling and acting, and cannot be made object. It can be known by experience but not localised and it is not a part of one's object-world, as it is not formed by our sense-experience and thoughts. This subjective consciousness is transcendent and cannot be influenced by the external world.

Conventional psychotherapy and traditional spiritual discipline both aim at the observation of mental processes and the separation of the subjective and objective self, i.e., separating the observing (subjective) self from thoughts, imaginations and automatic reactions. However, psychotherapy does not assimilate the self with consciousness but equates the self with the person, I or ego. The self gets a psychic structure analogous to an object, whereas consciousness in spiritual discipline is the essential origin of the experience of the Self and the observing self is not considered as the content of the psychic apparatus because it transcends every content. The individual is conscious beyond the world of senses and intellect. Through various techniques the observing self can be developed. Once it is sufficiently established, the awareness and knowledge of traumatic past experiences gets meaning and becomes useful. A. Deikman suggests that "the fundamental activity of psychotherapy as practised in the West is the release of the observing self from the content of consciousness. When we do that we'll see that we are the observer, not the content—the patterns of emotions, thoughts and imaginations which are responsible for our pain. By dis-identifying ourselves from automatic succession [of emotional reactions] we weaken its influence and create a free space in which we can select a suitable reaction. In this way, we realise autonomy where we previously felt overwhelmed and powerless. The scope of fear, depression and anxiety is restrained and weakened, even though they don't disappear completely."[15]

He does not want psychotherapy to abandon its attainments, but "to add and give priority to that which is already central and dominant in our experience—the basis of the experience itself."[16] For A. Deikman, the therapist could interfere to help the client detach the observing self from the area of selfish thoughts and create the possibility of a deeper knowledge of the self and the world. Through proper instruction the needs of the object-self can be reduced. Similarly, with the development of the observing self the extent of emotional reactions is reduced and the individual gains more freedom from emotional disturbances that were previously dominating one's consciousness. Consequently, the client gets a more intense contact with direct reality, a heightened perception of the surroundings and other people and a more intense satisfaction in daily life.

In Eastern disciplines the personal identity includes buddhi, ego, sense-mind and memory; it is not a distinct property of the mind and not tied to the ego. As discussed before, buddhi makes decisions, manas produces sensory input and coordinates them with motor responses and the ego is only a property of individuation and not an active decision making or thought-producing agent.

Eastern disciplines emphasise the development of buddhi for promoting growth. Sri Aurobindo recognises three gradations of the buddhi, beginning with the crude ordinary kind of judgements, then the more sophisticated level of discrimination, arriving at a clear concept of reality and a coherent *Weltanschauung* and, finally, attaining the highest buddhi development which is mainly concerned with the pursuit of pure truth, i.e., the transcendent laws of

God, life and nature.

When it asserts its authority over the instinctive impulses and habits and remains detached from the influence of sense impulses and memory traces, the buddhi allows them to simply pass away and dissipate. With its discriminative power, the buddhi permits the seeker to see through conflicting mental tendencies and is effective in disentangling oneself from all sorts of psychological problems.

In Eastern disciplines and Sri Aurobindo's integral sadhana, attention is directed towards the development of the higher buddhi rather than the workings of the manas. The Western psychotherapeutic emphasis on the workings of the manas and the mental and intrapsychic conflicts that dominate its activities neglects the study of the development of the buddhi which is able to separate itself from the effects and influences of mental conflicts.

NOTES

1. A. Watts; Psychotherapy and eastern religion, *Journal of Transpersonal Psychology,* Vol. 6, 1974, p.18.
2. F. Staal, *Exploring Mysticism,* p.141.
3. B. Cortright, *Psychotherapy and Spirit,* p.157.
4. Sri Aurobindo, *Letters on Yoga,* p.292.
5. Ibid., p.278.
6. Sri Aurobindo, *The Life Divine,* p.226.
7. Ibid., p.426.
8. Ibid., p.508
9. Sri Aurobindo *The Synthesis of Yoga,* p.242.
10. Sri Aurobindo, *The Life Divine,* p.689.
11. Ibid., p.692.
12. Ibid., p.755-756.

13. Sri Aurobindo, *The Synthesis of Yoga*, p.247.
14. A. Deikman, *Mysticism and Psychotherapy*, p.103.
15. Ibid., p.119.
16. Ibid., p.122.

Chapter Four

The Transpersonal Psychology Movement

TRANSPERSONAL PSYCHOLOGY

Transpersonal psychology, as a new discipline, does not seek to impose a new belief system or a new metaphysics, but attempts to expand the field of psychological inquiry including spiritual experiences. In the last fourty years, transpersonal psychology has moved beyond purely psychological investigation and now includes areas such as transpersonal sociology, anthropology and psychiatry. Its studies are no longer used only by transpersonal psychologists but also by social scientists, mental health practitioners and clinicians.

Transpersonal psychology became a separate discipline in the late 1960's, with the emergence of the transpersonal realm in psychology following A. Maslow's presentation of *The Farther Reaches of Human Nature.* He considered "Humanistic Third Force Psychology to be transitional, a preparation for a still higher Fourth Psychology, transpersonal, transhuman and centered in the cosmos rather than in human needs and interests, going beyond humanness, identity and self- actualisation."[1]

The initial stages of the transpersonal movement emphasised "altered states of consciousness" and "beyond the personal", the transpersonal realm far away from ordinary reality. But this emphasis left out certain aspects of the personal realm such as human suffering, pain and psychopathology. Later on, the movement focused its attention more on contemplative practices—which evoke spiritual experiences—in relation with psychotherapy but it also concentrated more upon the integration of spiritual practices and experiences with psychological, philosophical and theological disciplines. At present transpersonal psychology studies the spiritual realm as expressed in and through the personal in everyday life as well as the transcendence of the personal. With this wider perspective in view, the transpersonal psychological movement focuses nowadays also on the lower aspects of human functioning, including psychopathology within a spiritual context, i.e., various forms of psychopathology may create psychic opportunities for spiritual emergence and psychological healing.

B. Cortright defines transpersonal psychology as, "the melding of the wisdom of the world's spiritual traditions with the learning of modern psychology."[2] The former is concerned with the question of man's soul as a spiritual being, whereas the latter occupies itself with a self or ego as a psychological existence. Transpersonal psychology aims at the integration of man's outward experience and nature and the spiritual dimension of human existence. In its scientific pragmatism it reflects upon and integrates the spiritual realm within the healing perspective of the psychological realm, that is to say, spiritual issues are explored from a psychological perspective.

In the past, scientific approaches failed to deal adequately with human experience of the spiritual realm, i.e., higher entities, ultimate purpose, God, love, etc., either ruling out its validity or labelling it "pathological". The individual who has experienced Divine Grace but whose psychological condition is deteriorating cannot be labelled as psychopathological. This Grace or consciousness-force is a Divine Force and cannot be reduced to physiology or psychology. As will be seen later on, for Sri Aurobindo, consciousness is not in the body or in the mind but the body and the mind are in consciousness; so the potential to manipulate consciousness via the body or the mind will be limited. Sri Aurobindo assumes that Consciousness is Spirit.

The transpersonal psychologist insists that the various human experiences within the field of spiritual psychology are not incompatible with the essence of science, on the condition that science includes subjective experiences as part of its subject matter. The transpersonal psychological movement as a subject for scientific investigation affirms that the transpersonal realm is not the exclusive domain of priests, yogis or mystics but also of scientists; it is an open system undergoing a continuous development. In this development it brings together the ancient wisdom of all the great spiritual traditions of the world and the pragmatism of modern Western science. It maintains that life around us is only an outer form of spiritual processes which form the basis of reality and the higher spiritual urges or drives are indispensable for optimal health. As a science of consciousness transpersonal psychology considers the human psyche as an open and transcendental system of consciousness. It is based upon man in whom matter, life, mind and Spirit meet, i.e., the embodied Spirit in man.

The Latin prefix 'trans' often refers to 'beyond' as in the word transcendental but it also means 'across' or 'through'; the Latin root of the word 'persona' is related to a theatrical mask. The term transpersonal may be referred to as the development beyond the conventional, beyond the average, beyond the person, through the person, connecting all persons. S. Grof uses the term transpersonal as, "transcending the usual way of perceiving and interpreting the world from the position of a separate individual or body ego."[3] The person is seen as ultimately spiritual, in addition to one's physical, vital and mental dimensions. This spiritual realm involves a dimension of power and meaning, transcendent to the world of sensory reality.

Spirituality has its own rationale other than merely feeling or blind faith. It is based upon experience and intuitive knowledge and, unlike religion, is not received by means of dogma and external authority. The term spirituality signifies an individual's experience of a dimension of power and meaning transcendent to the ordinary sensory reality. These spiritual experiences may be associated with natural mysticism as well as with religious tradition and/or spiritual disciplines.

For Ken Wilber, "the word transpersonal simply means 'personal plus'. That is, the transpersonal orientation explicitly and carefully includes all the facets of personal psychology and psychiatry, then adds those deeper or higher aspects of human experience that transcend the ordinary and the average—experiences that are, in other words, 'transpersonal' or 'more than personal'; personal plus. Thus in the attempt to more fully, accurately and scientifically reflect the entire range of human experience, transpersonal psychiatry and psychology take as their starting point the entire spectrum of consciousness."[4]

According to F. Vaughan, "the term transpersonal does not deny the validity of the importance of individual uniqueness. 'Transpersonal' can be distinguished from transcendent in that it refers to the transcendental as manifest in and through the person."[5] Vaughan defines transpersonal psychology as "the psychological study of transpersonal experiences and their correlates. These correlates include the nature, varieties, causes and effects of transpersonal experiences and development, as well as psychologies, philosophies, disciplines, arts, cultures, life-styles, reactions and religions that are inspired by them, or that seek to induce, express, apply or understand them."[6] Transpersonal psychology seeks to understand how this transcendent dimension can be integrated in the seeker's life. Ordinary psychology contributes to an understanding of the nature of the self and its relationship with other selves; transpersonal psychology seeks to expand these psychological inquiries into the farther reaches of human nature. These farther reaches of human nature include wider relatedness between the individual's psychological and spiritual dimensions in relation with universal life principles.

In a holistic approach to psychological health, the spiritual dimensions of the person are affirmed as a vital aspect of human potentials and the transpersonal enquiry aims at unifying man's spiritual and psychological perspectives. Transpersonal psychology views all psychological processes within the context of spiritual evolution. Optimal mental health is considered as inextricably connected with the spiritual realm and the healing and growth of the psychological self is seen against the background of the self's spiritual dimension. The transpersonal psychologist attempts to cast the psychological realm into a spiritual frame, as it is the spiritual realm which gives meaning to the psychological realm.

Although transpersonal psychology is concerned with the study of man's highest potentials, the discipline does not tie itself to any particular religion, philosophy, specific worldview or metaphysics. As such transpersonal psychology as a spiritual psychology emphasises not so much human behaviour itself but the study of transcendental and spiritual experiences.

At present, there are two paradigms functioning within the transpersonal movement. The first paradigm is Ken Wilber's 'ladder model', where the personal merges into the transpersonal. In this 'height' psychological ladder model the individual begins his or her developmental process in a state of fusion not with the Self, but with the physical body. The more the ego develops itself, the more the body fades into the background and is often repressed. To find the Self, the individual is not compelled to regress but to progress in his or her development, so that body and ego are transcended in the spiritual stage of development. The second paradigm, S. Grof's and M. Washburn's 'spiral model', places spiritual development in a 'depth' spiritual context, i.e., spiritual development is the regression to the past and to something that is lost. In the spiral model, the ego disconnects itself from the Self and afterwards unites itself with the Self but at a higher level. During the first part of life, the ego has repressed the Self, and in the second part of life it has to remove this repression so that the Self can return to consciousness again. These two models are contradictory and exclude each other, and a controversial dialogue between the two approaches is still going on.

TRANSPERSONAL PSYCHOTHERAPY

Due to various intolerable mental pressures and a dehumanising society, many seekers in today's culture are attracted towards the spiritual and esoteric realms of mental healing. Transpersonal psychotherapy represents the beginning of a systematic comparative psychotherapy that builds upon the contributions of traditional psychotherapies; psychoanalytical, behavioural and humanistic. It includes many of their views, goals and techniques but places them in a larger and more expanded context. In addition to the goals of traditional psychotherapies, transpersonal psychotherapy aims at the disidentification and transcendence of these issues. It assumes that the behaviouristic, psychoanalytic and developmental schools are all more or less correct, as far as they go, but transpersonal psychotherapy aims at a more integrative, comprehensive psychology. B. Cortright is specific when he affirms that "transpersonal psychotherapy will never reach its full stature until it has synthesized into itself the most powerful insight and techniques that the behavioral, psychoanalytic and humanistic schools have discovered."[7]

Transpersonal psychotherapy is not primarily concerned with psychopathological symptoms and it does not directly aim at the relief of daily compulsions but in contrast it moves the client towards a wider field of human capacities, self-transcendence and, in its attempt at soul-searching, towards the understanding of one's complexities. Transpersonal psychotherapy holds that misery is not inherent in the human condition and it aims at the liberation of the root cause of misery. It is characterised by the acceptance of the spiritual and cosmic dimensions of the personality and the possibility for the development of consciousness. Its ultimate goal is related to the individual's fullest development of one's true nature as a psychological and a spiritual being. From this perspective, it becomes clear that transpersonal psychotherapy does not differ so much in its methods or techniques as in its contents and scope from traditional psychotherapy.

In its clinical practice the Transpersonal psychotherapist emphasises the direct transpersonal experience which has an immense therapeutic value and offers potential therapeutic possibilities. However, the therapeutic values of the transpersonal experience are not honoured as an end in itself; rather, they are accepted as meaningful and integrating aspects for human development: the transpersonal experiences of the seeker can be used as an impetus for healing when they are effectively integrated into daily life.

Transpersonal psychotherapy is an approach to healing through the integration of the physical, emotional, mental and spiritual aspects of the person. The spiritual dimensions and potentials of the seeker are explored from a psychological perspective. It tries to bring the individual in contact with the hidden dimensions of his or her personality. There exists a close connection between human personality and spirituality, and the latter is therefore seen as an intrinsic property of the psyche. In the process of transforming one's personality during the journey into the unknown, in which one continuously encounters newer elements, the seeker is encouraged to penetrate into the deeper levels of his or her being. In the course of therapy, the seeker moves from identification to disidentification to self-transcendence. Problems that seem to remain insoluble at the ego level may finally be understood when the seeker gradually becomes aware of the transpersonal dimensions of his or her being. In this inward developmental process, transpersonal psychotherapy accentuates the importance of one's own responsibility in one's relations and in the world; all life experiences are part of a learning process and transpersonal psychotherapy helps to integrate these experiences.

Earlier definitions of transpersonal psychotherapy were often defined in terms of altered states of consciousness, or spiritual and transcendental experiences. In 1972, A. Sutich defined transpersonal psychotherapy as "therapy directly or indirectly concerned with the recognition, acceptance and realization of ultimate states... with the psychological processes related to the realization, or making real, of states such as 'illumination', 'mystical union', 'transcendence' and 'cosmic unity'. It is also concerned with the psychological conditions or psychodynamic processes which directly or indirectly form barriers to these transpersonal realizations."[8] F. Vaughan defines transpersonal psychotherapy with the help of three parameters—content, process and context. The transpersonal content is related to the discussion of spiritual experiences that may emerge in psychotherapy; the transpersonal process deals with the development of non-traditional therapeutic techniques; and the transpersonal context presents the orientation out of which the therapist works, i.e., his or her beliefs, values and intentions. She emphasises the context which defines a transpersonal approach. For Vaughan transpersonal psychotherapy is "the aspect of therapy that goes beyond ego goals and bridges psychological and spiritual practice... it encompasses a wider range of human experience than that which has been the predominant concern of Western psychotherapy in the past."[9] Transpersonal therapy aims at the development of the awareness of the transpersonal self and questions beliefs about the nature of the self and reality. Vaughan relates the transpersonal dimension of human potentials to the integration of the transpersonal experience, which will lead to selfrealisation and transcendence. T. Weide describes transpersonal psychotherapy as "on the one hand, the employment of transpersonal energies during 'regular' psychotherapy and, on the other hand, as the utilization of 'standard' psychological knowledge for transpersonal purposes."[10]

All these definitions deal with the experience of an extension of identity beyond the usual limits of the ego, beyond space and time but they remain confined to the term "humanness", as they do not recognise any transpersonal self-substance beyond the limits of human consciousness. In this way transpersonal therapists appear to limit themselves to the evocation of highest human potentials, the full realisation of human possibilities. Ken Wilber relates the various levels of "the Spectrum of Consciousness" with the major fields of Western psychotherapy, assigning a particular school of therapy to each major level of the spectrum; he is concerned with the pathologies which may occur at any of these levels. For Ken Wilber transpersonal therapy aims at the level of "Unity-consciousness" but he runs into linguistic difficulties when he explores the highest level of the spectrum, the *Brahman* and *Atman* consciousness. The term "therapy" can be used in this level only as a concession to language. For B. Cortright, "it is customary in psychotherapy to differentiate between theory and practice... The defining character of transpersonal psychotherapy is the theoretical and methodological framework which informs the therapeutic process... The importance of theory, therefore, is that it is the overarching framework that defines transpersonal psychotherapy."[11] The practical aspects are related to the appropriate use of techniques within the transpersonal context.

The individual seeking help from a transpersonal therapist is expected to have a reasonable degree of mental stability and self-integration, so that the same individual is able to disseminate unconscious elements and bring these to the level of the conscious and thereby expand one's consciousness. In clinical practice, transpersonal therapists attempt to bridge the gap between the personal and the transpersonal. They show interest in the metaphysical aspects of psychology but do not presume to delineate any spiritual goal; this is left to the seeker. The therapist attempts to bridge the long-neglected and often difficult gap between emotional development on the one hand and spiritual maturation on the other hand; the instinctual and the sublime, the personal and the transpersonal. He or she tries to uncover self-deceptions and guides the seeker on the way to discovering and integrating the transpersonal experience, without excluding working on the everyday affairs of life.

The transpersonal therapist makes the seeker aware that reliance on sacred truths may discourage him or her from obtaining insight into self-defeating behaviours; consequently, one may fail in making efforts to use these insights to change oneself. However, the therapist does not exclusively focus on problem solving issues; one of his or her main tasks is to distinguish healthy spirituality from those spiritual practices that hide psychological problems. This does not mean that the therapist provides the client with clear-cut solutions or predetermined goals to resolve one's personal problems but enables the person to open up to inner resources or inner healing potentials. According to Vaughan, "the therapist does not cure an ailment for a patient but enables a client to tap inner resources and allow the natural healing or growth process to occur."[12] During the therapeutic process the transpersonal therapist brings into awareness the client's unknown latent capacities, supposed to have a healing potential. Nevertheless, as mentioned before, the healing effects of these experiences are often only temporary and for this reason the therapist does not aim at treating these experiences as ends in themselves but at integrating them effectively as meaningful aspects of the client's daily life. The role of the therapist is that of a guide rather than of an analyst. He or she does not attempt to interpret upcoming processes but is active in guarding the client against unconscious projections. The therapist examines the negative influence of psychological conflicts on spiritual development and the positive influence of spiritual practices on intrapersonal and interpersonal conflicts. In exploring the dark areas of the client's psyche, the therapist guides the client towards an integration of rejected aspects of the self. For the transpersonal psychotherapist the ordinary concept of the self and the everyday average consciousness are only limited facets of our more complex nature.

Summary

Transpersonal psychotherapy takes the metaphysical concept of Spirit as the basis of reality and in its therapeutic approach it concentrates on the restoration of the contact with the spiritual self. It tries to be a meeting ground for psychotherapy and spirituality by including the spiritual aspect of existence in the journey towards wholeness. Both are mutually enriching each other. Psychotherapy is also seen as a useful element for clearing-up old and repressed trauma and provides the seeker with a strong sense of the self which is helpful for spiritual development. By integrating spirituality and psychology, transpersonal psychotherapy aims at an underlying system for the enhancement of growth.

Transpersonal psychotherapy affirms the spiritual search for an increased contact with the Divine and emphasises the realisation of one's spiritual nature. Psychological life is seen in a spiritual perspective and the individual is more than a psychophysically conditioned self; the individual's true identity is a spiritual being which supports one's psychological life. According to B. Cortright, "much of transpersonal psychotherapy during its first two decades was simply an addictive mixture—adding psychology to spirituality without changing either one very much. But more recent formulations see this as a new synthesis in which both are changed and modified as part of a new whole. The challenges for transpersonal psychology are to be rigorous in developing and testing theory, to be steeped and grounded in both western psychological theory and spiritual tradition and to carefully attempt to put these two deep sources of wisdom together in a bold new vision. The hope is that this will result in a more psychologically-informed spirituality and a spiritually-based psychology."[13]

Transpersonal psychotherapy is still in its formative stages and is continuously developing. With its initial emphasis on ecstasy, mystical experience, transcendence, spirit, cosmic awareness, bliss, etc., it attempted to bring into focus such parts of human experience within the context of traditional scientific psychology. As an important aspect of human motivation, spiritual seeking for the Divine is no longer relegated to religion or metaphysical speculation but has become the central inspiration for transpersonal psychotherapy. An important issue which has come to the foreground in transpersonal psychotherapy is the appreciation of the difficulties which accompany many seekers when they move into the transpersonal realm.

To cite B. Cortright again, "More recently there has been a shift in transpersonal psychology to how the spiritual is expressed in everyday life. It has become clear that transpersonal psychology must include the whole not just the high end of human experience but the very personal realm of ordinary consciousness as well. With this larger viewpoint, we assume a different perspective even in the exploration of the 'lower end' of human functioning and psychopathology. For example, psychosis can be seen to be more than just pathological flooding of the ego by the id, it also becomes a psychic opening to vast cosmic forces and presents a possibility for spiritual emergence and psychological healing."[14]

As referred to previously, in *The Quest for the Inner Man,* this author questions a medical approach to "healing" within a transpersonal perspective; it may be argued that the very phrase "Transpersonal psychotherapy" appears to be a contradiction in terms. The transpersonal field has no finite limits; it is already whole within itself and needs no clinical healing as in psychotherapy. If the seeking of transcendence is the highest goal for the transpersonal psychotherapist, beyond self-actualisation, then it seems inappropriate to equate the transpersonal realm with therapy. Psychotherapy is concerned with the medical treatment of the 'arrest' of the individual's psychological problems, but this healing process stands in contrast to the wholeness or transcendental dimension of the transpersonal, which needs no medical treatment. It could be better classified as guidance towards a universal fulfilment for the transcendence of apparent human limitations. Transpersonal psychotherapy is, therefore, more closely associated with the concept of a method of self-perfection, rather than a method of medical treatment.

Spiritually oriented therapies are increasingly accessible to everyone; they provide growing opportunities for spiritual growth but they also present unique problems.

Many methods are relatively or even excessively specialised and focus only on one part of the overall process of self realisation. Such techniques may be effective but their effects are often only temporary.

Transpersonal psychotherapists increasingly try to infuse the world's spiritual traditions with their transpersonal ideas in the hope of discovering a universal "common core" in spirituality. This cross-cultural comparison of spiritual traditions may easily distort the specific spiritual tradition's uniqueness; the result of superficial inquiry may often lead to simplistic conclusions. In the words of Richard Mann, "transpersonal psychology's important goal should not be to amalgamate the systems of thought and practice that it explores but to create a common language for respectful inquiry and mutual appreciation."[15] Reformulating and adapting sacred spiritual systems to the language of modern psychology or vice versa often leads to confusion.

To go beyond the personal seems to suggest that the transpersonal psychotherapist would like to write and speak about the Spirit but it is difficult to study the Divine psychologically. The only thing transpersonal psychotherapy can study is the process and the effect of the Divine spark on the seeker, not the Divine itself.

TRANSPERSONAL PSYCHIATRY

During the last decennium transpersonal psychotherapists examined and treated an increasing number of seekers having a transpersonal crisis. These crises are interpreted within a psychological context. Sometimes transpersonal experiences erupt unexpectedly during a psychopathological process and this psychopathological process may function as a means of growth that results in increased psychological or spiritual wellbeing. At other times a transpersonal crisis arises due to lack of transpersonal experiences, described by A. Maslow as 'metapathology', the failure to gratify higher transpersonal needs. However, not all spiritual developmental crises result in psychospiritual well-being, often they complicate transpersonal development and some seekers can be left impaired.

It is sometimes difficult to distinguish spiritual awakenings from episodes of mental disorders such as a psychotic state. Both states are often associated due to the gap between the spiritual interest amongst mental health professionals and that of people in general. But spiritual problems should not be confused with psychopathological phenomena even though these problems may appear simultaneously with a psychological crisis or mental disorder. S. Grof and C. Grof make a clear distinction between a *spiritual emergence,* i.e., a gradual development of spiritual potentials without psychopathological interruptions and a *spiritual emergency,* i.e., an uncontrolled emergence of spiritual occurrences accompanied by psychopathological symptoms. Spiritual problems that may come up during long-term spiritual practice should not always be diagnosed as mental disorders as they could be more related to a spiritual crisis facilitating the improvement of one's total well-being.

Psychiatry originated in dealing with the treatment of disorders in mental functioning and could be defined as the science of reducing the suffering of mental illness and increasing mental health. R. Walsh and F. Vaughan define transpersonal psychiatry as "the area of psychiatry that focuses on the area of transpersonal experiences and phenomena. Its focus is similar to transpersonal psychology, with a particular interest in the clinical and biomedical aspects of transpersonal phenomena."[16] B. Scotton gives a more refined definition of transpersonal psychiatry, as "psychiatry that seeks to foster development, correct developmental arrests and heal traumas at all levels of development, including transpersonal levels.

It extends the standard biopsychological model of psychiatry to a biopsychological-spiritual one in which the later stages of human development are concerned with development beyond or transcendent of, the individual."[17] The transpersonal multidisciplinary approach of the biopsychosocial -spiritual continuum relies on the methods and findings of biology, psychology, sociology, theology and traditional spiritual disciplines. For the transpersonal psychiatrist the mystical experience can be transformative and healing, unlike the traditional psychiatrist, who has the tendency to pathologize spiritual issues. The transpersonal psychiatrist who treats individuals with a spiritual orientation acknowledges not only the linkage between the biological and physiological factors but also includes the spiritual aspects of man. Psychopharmacology has a potential role in transpersonal psychiatry, as neurochemistry and neurophysiology are important mediators of mental change. Medication lowers the excesses of psychotic states and, after the arousal is controlled, the transpersonal psychiatrist tries to convert the disruptive altered state into an impetus for spiritual growth.

Psychopathology

At present the medical model plays an important role in psychiatric theories whereby symptoms are seen as manifestations of a pathological process. By focusing its efforts on suppressing symptoms it equates the alleviation of symptoms with improvement. However, the emergence of the symptoms of a disorder that is not organic but psycho-emotional in nature is not always the onset of disease but may be the manifestation of the healing process. When the medical model of psychopathology is used for a clinical understanding of spiritual traditions or for the influence of certain aspects of spititual practices on psychological difficulties, then this does not mean that the importance of the transformative spiritual experience in its own right is diminished. Knowledge of the clinical presentation of spiritual phenomena helps to avoid misdiagnosing.

Recent psychoanalytic theory acknowledges three levels of psychopathology: psychotics, borderliners and neurotics. Many people suffering from one of these three types of psychopathology may have genuine spiritual experiences but they are unable to integrate them. The transpersonal psychiatrist promotes the integration of healthy parts of religious-spiritual experiences in psychopathology.

Psychotics

People undergoing a spiritual awakening may enter an altered state of consciousness which resembles a psychotic state. Psychotic states on the other hand may include spiritual delusions or self-aggrandizing attributions of spiritual insight. Psychotic breaks resulting as a negative effect of spiritual methods are most often due to ego disintegration brought about by spiritual practices. Psychosis is usually not caused by a disturbed childhood experience; its causes are to be found more in multiple factors such as heredity or biochemical, psychological, sociological and cultural factors.

In a psychotic state the sense of the I experience has disintegrated and this self-dissolution can take various degrees. It is difficult for the psychotic to distinguish reality and fantasy, subject and object, and the unity and integrity of the body's perceptions and sensations is broken. The various psychoses are characterised by the individual's incapacity to interpret one's thoughts and feelings; such people with low self-esteem or with a basic flaw of ego development and defects in egoboundaries frequently have problems in making realistic life plans and in properly evaluating various different situations. With the breakdown of the self, the world around the client also disintegrates, which may create severe anxiety usually experienced in the form of delusions, hallucinations or withdrawal, up to a state of catatonic trance.

In psychotherapy, for psychosis, the primary attempt for the transpersonal psychiatrist is to determine some strong aspects in the behaviour pattern of the psychotic, as the psychiatrist is more sensitive to the religious and spiritual dimensions of psychosis. The psychotic is trained to resume mundane aspects of day-to-day living. The transpersonal psychiatrist gradually aims at the promotion of the integrative and transformative potentials in psychotic patients. Psychopharmacological intervention as symptom relief is only recommended in severe psychotic states such as depression, disabling anxiety and agitation.

Borderliners

The borderline personality, who cannot be classified as a psychotic or as a neurotic, suffers from a character disorder; the client is easily offended or overwhelmed by feelings and fantasies and is often unaware of his or her limits. There is a certain primitive split of consciousness; the structure of the separate self-image is extremely weak and the person is constantly engulfed by one's environment. For the borderline personality the views and opinions of others are of utmost importance, making the other person all good or all bad alternatively. When confronted with an ambiguous situation the borderliner may get lost in a non-consensual reality, which expresses itself in delusions, paranoia or fantasies. The borderliners are often tormented by an obsessive belief system in which it is difficult for them to maintain other perspectives of reality. There are usually ego defects but the borderliner may also experience many areas of considerable ego strength. Although one does not experience the irrational thought pattern of the psychotic, yet the person is unable to direct one's aggressive impulses appropriately.

The therapy with borderliners is primarily focused on the rebuilding of ego strength through identification with an empathetic therapist.' Stress-producing techniques or insight therapies are not advised for such persons. Concentrative meditation may be used for strengthening the ego structure and increased capacities for self-observation, and it may also be useful to regulate aggressive impulses or to attenuate anger. However, insight meditation may be contraindicated as it legitimates the lack of self-structure.

Neurotics

In neurotic illness there is a conflict within the person, a struggle within the mind between conscious and unconscious fantasies and feelings. The client experiences one's inner world as fragmented and confused. The individual's interactions with the external objective world can be traced back to childhood trauma, and neurotic symptoms are variously characterised by anxiety, guilt and the lack of self-awareness about the existence of one's problems. Frequently, the individual's past and repressed unconscious stuff stands between one's self and one's outer world, i.e., there is an imbalance of biological need, psychological state and social influence. There is often a loss of the ability to make a proper choice or the neurotic is disturbed by compulsive patterns that turn him or her away from reality. The sense of reality is preserved and the sense of the I experience is undamaged. Although neurotic illnesses are not accompanied by ego defects, there are emotional fixations and problems in the areas of self-control and regulation of heightened aggressive impulses. This lack of emotional stability and self-control, as well as the inappropriate expression of aggression, often leads to excessive dependence.

In interpretive psychotherapy the therapist aims to uncover unconscious wishes and fears, and uses the therapeutic intervention to clear failures of empathy in childhood development.

Alongwithtraditionalpsychotherapy,thetranspersonal therapist may use. some meditative techniques. The breakdown of ego repression during progress in meditation may produce forgotten repressed material which can be worked out simultaneously in continuing psychotherapy. For the transpersonal psychotherapist, however, neurosis is not always related to past conditioning but may also refer to a future destiny which is prevented from emerging. When the libido is traumatised in its growth, the aborted destiny drives become conditioned. Psychotherapy attempts to go back to the point where the past conditioning was an indication of a failed future growth.

HEALING THE SPLIT

In his impressive approach to the transcendental Spirit, J. Nelson explores a wide range of non-ordinary states of consciousness and he clearly distinguishes those that belong to pathological conditions and those that are able to awaken spiritual potentials. In his fundamental philosophy, which is based on the study of Ken Wilber, S. Grof and M. Washburn, he maintains that psychotic alterations are not exclusively disorders of brain or mind or spirit but "are aberrations of consciousness itself, whatever their manifestation."[18] For Nelson the spiritually based therapeutic techniques, with their detailed maps of consciousness, lack practical application for human suffering and often exclude biological science in their approach to psychosis. He tries to reintegrate spiritual psychologies with modem medical science. In this work, Nelson attempts to clarify the essential differences between "1. severely regressive psychotic Altered States of Consciousness [ASCs] caused by inherited predisposition or early-life failure of self-boundary formation, 2. spiritual emergencies with benign regression in the service of transcendence and 3. genuine spiritual experiences of people who have mastered the tasks of the lower chakras and are naturally expanding into higher consciousness."[19]

Nelson starts his transpersonal perspective with the Spiritual Ground, a deep level of pure Spirit as a manifestation of divine nature. It manifests itself in the world as energy and as a field of consciousness which interacts with physical matter, even though it is a non-physical force beyond physical laws and entities. As life begins with a blissful communion with the Spiritual Ground, the child seals off this portion of consciousness from the Ground in order to form a self, a sense of I-ness to separate oneself from others and the Ground. However, the necessary gradual estrangement from the Ground is influenced by genetic endowment, parental relationships, and physical health and need not completely seal off its connection with the Ground. Mystics use this spiritual Ground as a vitalising presence, whereas the psychotic experiences it as a terrifying force that intoxicates one's unfortified self but that impairs the psychotic patient. Spiritual discipline aims at a gradual reopening of the self to the Ground in a "controlled" manner though this spiritual path can be dangerous as unplanned openings can create psychotic-like states.

Nelson defines psychosis as "any one of several altered states of consciousness, transient or persistent, that prevent integration of sensory or extrasensory data into reality models accepted by the broad consensus of society and that lead to maladaptive behavior and social sanctions."[20] The two major forms of psychotic ASCs are schizophrenia and manic-depressive disorder. The schizophrenic disorder is still awash in controversy, as there exists a multiplicity of theories. It is difficult to find a single specific cause for all schizophrenic psychoses; it ranges from biochemical to psychological causes and from heredity to environment. There are various stages in the pathogenesis of the acute schizophrenic psychotic: the destruction of the self-sense, the destruction of perception and affect, and the formation of delusions (beliefs that contradict the prevailing realitymodels of society) accompanied by hallucinations. The schizophrenic may initially feel hyper-functional, be in an elevated state of awareness or experience a qualitative experiential alteration in the contents of consciousness. Normal processes of logic and reason are suspended as all sorts of cognitive experiences overwhelm the schizophrenic. There is often a regression towards primitive modes of functioning, ego-loss or ego fragmentation and delusional ideation. Not all schizophrenics manifest each or every characteristic symptoms as described above. The transpersonal psychiatrist aims at restoring conditions for spiritual growth which includes antipsychotic medicines in the initial stages, a supportive personal relationship with the client, basic social skills training, rebuilding of ego-strength and some form of behaviour therapy.

Manic-depressive disorders are more related to an increased high velocity stream of ideas and activities accompanied by an uncontrolled energy inflow from the Ground, which finally leads to a breakdown of ego-functioning in varying degrees, along with the break up of consensual reality. After one has consumed all one's inner vital resources, what follows is depression, a loss of meaning in life and the retreat from the life-giving energies of the Ground. The art of healing focuses on the distinction between regressive psychotic states of consciousness and a breakthrough of a higher consciousness in spiritual unfolding. The first category requires level-specific, therapies, whereas the latter benefits from spiritual practice. Transpersonal psychotherapy for mania begins initially with *lithium* medication to soften the disorganised, incoherent and overactive symptoms. Once the ordinary state of consciousness returns, the transpersonal psychiatrist—being aware of the potentials inherent in the manic altered state of consciousness—helps the individual to establish a disciplined pattern of spiritual growth which includes bodywork and emotion-releasing strategies supplemented by insight- oriented psychotherapy.

Those people living in between the boundaries of psychotic and ordinary states of consciousness, who are neither, insane nor neurotic, are classified as having a borderline personality. Such people, "experience their indistinct selfhood as partially merged with other people and the Ground."[21] Their vulnerable sense of self forces them to be dependent on relationships to which they can surrender or which they can manipulate. In their chaotic existence they fill up their unreliable interpersonal lives with imaginations, delusions or just lies.

One's fragmented sense of self renders the borderliner vulnerable to spontaneous psychotic states whenever his or her weak sense of self is threatened. Some cardinal features of the borderline syndrome are described by Nelson: "A borderline individual maintains an intense, clinging dependency that reflects his need for exclusive and engulfing relationships... self-destructive acts such as drug overdosing and superficial wrist slashing are his way of exacting rescuing responses from others. He experiences extreme discomfort or panic at being alone. ... A stubborn type of restless depression and feelings of inner emptiness characterize his subjective state.... He often shows exquisite sensitivity to the thoughts and feelings of others.... He is notorious for his impulsivity.... He may display exaggerated acts of will designed to establish or fortify his self-boundary."[22]

In explaining the physical nature of psychoses, Nelson attempts to elaborate on the relation of brain anatomy to psychotic ASCs. Physical events within the brain do affect interactions with the Spiritual Ground; genetic influence, abnormalities in anatomical structures, biochemical fluctuations, psychological stress and social environment may all be conditions for psychotic states. In recent years, neurobiology has discovered certain chemical 'messengers' or neurotransmitters such as norepinephrine, dopamine and serotonin which play some role in the shifts of thinking and feeling in psychosis. According to Nelson, "psychotic altered states of consciousness are *psychosomatic,* a word that honors the wedding of the mental and physical aspects of our being.... Although it is easier to demonstrate that physically altering the brain changes subjective experience, there is mounting evidence that mental events also leave their imprints within the brain'[23] Certain spiritual practices may increase or decrease sensitivity to these neurotransmitters, which could predispose a person to temporary psychotic states that function as an opening to higher realms of the mind or into pathological domains.

Beyond the brain's anatomical and chemical-strata Nelson acknowledges consciousness as a force of the Spiritual Ground which interacts with the brain to give rise to the human mind. He does not want to reduce the complexity of the mind to elementary atoms or molecules in the search for the roots of psychosis but turns "to levels of activity and the dynamic relations between them." Nelson bases these levels of activity on a reinterpretation of the ancient chakra system, which represents deep structures imbedded within Ground-consciousness itself. In their psychological aspects these chakras create unique modes of experience that guides the seeker in his or her spiritual growth. Nelson uses the chakra system to contrast "the problem of distinguishing between malignant regression, adaptive regression, that precedes spiritual growth and higher states of consciousness that may be confused with regression."[24]

The Chakra System

Spiritual growth through the chakras involves a process of incorporating ever-larger areas of the Ground into the self. This view of human consciousness as developing through succeeding levels need not always proceed in synchronicity. In spiritual emergency there is a precipitous breakthrough of a higher chakra before the self has lived through the lower chakras. He distinguishes three kinds of derailment from the ideal progression through the chakras; "1). Fixations on a particular level, 2). repression on a particular level, 3). intrusions of energies from higher levels before the self can make useful sense of them"[25] Each chakra represents a state of human development and indicates distinct features. However, "transitions between *any* of the seven chakras can precipitate abrupt regressions to lower levels. These passages have a distinctive character at each level... he symbolically *dies* to his old life, to be reborn to a higher mode of functioning that subsumes the lower mode."[26] Before the smooth ascent to higher chakras takes place the individual is often confronted with certain barriers to further progress, which may cause some brief psychic disturbances. In order to avoid such encounters, the individual temporarily regresses to a lower level. These mini regressions are benign and are used as "a natural healing process that lowers defenses against confronting unresolved impediments to higher consciousness. It can take place during transits from any chakra to a higher one.... Arising from a stalemate in human growth... the ego initiates a life-or-death struggle to free itself from the ominous force it confronts... It can destroy his ego and degenerate into malignant regression. This is the supreme risk of any spiritual quest and it accounts for the many similarities between madness and mysticism... These upheavals at the very core of the self can be personally catastrophic, for they hazard a return of the repressed Ground in full fury. The outcome can be madness as well as enlightenment, disintegration as well as higher integration."[27] However, such a temporary regression should not be confused with schizophrenia.

In the first-chakra, there is free communion

between the individual and the Spiritual Ground. In this chakra consciousness can be distorted by physical and psychological events. The child in one's early stages of selfhood establishes an I/not I split to form one's own self-boundary away from the primal unity with the Ground. Disruptions of individuation, such as genetic predisposition or family influence, play important roles in some forms of malignant psychotic states and as such can be the soil for the roots of madness. This first chakra consciousness is often used by the maturing self while regressing from a higher chakra into this first chakra during a severe psychotic state; it takes one back to the primary needs of the infant's struggle for survival. People severely regressing to the first chakra consciousness are not capable of receiving intensive psychotherapy or spiritual techniques designed to enhance openings to the Ground but respond better by simple behaviour modification or the artful application of antipsychotic medicines.

In the second-chakra, the self develops from the instinctual level to the emotional realm and forms the ability to create a stable mental image without being immediately satisfied by the senses. The child gradually moves away from the Ground into a world of consensus, fortifying larger realms of emotion, increased self-autonomy and a coherent ego development. However, a complete separation of the self from the Ground cuts the self off from the vital power underlying sentient life itself. The separation of the self from the Ground should therefore be a partial and temporary one in order to avoid a complete disconnection of the self with its instinctual creative and spiritual roots. Partial openings to the Ground inspire the individual to continue the journey upward to higher chakras and back to its Source. Regression from higher chakras to the second chakra produces a confused ego and an absurd mismatch with consensual reality. The resurgent Ground energies are now perceived as not-self and invade the psyche as alien feelings and impulses or as psychotic hallucinations.

The third-chakra consciousness is related to the level of the intellect and the will and provides the individual with the power to manipulate one's mind and environment but it lacks a purpose beyond the self.

The adolescent no longer identifies one's self with Spirit but exclusively identifies the self with one's ego. Having lost its connection with the Ground and isolating oneself from the power of the Ground, the individual now turns to the social world to find gratification of one's desires. In doing so one banishes everything that is not connected with the ego to the subconscious, forgetting that the ego is not the whole self.

Psychotic (schizophrenic) regression from a higher chakra consciousness to the third chakra consciousness is characterised by the person's loss of the rational and logical aspects of one's psyche and its consequent loss of consensual reality. A delusional world is often substituted in its place. The loss of abstract thinking takes away insight and the ability to focus on long-term goals. "As regression sinks the self deep into second-chakra consciousness ideas adhere to each other not through incoming stimuli, or through logical association but through a private *emotional* link that is generally inaccessible to an outside observer."[28] Regression may continue into first chakra consciousness where the abstract-conceptual is replaced by the concrete-conceptual nearing the preverbal realm of the primitive emotions of the toddler. Unlike a person in the psychotic state, the person in a manic state does not regress in the early states of the ego's arousal: the ego untimely inflates into previously unknown higher areas of the Ground without being able to integrate these. Initially, a manic state may induce a quantitative expansion of consciousness within the individual but soon after the unfocused psychic energy engulfs the self. Often neuroleptica is the only way to control the excesses of a manic state and afterwards psychotherapy is able to help integrate higher realisations into the context of an individual's life. Most people who are on the level of the third chakra consciousness experience great resistance to move upwards to the fourth chakra and many who cannot resist the call of the larger self step back from the ego-threatening dilemma into numbing addictions or other escape mechanisms. The strong ego renders the psyche relatively impermeable to the energies of the Ground and often retains its supremacy in consciousness much longer than necessary.

In the fourth-chakra consciousness, which is connected with the opening of the heart, the self rises above its selfish motives into universal love and compassion. At the heart chakra, love is no longer based on craving or possessiveness; there is an urge for commitment beyond the ego. Often the individual must travel on this path without support from the outside world. Because of unfamiliarity with these sublime energies the individual may be overwhelmed by empathy and then by depression. After confronting one's resistance to the Ground and complete surrender to it, one's larger Self experiences the Ground as a healing power and a source of inspiration. However, when the ego refuses to accept inner changes and growth and is unable to integrate these into a higher consciousness, a spiritual *emergency* may take place. When the less-prepared person who lacks grounding in the lower chakras encounters an inrush of spiritual energy and non-ordinary reality, one may be confronted with a disruption of the ego. This spiritual crisis differs from schizophrenia "in that the self neither regresses nor retreats in any other way but actively engages the process even though it temporarily forfeits its ego-based ability to function comptntly in the social world."[29] If the spiritual emergency is successfully resolved by the practice of meditation and the guidance of an artful healer who is able to reorganise and validate the symptoms of the uncontrolled spiritual emergency, the individual is able to surrender one's resistances, which results in a genuine growth of one's personality. The ego, though still operative, dwells within the larger realm of the illuminative heart chakra and encompasses all universal and human love. But this state is hard to sustain, as the individual is confronted with the hard facts of life and after some time one's ego starts repressing the Ground again. "Just as during regressions that attend transitions from the lower chakras, a person who has a vision of higher consciousness cannot peacefully return to his old state. The memory of the beauty and power of the Ground haunts him, despite the ego's halting efforts to suppress it. The ego is simultaneously drawn to, and apprehensive of, the great power it recognizes as its superior."[30] This 'dark night of the soul' is only part of a purifying procedure, a natural process of renewal and, once the individual completes this purifying process, the ego becomes a willing instrument of the Spirit.

The fifth-chakra is characterised by creative inspiration, a higher self, a balance of self-control and surrender, discipline- and freedom, individuality and unity. One is guided by one's intuition and is able to observe untempered rationality. By now the individual becomes accustomed to communicating freely with the Ground and surrenders to the power and the wisdom of the guiding hand. "Just as there may be uneven regression in psychoses, there may be uneven progression in normal development. Breakthrough of higher energies into the awareness of people centered in the lower planes of consciousness cause most of the confusion between higher and lower states of consciousness."[31] People who have fully actualised this fifth chakra are fare but glimpses of breakthroughs of this chakra are common and, like the fourth chakra consciousness, these glimpses may torment as well as enlighten its recipients. The creative impact of this fifth chakra can be realised only by those who have understood and mastered the first four chakras. People with extraordinary creative vision are able to convert that vision into a new reality. The genius and the psychotic have much in common but the former is able to make productive use of psychotic states such as mania and depression, whereas the latter is crippled by them. The schizophrenic whose psyche has regressed to a second chakra consciousness, with a loss of consensual reality, can hardly be creative. The genius possesses a mature ego and can therefore dedicate oneself to an act of creation, whereas the schizophrenic without 'a proper' working ego to integrate the opening with the Ground only gets intoxicated by the same Ground. There is more similarity between madness and genius in manic states than in schizophrenic states. "Many people who inherit a predisposition to manic ASCs are blessed with healthy personalities prior to their first episode, with egos comfortably nested in third-chakra consciousness. ... The chief danger of the hypomanic state is that an immature self is vulnerable to bombastic inflations of self-esteem."[32]

The sixth-chakra consciousness, which is often accompanied by paranormal phenomena, involves the transcendence of the ego and the realisation of one's divine nature. The individual enters a subtle realm which transcends worldly compassion and simultaneously cultivates intuition in order to gain direct experience of a reality beyond the personal and physical realm. "But if such an expansion of consciousness were to occur precipitously, even to one who had mastered the tasks of the first five chakras, the result would be spiritual emergency of the first magnitude. ... The reason such crises are uncommon in the Western world is that few individuals ever attain sixth-chakra consciousness, or even risk approaching it. It is far more likely for people centered in the lower chakras to experience *partial* openings to this realm. ... In contrast, Eastern cultures take pains to prepare their members for this transition."[33]

The seventh-chakra consciousness, the experience of mystical unity, when fully integrated indicates the completion of the journey, i.e., the culmination of the divine perfection of humanity. This consciousness is without an ego or separate self and its perfect unity pervades everybody and everything with its divine presence. In this pure consciousness, the individual directly realises the Ground. Nelson relates this state of consciousness to the term *Sat-Chit-Ananda:* pure being, pure consciousness and pure bliss. Even though both are non-rational, the state of seventh chakra consciousness should not be confused with the schizophrenic state. The pre-rational schizophrenic state lacks the ego strength and the power of logical reasoning to integrate the spiritual energies of the Ground, whereas the trans-rational state of the mystic transcends ego and reason but remains fully capable of returning to consensual reality, while integrating new insights into an expanded worldview. Nelson writes that, "Endowed with the power to re-create reality, both madman and mystic feel themselves to be godlike creators of the world. At that point, the mystic surrenders the last vestiges of ego and recognizes that all sentient creatures are also godlike, even if they don't yet know it. The schizophrenic, however, desperately clutches his ego and expresses his power over reality as the quintessence of madness: 'I am God but you are not!'"[34] The essential difference between the transcendental mystical state and the regressed schizophrenic state is related to the loss of the ego. While the schizophrenic is unable to manage one's life without a proper functioning ego, the mystic is able to tolerate one's ego loss with equanimity and comes back to ordinary life activities with an expanded perception.

In manic states, self expands into higher states while it is at the same time flooded by the energies of the lower states. Intermediate stages are evaded, which consequently hinders the integration of the higher ones and finally the lower ones begin to predominate. Mania is not only a regression but also has spiritual dimensions which return as the manic comes back to the normal state.

Conclusion: Healing the Split

For Nelson, healing requires more than medicines and psychotherapeutic techniques; he considers the exchange of spirit from healer to patient and vice versa as more essential. All psychotic states disrupt the dynamic relationship between individual consciousness and the Spiritual Ground. Therefore, healing takes place through the medium of consciousness. After having gained an appreciation of the state of consciousness of the client, the healer collects information about the client's personal history and, where necessary, prescribes antipsychotic medicine in the initial stages of the psychotic state. The healer then guides the psychotic into the investigation of his or her external environment. Quiet surroundings away from the stress factors that precipitated the acute psychosis are often all that is necessary to handle the crisis. By now the healer is in a position to determine if the client is facing a spiritual emergency or a severe psychotic regression and is also able to distinguish a malignant from a benign regression. "In any case, the goal of any treatment for acute psychotic ASC's should be *restoration of the patient to a condition in which spiritual growth can resume.* For some this means surrendering the ego; for others, fortifying it."[35]

As a crisis, a spiritual emergence is often accompanied by an altered state of consciousness resembling severe forms of psychosis. When the ego in its urge toward greater unity and the unfolding of higher consciousness is thwarted and hindered by impediments from within or without, it develops a spiritual crisis. When such development occurs with an explosive force it takes the form of a severe psychosis though often it develops gradually. During these periods the seeker is unable to participate in daily activities and risks damage to his or her personality. For the therapist it is important to avoid the error of confusing regressive ASCs—requiring level-specific therapies—with transcendent ones, which are benefited by consciousness-expanding strategies. The artful healer learns to distinguish between a natural and timely spiritual emergence into higher levels of awareness beyond the ego and an uncontrolled abrupt and confusing spiritual emergency into regressive states of fragmented ego disruption. For Nelson,"A transpersonal approach to spiritual emergencies is radically different from orthodox therapies, which aim to 'readjust' an individual to the limited consciousness of third-chakra societies... In contrast, a transpersonal approach holds that unhappiness is not inherent in the human condition and strives to help the patient to liberate himself from the root cause of unhappiness: alienation from his larger self and from the Spiritual Ground."[36] Throughout this work .Nelson attempts to reintegrate spiritual psychologies with modern medical science, i.e., he affirms the power of consciousness in determining health or sickness, without simultaneously excluding or over-interpreting biological science.

INTERFACE BETWEEN MEDITATION AND TRANSPERSONAL PSYCHOTHERAPY

Meditation is a very complex subject and has been thoroughly investigated by the transpersonal psychotherapeutic movement. Is meditation used in transpersonal psychotherapy as a mere by-product of a larger psycho-spiritual enterprise or does the transpersonal therapist employ meditation as just another present-day technique? Does a combination of psychotherapy and meditation make each more dynamic and meaningful? Meditation as a tool for relaxation and personal growth aims at enhancing awareness through the conscious direction of attention. The mind becomes receptive rather than reactive. As a tool for spiritual growth meditation unveils new dimensions of existence; the seeker enters into communion with deeper levels of Being, the ultimate Ground of all existence.' This presupposes a prepared and mature frame of mind, which is capable of comprehending various human capabilities. In the process, the seeker may develop a vision that transcends everything human.

Meditation in spiritual discipline aims at an altered mode of perception and is in essence a state of passivity combined with an apparently paradoxical state of expanded awareness. As an enhanced perceptual ability, it allows and stimulates more insight into the psychological processes and habitual deep-rooted patterns of behaviour as well as increased capacities—creativity, empathy, self-control and perceptual sensitivity of the meditative practitioner. During the process of increasing self-awareness, when deeper resources become available, the seeker usually undergoes a rigorous discipline in order to prepare him or herself to integrate the spiritual experience. Meditation in spiritual discipline is used as a technique for intensive self-exploration and transformation; it is often accompanied by a shift in attitudes, motivation, thought pattern, awareness, identity and life-style.

As a means of psychological self-discovery, meditation can be a process of learning to still the disturbances of the inner and outer life of the meditative person. The practice of meditation, if used to expand the seeker's attention beyond ordinary concerns, allows the person to investigate the processes of one's own consciousness, to discover the underlying qualities of one's existence and to become free from habitual conditioning and impulsive behaviour. Through various techniques the meditative practitioner's attention is freed from immediate and distracting sensory stimuli, so that his or her awareness shifts to more unconscious processes.

As an area of psychological study, research focuses on the beneficial psychological and physical effects of meditation. As psychological correlates of meditation, investigators have reported "the reduction of non-specific anxiety, release of stress and the helpful intervention in treatment of specific phobias, drug and alcohol addiction and the enhancement of self-esteem, self-control and self-actualisation. Meditation also has psychosomatic and physiological benefits, as in the treatment of bronchial asthma, hypertension, high blood pressure and myocardial infarction."[37] Additional therapeutic effects of meditation, when used in a clinical context, include a marked reduction in the metabolic rate, desensitisation to stressful stimuli and modification of hormone levels and blood chemistry.

Meditation does not seek to destroy the ego. The practitioner experiences the finiteness of ego-consciousness, which is only a contemporary construct. When practiced regularly, meditation disengages the ego's attention from external involvements and internalises awareness. In the initial stages of the practice, repressed inner subjective stimuli from the unconscious may come to the foreground of the ego-consciousness but in the course of sustained practice meditation arrests ego-activities and ultimately transcends the ego. In overcoming the limitations of the ego, the latter is not fragmented but left intact to function in the world when it is appropriate for it to do so. Ego consciousness is, therefore, not given up so that one can drift away in a state of self-dissolution but to enable the seeker to grow into a new, higher and profounder consciousness. In a deeper awareness of one's psychological functioning, where egocentrism is transcended, the meditative person gradually becomes free from past distortions and future anticipations and lives increasingly in the present. Various meditation techniques do not aim only at increased awareness in the present but also at detached observation, in which thoughts are not prevented but allowed to pass on without elaboration. As a procedure in spiritual discipline, meditation has as its end-state a goal far beyond the scope of psychotherapy.

B. Cortright gives a detailed and meaningful description of various meditation techniques without limiting its scope to particular dimensions of spiritual experience in the world's perennial traditions. He distinguishes five major psycho-spiritual practices that are utilised in spirit (non-dual) and soul (dual) paths.

1. In Buddhist 'insight meditation', a technique used for the expansion of awareness, the seeker observes the contents of consciousness without attachment and without identification. Thoughts are not prevented but are allowed to pass without elaboration. One is thus able to observe the process of awareness itself. During insight meditation the person gets to look through the shifting contents of his or her awareness of changing physical sensations, mental states and thoughts without reacting. Thus, insight meditation is the practice of sustained non-selective awareness: whatever emerges in the mind is observed crisply but without being reacted to or acted upon.
2. In 'soul paths', the meditative technique based on the dualistic aspects of being, the meditative person uses prayer, devotion, surrender and faith to develop a personal relationship with the Divine Being or Presence. This Divine being may be experienced within the meditative person oneself—one's individual soul as a spark of the Divine—or the meditative person may experience the otherness of the Divine without.
3. In 'evocative practices', certain aspects of consciousness are activated and purified through shifting attention to spiritual objects or symbols, in order to become more receptive to soul or Spirit.
4. In 'suppressive practices', impure or undesirable states of consciousness are suppressed i.e., impure negative states of mind are replaced by more pure positive mind-states.

5. In 'concentration practices', the meditative person gradually learns to focus steadily on a selected aspect of experience, which enhances one's concentration so that one's mind is no longer dispersed in many directions. The evocative, suppressive and concentrative practices are shared by both the spirit and soul paths.

B. Cortright elaborates on the convergences and divergences of the various meditation practices in relation to psychotherapy, as well as the dangers of various meditation techniques.

Insight practice, like psychotherapy, aims at an increased awareness, although "they work with awareness in different ways." Both approaches focus on the depths of being and openness to the here and now. Differences are mostly related to the different degrees and values of identification with the contents of consciousness. In insight meditation the meditative person detaches oneself from one's normal identification with the content of awareness, whereas in psychotherapy the individual actively identifies oneself with the contents of awareness in order to understand its meaning. Some of the other differences are related to the interpersonal situation, verbal and non-verbal experience and to the different goals of insight meditation and of psychotherapy. Psychotherapy as an art of healing aims at the growth and actualisation of the ego, whereas insight meditation aims at the awareness of the illusion of the ego.

Insight meditative practice can entail some risks when the self is not sufficiently integrated or stabilised. This technique often brings painful recollections and psychological dilemmas to the surface. It can expose the practitioner to the primordial contents of one's subconscious. Initially, the practitioner may be confronted with repressed unconscious material and the seeker is bound to encounter all kinds of resistances, his or her limitations, fears, pains, uncertainties and frustrations. It is not necessary to be too cautious about these distractions and the meditating subject is advised to observe them and return to the object of meditation. But sometimes these negative feelings are so deep-rooted and locked up in the past that 'insight meditation' may bypass them. In such cases, insight practices can be used *to avoid* unconscious emotional and psychological issues, because its goal is related to the disengagement of identification with psychological contents; moreover, it is often extremely difficult to integrate the realm of the transcended ego into the ordinary psychological realm of everyday life. Psychological problems need not always be resolved by the spiritual realm and often need to be dealt with at the psychological level.

The soul paths that one's being traverses and psychotherapy aim at the widening of the individual's identity by surpassing his or her outer surface self and reaching the deeper ground of being. Both approaches are concerned with the reduction of fear, anger and anxiety caused by resistances and defences. However, this form of spiritual practice has also its limitations and risks.

There is always the possibility that the inner opening does not touch the outer personality, which remains in its habitual patterns of behaviour. Moreover, there may arise a confusion of the witnessing subject with the neurotic superego "should" attitude, in which the latter represses or denies certain negative aspects of one's being. In transpersonal language this process is referred to as "spiritual by-passing", i.e., the seeker is committed to a dogmatic clinging to a spiritual path for defensive purposes in order to evade specific inner explorations. The seeker tries to avoid or prematurely transcend basic human needs or developmental tasks. One uses spiritual concepts in the service of repression and defence, as described by B. Cortright: "It is the use of spiritual content for psychological purposes, in the service of neurotic conflict."[38] These moral 'shoulds' fortify old repressive negative aspects of the psyche and allow only positive aspects to come to the surface. In such cases, the neurotic personality misuses spiritual aspiration for solving psychological conflicts by manipulating them "into a new version of our old patterns." This does not mean that meditative practices have no effect at all on these neurotic inner splits but such practices do not eradicate the inner splits. Psychotherapy is more sufficiently capable of dealing with these distortions and restoring the integration process of the disintegrated surface structures of the self.

Meditation used in a clinical model and as a therapeutic technique to reduce psychological disturbances may be useful for relaxation and self-control. As a therapeutic means in transpersonal psychotherapy, it is a healing experience because it transcends the limitations and distractions of the ego and brings the seeker in contact with his or her transpersonal self. Meditative techniques in transpersonal psychotherapy are also used for realising transpersonal potentials and the development of direct intuitive insight and psychological well-being. Unlike psychotherapy, meditation does not always pinpoint unconscious conflict areas nor does it try to stimulate the reorganisation of the ego functions. For Ken Wilber and some transpersonal psychotherapists meditation need not necessarily be a technique for uncovering the psychodynamic unconscious, although it may come into play during meditation. On the contrary, it may function as a technique to allow the emergence of higher domains of consciousness while bypassing the lower repressed unconscious. Seen is this perspective, meditation is more conducive to a sustained growth or an orderly unfolding of successively higher-order unities than to the lifting of repressions from the past. The changes brought about by meditation are more of a universal nature and often bring about changes in non-specific adjustments. It is for this reason that it may leave out specific inner conflicts and their psychological solutions.

Questions arise: are meditative practices powerful enough to keep defences against unpleasant feelings intact? Is it possible that neurotic symptoms are sometimes bypassed? Meditation tries to change the quality of experience and as mentioned before it is not specifically focused on the traumatic experiences of the past or problem solving issues. If these mental disturbances are excessively present, the seeker may develop spiritually in the course of spiritual practice but these mental limitations are then often pushed back, further into the unconscious, where they remain untouched. The psychotherapist is able to help the client to detect those spots, and thereafter concealed underlying problems can be dealt with. In meditation such self-confrontation problem areas are often avoided and these unresolved, unmanifest psychological issues could become important barriers later on in the development of spiritual discipline. It seems reasonable to deal with these unresolved issues first, before general positive changes are brought about by meditation; or the impasse can be solved when meditation is accompanied with the guidance of a psychotherapist who guides the seeker towards insight into the various resistances which are the cause of one's unconscious psychological conflicts. Those meditative practitioners with an inclination toward ego fragmentation may dissolve precisely what needs to be strengthened. Psychotherapy can have a supporting function in such cases so that the release of ego tendencies can be realised. In cases where the unruly self needs to be controlled and disciplined, the results obtained by spiritual discipline are bound to be shallow and psychotherapeutic intervention may offer a better solution in the seeker's quest for reunion with the Divine.

Conclusion: Meditation and Psychotherapy

Meditation allows the practitioner to open up to a consciousness of inner realms and consequently to an enhanced awareness of psychological issues, but it can also be used as a means of avoiding psychological problems by escaping into an inner world which is partly real and partly imagined, dissociated from the psychological level. Meditation allows the practitioner to investigate the process of one's own consciousness, to discover the underlying qualities of one's existence and to become free of various habitual impulses and conditioning. Giving up habitual compulsive conditioning and the seeker's self-created identity is often a painful process. As a technique related to self-improvement and used for 'mastery over the world' or, on the contrary, as a passive withdrawal into the seeker's inner realm, meditation is often based on misconceptions about meditation as a spiritual practice. Traditionally, meditation in spiritual discipline is employed as an essential practice for advanced psycho-spiritual development and self discovery. In recent times, meditation has also been used by Western psychotherapists for reducing specific psychological or psycho-physiological disorders, as well as by healthy non-clinical individuals for a heightened sense of psychological well-being. Although the beneficial influence of meditation on one's physiological and psychological functions has been proven in the laboratory, not much is known about the importance of the context in which a particular method of meditation was originally practiced, its objectives and the conditions for its correct application.

Although psychotherapy and meditation both focus on heightened states of self-observation, they differ in their aims. It is easy to confuse the absorption in and analysis of the *contents of awareness* in psychotherapy with the attendance to and observance of the *process of awareness* in meditation. When used as a clinical intervention for self-regulation and self-exploration or as a possible adjunct of psychotherapy, meditation often extracts the content of the meditation techinque from its original context. To eliminate the metaphysical setting of meditation, reducing it to a mere psychological self-help device, may easily lead to the omission of the spiritual roots of its tradition. As a procedure in spiritual discipline, meditation has as its end-state a goal far beyond the scope of psychotherapy. When meditation is extracted from its original context and offered as a consumer's item, like a kind of vitamin, it may increase tranquillity, and enjoyment and improve efficiency but may not lead to increased wisdom.

Meditation can have certain therapeutic aspects and may sometimes be used as a support in psychotherapy but, nevertheless, there exists a fundamental difference between the two. A similar view is expressed by P. Carrington: "Meditation differs clearly from conventional psychotherapy. The latter seeks to pinpoint conflicts and problem areas (often of an unconscious nature) and to bring into play the conscious integrative functions of the ego. Meditation, on the other hand, does not provide any conceptual' 'handle', which can be used to reorganise one's cognitions of self. The rational elements of the psychodynamic psychotherapies are consciously absent in meditation and the interpersonal elements take a back seat as well. ... Meditation appears to bring about complex but *nonspecific* adjustments. Because of this it may in fact leave intact *specific* inner conflicts and their psychopathological solutions."[39]

Psychotherapy cannot replace meditation and the reverse is also true. Meditation as a clinical utility may provide a general psychological pattern of positive mental states but need not provide a response to any particular underlying problem. When meditation is practiced alone without a referential background it can have notable positive effects on the individual but, when the same individual lacks a concern for spiritual fulfilment, meditative therapy remains only a strictly symptomatic cure. Clinical symptoms may be alleviated temporarily or replaced by others, but as it is strictly a symptomatic approach it is not advisable for the alleviation of deep-rooted complex unconscious conflicts.

Meditation used in spiritual discipline, as a technique for self-transformation, is usually accompanied by changes of identity, backed up with a major reorientation in life; the means for attaining psychological health is related to non-attachment, calmness, control, purification and the reduction of aversion and ignorance. Detachment allows the seeker some form of contemplation that is consistent with most forms of psychotherapy, which uses the method of-self-examination. But in psychotherapy detachment is only a temporary means of solving a psychological difficulty, whereas in meditation the seeker aims to gradually develop the state of involved detachment so as to remain in that state of detached observation.

The meditative practitioner, turning one's attention away from bodily striving, is able to control (aggressive/sexual) impulses but, as mentioned before, in these altered states of consciousness the seeker may bypass his or her neurotic tendencies. However, a breakthrough in neurotic symptoms requires more than meditation; it demands not only the discipline to control the unruly self but also a coherent relationship between truth and belief.

Psychological difficulties may appear at any stage of the practice but it seems that the beginner meditative person encounters different psychological problems during meditation than the intermediate and more advanced meditative practitioners. When meditation effects changes in the higher states of consciousness it need not always bring about changes in the lower unconscious contents. In such cases psychotherapy can be very helpful as a preparative method for psycho-spiritual growth. However, the various kinds of psychological problems as discussed in this chapter need not always be applicable to all meditative persons with a fragmented ego structure. Some practitioners do not face any major psychological disruptions during long term meditative practice and when they experience higher states of consciousness, these states have no or little effect upon the re-awakening of the contents of unconscious or defence mechanisms. On the contrary, when meditation activates these higher or inner states of consciousness, they themselves purify and transform the surface consciousness. Difficulties and problematic issues of the surface consciousness are not eliminated but absorbed and transformed by the inner/higher consciousness. Their significance is changed because the old patterns of the surface consciousness are reorganised and transfused into a greater consciousness.

NOTES

1. A. Maslow, *Towards a Psychology of Being,* p. Ill - IV.
2. B. Cortright, *Psychotherapy and Spirit,* p. 8.
3. C. Grof and S. Grof, *The Stormy Search for the Self,* p. 40.
4. B. Scotton, A. Chinen and R. Battista, *Textbook of Transpersonal Psychiatry and Psychology,* p. xviii.
5. F. Vaughan, *The Inward Arc,* p.39.
6. R. Walsh and F. Vaughan, *Beyond Ego,* p.3-4.
7. B. Cortright, *Psychotherapy and Spirit,* p.22.
8. A. Sutich, "Transpersonal Psychotherapy; History and Definition". In Boorstein, Ed.; *Transpersonal Psychotherapy,* p.9.

9. R. Walsh and F. Vaughan, *Beyond Ego,* p.161-162.
10. "Varieties of Transpersonal Psychotherapy", *Journal of Transpersonal Psychology,* Vol. V, No.l, 1973, p.7:
11. B. Cortright, *Psychotherapy and Spirit,* p.15.
12. R. Walsh and F. Vaughan, *Beyond Ego,* p.182;
13. B. Cortright, *Psychotherapy and Spirit,* p.22-23.
14. Ibid., p.13-14.
15. R. Mann, *The Light of Consciousness,* p.119.
16. R. Walsh and F. Vaughan, *Paths beyond Ego,* p.4.
17. Bruce Scotton, Allen B. Chinen and John R. Battista, *Textbook of Transpersonal Psychiatry,* p.4.
18. J. Nelson, *Healing the Split,* p. ix-x.
19. Ibid., p.360.
20. Ibid., p.3.
21. Ibid., p.54.
22. Ibid., p.55-56.
23. Ibid., p.129.
24. Ibid.,p.l62.
25. Ibid., p.166.
26. Ibid., p.246.
27. Ibid., p.247.
28. Ibid., p.240.
29. Ibid., p.266.
30. Ibid., p.276.
31. Ibid., p.290.
32. Ibid., p.304-305.
33. Ibid., p.313.

34. Ibid., p.349.
35. Ibid.,p.402.
36. Ibid., p.407.
37. Benjamin Wallace and Leslie Fisher, *Consciousness and Behaviour*, p.149.
38. B. Cortright, *Psychotherapy and Spirit*, p.213.
39. Carrington, Modem forms of meditation, *in Transpersonal Psychotherapies*, p.253

Part II:

Ken Wilber's Integral Psychology and Sri Aurobindo's Metaphysical Yoga Psychology

Chapter Five

A General Introduction to Ken Wilber

Ken Wilber's systematic multidisciplinary theories characterise the mainstream of transpersonal psychology. As one of today's best known transpersonal theoretical psychologists, he tries to develop a synthesis from various disciplines and attempts to integrate apparently conflicting outlooks from Eastern and Western thought. His works are remarkable not only for their wide scope but also for their exceptional depth of understanding.

Doing justice to the rich contents of all of Ken Wilber's works seems to be an impossible task; rather than providing a full-length representation of all of Ken Wilber's ideas, the author here only attempts to give the reader a general view of his main works, omitting certain essays, such as *Holographic Paradigm and Other Paradoxes, A Sociable God, Quantum Questions, Spiritual Choices,* and *Grace and Grit.*

Ken Wilber's developmental views have many similarities with Sri Aurobindo's vision of evolution. Ken Wilber traces common patterns that occur at each stage of evolution to contemporary fields of biology, anthropology, psychology, philosophy, theology and ecology. He does not develop metaphysical arguments to clarify his model, but uses accessible data and currently accepted general theories drawn from various contemporary fields of inquiry.

In his attempt to reconcile contemporary psychological theories with the wisdom of perennial philosophy, he uses the *'Great Chain of Being'* as the first principle of his unifying vision; Reality is composed of several different levels which form major links in the chain of body, mind and Spirit. Its developmental sequence seems to correspond to the movement from nature to humanity to divinity or from pre-personal to personal to transpersonal. The sequence constitutes a settled hierarchy—a classification of phenomena according to their holistic capacities; each successive level representing an increase in 'wholeness' and integrative capacity. Human beings are explicable not only in terms of the physiosphere and biosphere (the realms of body and life) but also in terms of the noosphere and theosphere (the realms of mind and Spirit).

In his first book, *The Spectrum of Consciousness,* he uses a metaphorical model of consciousness, called the Spectrum, whose innermost centre is constituted by an infinite, eternal and timeless entity. The various other levels of the spectrum represent a different sense of individual identity, i.e., different schools of psychology represent different levels of the Spectrum. In his next book, *The Atman Project; A transpersonal view of human development,* he provides a developmental psychology of human growth, from the lowest development—instinctual and libidinous—to the highest level, *Atman* consciousness. Ken Wilber describes different Eastern and Western theories of development and. integrates them into a unified view. In *Up from Eden; A transpersonal view of human evolution,* he applies the developmental Scheme from the *Atman Project* to social human evolution. Ken Wilber then wrote *Eye to Eye; The Quest for the New Paradigm,* in which he explains the relative merits of competing worldviews. He maintains that the three different "eyes of knowledge", the sensory, intellectual and contemplative, each have their own data, facts and domain. To confuse these realms, mixing up the intellectual understanding with contemplative knowledge is to lose the unique information of each domain. The transpersonal researcher no longer uses only the model of natural sciences in studying the structure of consciousness, but its methodological pluralism includes the three eyes of knowledge, each with its own distinctive standards of rigor. A truly scientific approach to the psyche involves such multiple perspectives. In *Transformations of Consciousness* Ken Wilber refines the developmental stages and connects them to specific pathologies and therapies. For him, each stage of development is predisposed to specific types of pathology, which needs corresponding treatments.

Sex, Ecology, Spirituality: The Spirit of Evolution, the first volume of a planned three volume series, aims to trace physical, biological and human evolution and place them within the context of perennial wisdom. He relates human evolution—physical, mental, social and cultural—to philosophy, religion, ecology, biology, sociology and psychology, all in accordance with the facts of contemporary fields of research. In *The Eye of Spirit; An integral Vision for a World Gone Slightly Mad,* he includes a summary of his previous works and responses to the various criticisms he has received in reference to *Sex, Ecology, Spirituality. The Marriage of Sense and Soul; integrating Science and Religion* elaborates upon the relationship between science and religion and Ken Wilber attempts to integrate them with the help of ancient wisdom and modern scientific knowledge. In *One Taste: The Journals of Ken Wilber,* he offers a further exploration into his theoretical vision on the perennial philosophy and a reflection of his work and that of others in the field of transpersonal psychology. *One Taste* also includes his daily personal experiences as well as various details of his own spiritual practice and the correspondence with leading spiritual and transpersonal theorists. His next-to-latest work, *Integral Psychology,* presents an integrative model of consciousness, spirituality, psychology and therapy. This integrative model attempts to include and integrate some of the more enduring insights drawn from premodern, modern and postmodern sources. However, he also published this book to initiate a discussion and motivate others to correct some of his mistakes and clear up any inadequacies. In his latest work, *A Brief History of Everything: An integral vision for business, politics, science and spirituality,* he gives the reader a diagnosis of the evils of the present age and a remedy based on his integral vision. He also outlines the many applications of his integral model varying from medicine to management and from science to education and spirituality.

To get a better understanding of Ken Wilber's multi-disciplinary approach, before proceeding to compare some of his unified views with Sri Aurobindo's integral vision, it is advisable to explore in detail his integral views as exposed in his writings.

KEN WILBER'S MAIN WORKS

The Spectrum of Consciousness

The Spectrum of Consciousness describes a universal view on human consciousness. The centre of this model, man's innermost consciousness, is identical to the absolute and ultimate reality of the universe and the human personality is a "multi-levelled manifestation or expression of this single consciousness." *The Spectrum of Consciousness* represents a pluri-dimensional approach to man's individual identity and each level of the Spectrum is addressed to a major school of psychotherapy. Out of the various levels of consciousness Ken Wilber selects five major levels and attempts to synthesise these with the insights of different schools of psycho- therapy. Each school, focusing on one major level of the spectrum, is not contradictory to the other schools but complementary.

The deepest level of the Spectrum, the "level of

Mind", is not really a deep level but an all-inclusive yet dimensionless reality which is infinite, timeless and eternal. On this cosmic level, man is identified with the universe, i.e., the experiential self—existing as a non-dual mode of consciousness—is without divisions and fragmentations and thus the universe is not split into the 'seer' and the 'seen'. Eastern spiritual disciplines are generally concerned with this level; for at this level the seeker aims at the attainment of liberation or the complete release from the root-cause of all suffering primarily through a set of experiments rather than a set of theories or philosophies. In the process of self-transcendence, Eastern spiritual disciplines tend to ignore other levels of the spectrum because their goal aims at the realisation of Reality beyond the ordinary levels.

Ken Wilber maintains that "Reality is not ideal, it is not material, it is not spiritual, it is not concrete, it is not mechanistic, it is not vitalistic—*Reality is a level of consciousness* and this level alone is Real ... that *Reality is what is revealed from the non-dual level of consciousness that we have termed Mind.*"[1]

This level of non-dual awareness, called Mind or God or any other title, alone is Real, and though indescribable and inexpressible, it can nevertheless be experienced.

How does the evolution of the Spectrum originate? What initiates the movement of Mind into a world of phenomena? Because we are unconscious of the ways in which we observe Reality, we divide reality and forget that we have divided it, i.e., we have forgotten Mind. In order to remember this first level of consciousness the individual has to undertake a steep journey into the present. The level of Mind, being timeless and spaceless, does not itself actually evolve. However, the initial movement of Mind into a world of phenomena is initiated through the illusory creation of a dualistic and divisional process; man mistakes these unreal dualities for real and at this point a fragmentation through duality takes place in which the individual shifts from a cosmic identity with the 'All' to a personal identity with one's organism. One imagines this split, this primary dualism, to be real and it is, therefore, the initiator of the Spectrum of consciousness; each level of the Spectrum is a variation of this primary dualism. This seeming imposition of several dualisms upon Mind generates a distinctly narrower level of the Spectrum and each shift in one's level of consciousness corresponds with a shift in one's sense of identity. According to Ken Wilber, "dualism to the extent that we forget its 'underlying ground' of non-duality *represses* that non-duality and then *projects* it as multiplicity... Thus each dualism is accompanied by a *repression* and a *projection;* a dualism *represses* its 'uritary' character, and *projects* that process as two apparently antagonistic opposites."[2]

The second level of consciousness arising out of dualism generates the Transpersonal level, an area of paranormal occurrences, Jung's collective unconscious and Maslow's plateau-experiences. The separation between self and not-self has not taken concrete form, but this level does not represent Absolute Reality. Some subtle form of primary dualism is still present, but often it is more or less harmonised. "The transpersonal Bands represent a point where the individual *begins* to touch Mind. He does not yet directly realize that what he is, *is* Mind, but through insight and experience he understands indeed that there is within him that which goes beyond him."[3] The transpersonal view aims at a universal perspective and the individual is no longer exclusively identified with a separate self-sense and one's personal problems.

When the fragmentation continues through a secondary dualism, man arrives at the Existential or Centaur level, where the individual finds oneself exclusively identified with his or her entire organism against one's environment, i.e., the organism, which comprises one's basic sense of existence is distinctly separated from the environment.

In this existential awareness, the awareness is exclusively centred on man's separate existence in space and time, and the major dualisms present at this level are the self and the other, and life and death. Nevertheless, man is still in touch with one's total organism and still feels oneself as an undivided psychosomatic unity. At this level, man begins to develop rational thought processes and a personal will.

Further fragmentation originates the Biosocial level, which represents the upper limits of the Existential level. On this level each individual encounters the sum total of all the 'internalised' social conventions that the organism has accumulated. The individual learns to translate reality into the social terms held in common with others, such as cultural premises, social laws, ethical views, family structure, etc. In this socialization of existential awareness, one learns to respond to the world according to the beliefs of others. All of those aspects of reality which do not conform to society's views of the world are repressed and rendered unconscious to form the contents of the biological unconscious. This biosocial level also initiates the core feeling of being a separate being and functions as a reservoir for the formation of the ego-level.

Continuing the shift from the identity of the organism as a whole, man generates a tertiary dualism of the psyche and *soma* which triggers the emergence of the Ego-level. Man is no longer in touch with his 'organismic' awareness; in its place, one substitutes intellect, imagination and memories, and by now has formed a mental picture of one's ego. "The Ego level is that band of consciousness that comprises our role, our picture of ourself, our self-image with both its conscious and unconscious aspects."[4]

When the individual finally shifts one's identity from the ego, and imposes a split upon one's own ego, the last level of the Spectrum is generated, the Shadow-level. This shift, which creates an inaccurate self-image due to the identification of only parts of the ego, is called Persona, whereas the rest of the undesirable tendencies which are alienated form the contents of the Shadow. It contains all sorts of unwanted aspects of one's personality which the individual tries to push away but which nevertheless follows him or her as a Shadow.

"Each level of the Spectrum represents an increasingly narrowed sphere of identity, from the Universe to a facet of the universe called organism, from the organism to a facet of the organism called psyche, and from the psyche to a facet of the psyche called persona."[5] Through these successive dualisms the various levels of the spectrum evolve.

The model as described above does not fully represent the interactions between the various levels. It must be clear that these levels are not separate layers but mutually overlap each other and man is rarely confined to one level.

Ken Wilber also maintains that the evolution of the individual levels themselves does not occur only in a vertical movement, but "also do the individual levels themselves evolve and 'expand' in a type of horizontal movement."6 In the *Atman Project* he refers to this horizontal movement as 'translation'.

Psychotherapies related to the various levels of the Spectrum

Ken Wilber assumes that each school of psychotherapy addresses a different level of the Spectrum, and each school is more or less correct when addressing its own level.

For Ken Wilber, consciousness is pluri-dimensional and he supposes that pathology can occur at any of the levels of the Spectrum, except Mind, and that these pathologies become more intense as one ascends the Spectrum. This means that each level has its own characteristic set of potential psychopathologies. Psychotherapy aims at healing a major dualism at each particular level through a twofold process of conscious contact and then re-integration. This therapeutic principle is used on every level and is described by Ken Wilber as follows: "Now because the common thread running throughout each level is the process of dualism, then repression, then projection, the therapies of each level also share a common characteristic—*they reverse this process* (on their particular level) *by helping the individual contact the alienated and projected aspects, re-integrate them, and thus 'heal', 'make whole', and 'unify' that level* ... Anytime an individual completely reverses this process, heals and wholes the major dualism of any level, then it follows that he *automatically and quite spontaneously descends the spectrum to the next level,* to the level that 'includes' both poles of the 'old' duality, to the level of which the one above was merely a fragmentation.[7]

"This suggests that, in one sense, the descent of the spectrum of consciousness is a progressive process of *disidentification* from a 'narrower' sense of pseudo-subject to a 'broader' one, a process which brings an expanded sense of freedom and control... if each successive shift down the spectrum is a process of disidentifying with the 'old' pseudo subject, then it is also a process of discovering a 'new' identity on the level beneath it... which harmonizes what were once thought to be antagonistic opposites... Disidentifying with the 'half', he spontaneously identifies with the 'whole'... Because the 'old' level was actually created by a splitting of the level beneath, it its 'healing' automatically results in the restoration of that prior unity. This process occurs each time the individual descends a level."[8]

In discussing the various levels of therapy, Ken Wilber starts with the therapies aimed at moving from the Shadow level to the Ego-level up till the descent into the level of Mind, the return to the Source, i.e., the reverse order in which the levels themselves evolved. This descent is a simple dissolving of dualities, accomplished by re-owning a projection at each step of the descent.

The Shadow-Ego level: The Shadow contains all one's ego potentials, the bad ones (evil) as well as the good ones (godlike) but with its final dualism—repression/projection— the Ego's unity is repressed. Even though repressed, these qualities remain our own and continue to operate, but we project them onto the environment where they threaten our being.

Therapies on the Ego-level, such as psychoanalysis and the plethora of ego psychotherapies, aim at the restoration of and re-identification with one's alienated qualities and at reuniting them with one's Shadow. This undoing of a projection indicates a shift downwards from the Shadow to the Ego-level, as the individual enlarges one's area of identification, i.e., the individual takes responsibility for one's own projections and sees them no longer in the environment. To be aware of one's Shadow, a real facet of the ego, one need not necessarily include the will to act on its qualities; one only realises that symptoms, which the Shadow seem to inflict on the individual, are in reality symptoms the individual inflicts upon oneself. The whole process of the descent from the Shadow-level to the Ego-level is accompanied by a progressive expansion of identity, in which the individual is able to develop an accurate selfimage.

Biosocial therapies, such as family therapy, interpersonal and transactional analysis are concerned with dualisms most prominent at this level, organism and environment, and life and death. On the Ego-level, therapies are concerned with the I, but on the Biosocial level therapies are related to I and you (sociological factors). The Biosocial therapies aim at restoration of all the repressed (unconscious) aspects of experiences which are not conforming to the pervasive social make-up, and are obviously working on a "deeper" level than the purely individual repressions. For Ken Wilber "our social maps, in establishing meaning, dichotomize existence and hence screen or filter awareness, a process that results, at this level, in the bio-social unconscious."[9] These biosocial unconscious contents are formed by those aspects of awareness which are not embraced in the social framework, and as a consequence create dualism. The biosocial therapies strive to make these unconscious social fictions conscious. Through insight, the individual is able to go beyond these inappropriate dualisms and no longer takes these fictions as real.

Therapies on the Existential level aim primarily at our total organism by healing the split between the mind and body, the mind-body dualism. The descent from the Biosocial level to the Existential level is accompanied by a progressive expansion of identity which includes all the aspects of one's total organism which were previously threatening or were not under control. The therapist who works on this level guides the individual in the process of discovering one's authentic self, i.e., the integration of mind and body, or thoughts and feelings into a harmonious higher level. Ken Wilber divides these therapies into two classes: those proceeding primarily through the mind —logotherapy, humanistic therapies, and those that proceed through the body —bioenergetic analysis, Hatha Yoga or polarity therapy. Ideally, however, a combination of the two is highly desirable, as for every mental problem there is a corresponding physical problem.

Therapies on the Transpersonal level, such as Jung's Analytical psychology or Assagioli's psychosynthesis, aim at the suspension of all dualisms except some form of primary dualism which is still present in potential form— the split between subject and object. The individual can look at one's emotional and rational complexes and he or she is therefore no longer exclusively identified with them. However, one has still access to all levels above it—

from the Existential self to the Shadow, but they become instrumental and one is no longer limited by these levels. The individual's awareness gradually shifts from one's 'organismic' consciousness to a universal perspective, i.e., the transpersonal self, transcending space and time.

Level of Mind therapies do not aim at creating a healthy ego, but at a transcendence of the ego where all dualities are totally removed. Therapies, this term is used only as a concesion to language, addressing this level include Mahayana Buddhism, Taoism, Vedanta, Sufism and certain forms of Christian mysticism. The isolated soul here is confronted with an alien universe, and it is at this stage that Western psychotherapy may be able to offer some release from suffering for the individual. But for Ken Wilber, various Western psychotherapies could also be helpful as a preliminary preparation or concomitant aid when the seeker aims at liberation.

However, he is cautious regarding therapeutic measures on the upper levels of the Spectrum; they may facilitate the descent to the lower levels, but the descent to the Transpersonal level or Mind level does not always require upper-level therapy. Lower-level therapies may be able to reduce the work that has to be done on the upper-level therapies. He warns the seeker on the way to the Mind- Level not to overdo "this shuffling of therapies since a person might likely become enchanted with the games of an upper- level' instead of putting that level in order so as to more easily drop it."[10]

Conclusion

Like the transpersonal psychotherapists, Ken Wilber tries to synthesise a combination of various traditional psychotherapeutic systems and he pays simultaneous attention to the transcendental areas of the psyche. In doing so, his spectrum model attempts to bridge the gulf between Western psychotherapy and the *psychologies perennis,* a universal view regarding the nature of human consciousness.

Ken Wilber's spectrum psychology does not try to describe the complete spectrum of human experience within one psychological system. He creates an interpretation of human consciousness which is a psychological formulation of the fundamental insight of various Western and Eastern spiritual philosophies.

Ken Wilber maintains that the psyche is formed by various domains and levels of consciousness, which have their own characteristics and laws. It is, therefore, not possible to reduce all phenomena of the psyche to simple and suitable principles. Each form of psychotherapy is concerned with a different level of the Spectrum of consciousness, i.e., each therapy can be applied only to a certain level of the Spectrum, and each Western psychotherapeutic approach is more or less correct as long as it concentrates on its own level. The mistake of the conflicting schools is based on the fact that each school generalises its own approach and applies it to the whole Spectrum.

No Boundary: ***Eastern and Western Approaches to Personal Growth***

No Boundary, as a simplified popular version of *The Spectrum of Consciousness,* elaborates upon the various boundaries the individual creates in one's experiences, which result in a limitation of consciousness.

In the ultimate reality where there are no boundaries the opposites are harmonised and unified into unity consciousness. When there are no boundaries the individual experiences all things and events as mutually dependent and interpenetrating. The different identities, dualisms, are now referred to as different boundaries, and the primary boundary of the self and not-self is just like the primary dualism of unity consciousness and individual consciousness as described by Ken Wilber in *The Spectrum of Consciousness.* This primary boundary creates the opposition of me as the organism versus the world and the environment. By discovering unity consciousness, the individual transcends opposites and becomes free from all boundaries. "When the opposites are realized to be one, discord melts into concord, battles become dances, and old enemies become lovers."[11] The principal idea behind this book is that man unnecessarily limits one's sense of identity by putting up boundary-lines between psyche and body or organism and cosmos. By eliminating these boundary-lines, the individual reaches the level of cosmic consciousness. At each separate level of this spectrum, we have at our disposal a characteristic form of a sense of identity and, at each level, typical forms of psychopathology may arise which need a specific form of therapy or meditation at that level. As such, the spectrum model functions as an integrative model for all the different schools of psychotherapy.

The Atman Project: ***A Transpersonal view of Human Development***

In *The Atman Project*—the drive of God toward God through the instrument of the human psyche—Ken Wilber describes the individual's growth from infancy to adulthood, which is like the microcosmic reflection of universal growth on the whole. This psyche is a pluri-dimensional entity, composed of successively higher order wholes which show themselves in the human psyche as growth, i.e., the whole of any level becomes only a part of the whole of the next level, and at each stage the different parts are integrated into higher wholes. The various levels of 'conscious evolution' resemble an overall life cycle from subconsciousness (pre-personal unity) to self-consciousness (personal) to superconsciousness (transpersonal unity).

At birth, the primitive level of consciousness, the self

and the material cosmos are undifferentiated and the infant does not have an ego. Ken Wilber refers to this stage as the pleromatic self in which awareness is spaceless, timeless and objectless. This kind of pre-personal perfection should not be confused with a transpersonal one. The difference between the two lies in the entire life cycle of consciousness. New Age critics often confuse the two and don't differentiate between the pre-egoic or pre-rational and the trans-egoic or trans-rational, thereby confusing transcendence with regression. A more detailed analysis of the "pre/trans fallacy" is described in *Up from Eden* and *Eye to Eye.*

The next level—the uroboric self—is still characterised by the pre-personal in which the physical and psychical are not differentiated, but it already possesses some sort of ego boundary.

With the emergence of the body-self or body-ego—the typhonic self—the development of instincts, somatic processes and emotional-sexual impulses takes place. Initially, the body ego differentiates itself from the material environment, then transcends that environment and is now able to operate upon that environment.

By the time the child acquires a language and moves to the membership-self, one can perceive a particular type of descriptive reality. When the mental self emerges, it starts to differentiate itself from the body. The child is now able to control, postpone and transcend one's impulsive drives, but at the same time the growth of consciousness involves a loss of the paradisiacal state of ignorance into the world of separation.

The ego level is characterised by a more or less "correct self-concept", which gradually learns to internally differentiate the ego structure into various segments, such as interpersonal relations of the child with the parents. During the ego's development various aspects of the self that are threatening to the establishment of the super-ego can be suppressed; these suppressed aspects Ken Wilber calls the 'Shadow' and the resultant inaccurate self-image due to split-off facets of the ego-self, he calls the 'Persona'. When the ego-structure becomes more mature the individual masters one's various personae and starts to disidentify with them. By transcending them the individual tends to integrate all one's various personae into an integrated ego.

At the later stages of ego development, after having integrated all one's personae into a mature ego, the individual starts to disidentify with the ego altogether. Ego transcendence does not mean a loss of all egoic consciousness; it only reconnects the ego with the rest of nature, cosmos and divinity. This integrated self where the body, persona, shadow and ego are all integrated into a higher order, Ken Wilber relates to the 'Centaur'. The individual begins to transcend these lower elements and ceases to exploit them. However, in transcending language and ego, the individual does not transcend existence and, therefore, still does not enter the transpersonal realm of being.

Beyond the gross realm, (the gross body and the gross ego as discussed above) Ken Wilber explores the subtle and causal realms. The subtle realm—as an intermediate realm like Maslow's farther reaches of human nature—includes astral and psychic levels of consciousness (lower subtle realm) as well as the universal realm of religious intuition (higher subtle realm).

As development proceeds the individual enters the causal region which represents God-consciousness (lower-causal) as well as the release into Formless consciousness, the Ultimate Unity (higher-causal). This perfect integration of all prior levels is not a transcendence from the world but a transcendence as the world, the *Turiya* state as described in the Upanishads.

The Process

How does psychological development between various temporary levels takes place? For Ken Wilber, psychological growth aims at Atman (God) and the drive to actualise Atman is a part of the Atman project. But the other side of the Atman project is the struggle of the soul to seek unity through the constraints of the present stage, i.e., "each stage or level of growth seeks absolute Unity, but in ways or under constraints that necessarily prevent it and allow only compromises: substitute unities and substitute gratifications."[12] The superimposition of an illusionary self-boundary obscures the prior Wholeness of Atman, and even though man aims at the re-discovery of Atman one simultaneously fears the loss of one's separate 'self-sense'. Due to this conflict, man seeks transcendence in ways that actually prevent it, through the formation of symbolic objective substitutes like sex, power and money or the subjective substitute of a separate self. In the words of Ken Wilber, "all a person wants is Atman; all he finds are symbolic substitutes for it. This attempt to regain Atman consciousness in ways or under conditions that prevent it and force symbolic substitutes—that is the Atman-project."[13] For Ken Wilber, the Atman project is an intermediate substitute for a true Atman and, as a consequence of this process, the individual creates a separate self as substitute and substitutes this ego for Atman or, instead of being one with God, the individual him or herself as an ego tries to play God. These substitutes for Atman necessitate the creation of successive structures of consciousness which are later abandoned when they fail and then transcended.

Transcendence

In order to understand Ken Wilber's concept of evolution through the various levels of consciousness, it is essential to analyse the form of psychological development. He explains a triadic form of development through the process of differentiation, transcendence and integration.

Psychological development proceeds level by level, stage by stage, with each successive level superimposed upon its predecessor; each newly-emergent structure has to be consolidated with its predecessors, i.e., it includes but transcends its predecessors. At each stage a higher, more complex structure emerges through a differentiation of the preceding lower level. The lower eventually disidentifies itself with its present structure and identifies itself with the next higher-order emergent structure. The present structure detaches itself from its exclusive identification with that lower structure, without throwing away that structure. By transcending that structure, it can operate on the lower structure by using the means of the new structure. To formulate this characteristic form of psychological development, "we find; (1) a higher-order structure emerges in consciousness; (2) the self identifies its being with that higher structure; (3) the next higher-order structure then eventually emerges, the self disidentifies with the lower structure and shifts its essential identity to the higher structure; (4) consciousness, thereby transcends the lower structure and becomes capable of operating on that lower structure from the higher-order level; (5) all preceding levels can then be integrated in consciousness. Each successively higher-order structure is more complex, more organized, and more unified-and evolution continues until it reaches a complete unity or integration."[14]

For Ken Wilber each of these five points of development is a definition of transcendence and he equates development and transcendence as the very same process.

Integration

With the emergence of a higher structure, the lower structure is subsumed under it, i.e., the lower levels are not destroyed or annihilated but the individual ceases to identify exclusively with them. As consciousness begins to transcend a lower level and is no longer identified with any of the various elements of that level, it enables consciousness to operate upon and integrate all of the lower levels with the newly-emergent higher level. Failure to integrate the lower levels in the higher often results in repression of the lower levels (neurosis), but the lower structures can also overwhelm the higher ones.

Such is the ascent of consciousness and it continues until there is only Atman itself, where the utter transcendence into Formless Consciousness—the Ultimate Unity—reaches the radically perfect integration of all prior gross, subtle and causal levels. In the Ultimate transcendence, the various levels are not annihilated but are all included in Spirit, they serve Spirit rather than observing Spirit.

In the last chapter of *The Atman Project* Ken Wilber relates the movement of evolution to involution, a movement from the higher to the lower, as a process of pure creativity. Whereas evolution moves from the lower to the higher, involution moves from the higher to the lower. For Ken Wilber evolution occurs only because the higher structures are already enfolded as undifferentiated potentials in the lower ones, and "involution is simply the story of how the higher modes came to be lost in the lower... Involution, or the enfolding, of the higher in the lower, is the precondition of evolution, or the unfolding of the higher states from the lower."[15]

In involution, the soul constructs, step by step, substitute formations into lower states of consciousness or more restricted modes of identity and less Atman. However, the higher levels are present in the lower but are rendered unconscious, and "development or evolution is the unfolding (awakening) of these enfolded (forgotten) structures beginning with the lowest and proceeding to the highest."[16]

This does not mean that the higher comes from the lower, but the higher separates itself out of the lower and thus comes after the lower. The higher is not constituted by the lower but passes through it; the lower levels form the substratum for the higher exchange, and they interact and are interconnected with them. The integration of the lower and the higher strata occurs through the triadic form of development as described previously, i.e., differentiation, disidentification of the lower and the higher, and transcendence of the lower.

Ken Wilber maintains that all the lower levels are taken up and preserved in the higher levels and as such the higher preserves or integrates all lower stages. However, he is also aware that the lower can disturb the higher when the lower erupts which disrupts higher functioning, or a distortion in the lower predisposes similar distortions in the higher. Nevertheless, Ken Wilber does not elaborate on what remains left of the lower after it is integrated in the higher, but he will explain this later (Eye *to Eye)* in his more comprehensive model of consciousness.

Transformation

Ken Wilber stresses the transformative aspect of evolution, whereby each emergent stage of evolution is not so much a total negation of the previous level but a transformation upward or ascent of it. He makes a meaningful distinction between transformation and translation in the process of the evolution of consciousness. Each level of consciousness consists of a deep structure and a surface structure: "the deep structure is the defining form of a level, which embodies all of the potentials and limitations of that level. Surface structure is simply a *particular* manifestation of the deep structure."[17]

The horizontal movement of this surface structure Ken Wilber relates to translations and the vertical movement of deep structures he calls transformation, i.e., transformations are movements from one level to another level, whereas translations are the movements of the elements within any given level. Development is a series of transformations upwards or changes in deep structures, which involves the emergence of a higher level mediated by the unfolding of surface structures. Once a new level of evolution is created by a vertical transformation of the deep structure of the previous level, then a new level comes into existence through horizontal translations which integrates the surface structures of that stage into a higher level. These translations continue to develop surface structures of the new level till they are found inadequate and transformation follows.

These transformations can be either progressive or regressive depending on the success or failure in the process of transformation. If a specific level in the process of transformation encounters severe repression, then ascent to a higher level cannot be completed. Regressive transformations into the lower or pre-personal level may cause a psychotic break in the lower structure in which the individual loses contact with the normal or upper levels.

To sum up, when one translation fails to exclusively dominate consciousness then transformation to a higher level ensues with a new deep structure within, which enables new translations to develop. A transformation helps to create new types of translations and these translations help to maintain that transformation.

In *The Atman Project,* Ken Wilber realised that his Spectrum model, as a complete developmental process of consciousness, confused prepersonal with transpersonal levels. Whereas in the Spectrum model development is more based on the 'depth' psychological model, i.e., the descent of the personal to the transpersonal, in *The Atman Project* development is more based on the 'height' psychological model, i.e., the ascent from the prepersonal to the personal to the transpersonal. In the old Spectrum model development takes place in one direction, from the body to the Self; however, in *The Atman Project* linear development does not start with the full-grown personality of the adult individual but with the newborn child, whose personality still has to be formed. The personal (ego) is no longer the 'enemy' of the Self, but an important step towards the Self; the body (prepersonal) and Self are now the two extremes of the spectrum of consciousness. The various stages of human development are, from the beginning to the end, a journey to the Self. It starts from the physical level (the newborn child) to the mental level to the spiritual level (the enlightened Buddha or Atman). In *The Atman Project,* Ken Wilber attempts to integrate the contemplative structuralistic developmental approach of Eastern traditions in the areas of the Superconscious and the detailed phenomenological structuralistic developmental approach of Western psychology in the areas of the unconscious and waking consciousness.

Up from Eden: *A Transpersonal view of human evolution*

In *Up from Eden,* Ken Wilber applies the developmental scheme of T*he Atman* project to human social and cultural evolution. He emphasises the various structures of consciousness within the context of man's past, present and future history. He maintains that *The Atman Project* moves history, evolution and man's individual psyche. For Ken Wilber, history is the unfolding of man's basic nature, i.e., the unfolding which proceeds from and returns to the ultimate wholeness itself. History, as a slow path to transcendence follows the Great Chain of Being (hierarchic levels of increasing consciousness) and moves from the lower structures (matter or subconsciousness) to the higher structures (spirit or super- consciousness).

The earliest period of human evolution and the first structure of consciousness is referred to by Ken Wilber as the pleroma-uroboros stage, which stands for the symbol of primitive awareness.

The term uroboric indicates the image of the serpent that swallows its own tail. It represents matter and nature and is related to the lowest levels of the Great Chain. This uroboric period is characterised by a "biblical paradisiacal primal state" with a complete lack of distinction between the individual and the natural environment. This primal prepersonal infantile-like unity was dominated by unconscious nature, instincts, biological drives, and was pre-personal. This primal Eden of instinctual harmony with physical and biological nature was largely governed by the physical and biological realm.

Ken Wilber assumes that about 200,000 years ago, when the Atman Project in the urobic stage began to intensify, the next major stage of unfolding, the typhonic level, came into existence. The self distinguished itself from the natural environment and transcended its embeddedness in the physical and natural world. However, the self remained mostly body-bound, like Freud's infantile body-ego, and was not a mental ego. A residue from this stage can surface again in modern times as neurotic behavior. The emergence of the typhonic men necessitated culture as higher needs in the ever-expanding Atman Project. Intersubjective cultural activities allowed larger groups to take part in this Atman Project.

From the tenth millennium B.C. until 1500 B.C., when the substitute gratifications of the typhonic level were no longer effective for the Atman Project, the next stage in evolution, the mythic-membership level, the verbal mind emerged and evolved. With a higher form of unity, the verbal or membership-self could transcend the body and the present (with the development of language) and look into the future. The same language was responsible for mental goals and the new verbal self gained a relative freedom from the body's instincts and drives. It could postpone instinctual discharges and differentiate itself from the typhon body; consciousness was expanded beyond the empirical physical entities and started to operate on an inter-subjective plane through a network of inter-subjective memberships and communications. Language also provided the mechanism for a harmonious coordination of various social roles that came into existence with large societies. However, during this verbal-mind stage, money and war functioned as the cultural substitute gratifications in the Atman project.

The emergence of the next stage, roughly from 500 BC till the present, the mental-egoic stage brought a new reflective, self-conscious and higher mentality. The breakdown of the membership structure and the emergence of the egoic structure unfolded the possibility of rational and logical thought; the self became introspective with the capacity for self-analysis. But it also repressed or escaped the previous subconscious stages and had a strong tendency to resist future 'superconscious' stages.

According to Ken Wilber "it is one thing to gain a freedom from the fluctuations of nature, emotions, instincts and environment—it is quite another to alienate them."[18] Instead of the process of identification, differentiation and integration, the egoic self turned transcendence and differentiation into repression and dissociation. Differentiation between ego and nature, mind and body, became dissociations. In the meaningfully evolutionary steps toward Atman, the ego was not only repressing the body, but it was also leaving God's name out of the renovation of the universe, the ego-self became fully responsible for its renewal. With increased dissociation between the body and the ego, the ego claimed compulsive emphasis of the obsessive drive for power, and it repressed the body, reducing it to a mere mechanism, i.e. "the rational ego and the mechanistic body." The new power of the ego resulted sometimes in exploitation and slavery of the masses, hedonistic overindulgence and other exaggerated substitute gratifications. This new ego and its prosperity, however, was only a new distortion in the Atman project, and it seems that for many individuals the ego became the sole permanent self rather than a temporary movement in the Atman project. "And mankind will never, but never, give up this type of murderous aggression, war, oppression and repression, attachment and exploitation, until men and women give up that property called personality. Until, that is, they awaken to the trans-personal."[19]

Ken Wilber in his approach to evolution assumes that in each area and period of evolution there have been two parallel strands of evolution; those individuals who evolved along the average mode of consciousness and those who evolved along the most advanced mode of consciousness. When the average mode of consciousness reached the typhonic level, the advanced or fully evolved individuals (like *shamans)* reached the intuitive-shamanistic trance level with psychic capacities.

During the mythic membership level, the advanced mode reached the subtle realm level. On the mental-egoic level, the modern area of evolution, a few seers, like Buddha, Christ and Krishna, reached the Absolute Brahman/Atman level. These highly advanced sages made the evolution of the superconscious possible. This development of the successive levels of the superconscious sphere—from the subtle realm (transcendent oneness to the soul) to the causal realm (the soul becomes oneness)—is not only a historic movement, but is also related to the whole path of future evolution. For Ken Wilber, "Future evolution on the whole (i.e., the average mode of consciousness) will likely follow the same hierarchic path first glimpsed, stage by stage, by the successive transcendent heroes of the past *just as* meditation today follows the same hierarchic path, because what all three—past transcendent heroes, present-day meditators, and future evolution on the whole—are following is simply *the higher levels of the Great Chain of Being.*"[20]

For the future evolution Ken Wilber distinguishes another level of consciousness beyond the egoic level, the Existential or Centaur level, which he has described already in more detail in his *Atman Project*. In his opinion the Centaur level was first reached by the most advanced modes of consciousness in those individuals with a humanistic understanding of man, in the early 1600's; "this centaur period (really just starting) roughly corresponds with the first true and complete understanding of the Svabhavikakaya ... which is peaking with modern-day sages, especially Sri Ramana Maharshi, Bubba Free John, perhaps Aurobindo."[21]

Ken Wilber suggests that the future of humanity will eventually carry the evolution of consciousness beyond the egoic level into the level of psychic intuition or eventually to the subtle realm, the causal insight or the Atman level. However, he is also aware that "the vast majority of the present-day humanity has not yet stably reached the rational-egoic level",[22] and the most intensive transformation at present would occur if everybody truly evolved to a mature rational ego.

In *Up from Eden*, based on the idea of social evolution, Ken Wilber describes the complex history of human consciousness. Eden refers to the ignorant prepersonal level and not to the paradisiacal blissful transpersonal stage. For him, it seems that the New-Age movement mistakes the narcissistic prepersonal for the mystical transpersonal realm.

Eye To *Eye*: *The Quest for the New Paradigm*

In *Eye to Eye*, Ken Wilber attempts to present some fragments of a new and comprehensive paradigm in a full-spectrum approach to human consciousness, and to specify some of the major obstacles which prevent its emergence. He does not aim at a final view, but only endeavours to give some fragments of what a comprehensive model of consciousness might eventually look like.

In developing such a comprehensive model, he

examines three realms which offer themselves to the final structure of knowledge. These three modes of knowledge would unite science, psychology, philosophy and religion. The three realms are: the empirical realm of the senses, the rational realm of the mind and the contemplative realm of Spirit.

The three different modes of knowing, also referred to as 'the three eyes' according to the mystic philosopher St. Bonaventure, are related to (1) the empirical realm of the flesh which discloses the world of sensibilia, the external world of objects, (2) the realm of mind which reveals the world of intelligibilia by which the individual attains knowledge of science, philosophy, etc., and (3) the transcendental realm of contemplation which illumines the world of transcendelia. These three worlds are three different aspects of one world, disclosed by different modes of knowing and perceiving. The three realms are differently described by psychologists and philosophers as the gross-material, prepersonal or subconscious; the subtle-mental, personal or conscious; and the causal transcendental, transpersonal or superconscious. Ken Wilber assumes that each and every human individual possesses an empirical, rational and transcendental realm, that each level has its own object of knowledge (sensory, mental and transcendental) and that each realm is valid and useful in its own field. A truly comprehensive paradigm uses all the three realms, a synthesis and integration of the eye of flesh, the eye of mind and the eye of contemplation.

One of the major obstacles for the development of a comprehensive paradigm is related to the 'category error', when one realm is reduced or explained in terms of another realm. In the words of Ken Wilber, "category error occurs when one of the three realms is made to wholly substitute for another realm or we might say, when things (flesh) are confused with thoughts (mind) are confused with transcendental insight (contemplation).[23]

The empirical realm is not able to disclose the transcendental realm; the truth of the world of intelligibilia can be verified only with the eye of reason, but the eye of reason is not able to verify the truth of the eye of contemplation. "Sensation, reason, and contemplation disclose their own truths in their own realms, and any time one eye tries to see for another eye, blurred vision results."[24]

Till recent past, religion tried to be scientific and science tried to be philosophic, confusing the various realms of reason with contemplation, as reason is not able to grasp the transcendent reality. Proof of higher transcendental states are contemplative and not empirical; the methodology of empiric-analytic science cannot be applied to the contemplative realm; this does not mean that empirical data are not useful, but they are not essential. Ken Wilber concludes that his overall comprehensive paradigm should include and integrate all three realms and avoid confusing any of the three realms by delineating the respective roles of each. Each realm on its own has its respective role but cannot form a complete worldview; in other words, each part cannot play the whole.

When science includes any discipline that follows valid data accumulation and verification in all the three realms, and when it is obedient to the methodology of the three realms themselves, only then can someone speak of the science of sensibilia, intelligibilia and transcendelia, e.g., when the data comes from the domain of the transcendental one can speak of contemplative science. Ken Wilber attempts to include all these three kinds of sciences in his comprehensive paradigm. However, a premature attempt to integrate science and mysticism may be misleading. Science and metaphysics are not two different approaches to the same reality but the two realms involving two different levels of reality.

But, unfortunately, Ken Wilber, when admitting

sensory, intellectual and spiritual experiences in the physical, mental and spiritual realms respectively, advises transpersonal psychologists to restrict the term empirical to its original meaning "knowledge grounded in sensory experience"—to avoid ambiguities with strict empirical scientists who otherwise would reject their results. In bringing on par transpersonal psychology with the modem scientific' methodical approach it may seem that Ken Wilber mixes up the contemplative realm with the empirical realm in order that the former be accepted by the latter, forcing an artificial reconciliation of the eternal transpersonal realm with the temporary (sensory) realm. But later on he admits that "mysticism itself is too profound to be hitched to phases of empirical scientific theorizing."[25]

One of the other obstacles to the emergence of a truly comprehensive paradigm is related to the confusion of the "pre/trans fallacy", i.e., when the transpersonal realm is reduced to the prepersonal state or when the prepersonal realm is glorified as transpersonal.

The overall sequence of development, from nature to humanity to divinity, from prepersonal to personal to transpersonal, begins with the lowest realm, the realm of matter or physical sensations which Ken Wilber relates to the prepersonal. As development moves on to a self-conscious stage, that realm is related to the personal and finally development culminates in the transpersonal realm. The prepersonal subconscient level is the realm of irrational and simple bodily sensations and perceptions; the personal conscious level is the realm of mental awareness and the transpersonal or superconscious level culminates in the realm of Spirit. The prepersonal and transpersonal are both nonpersonal and therefore tend to appear similar to the untrained eye, but this leads to a confusion of transpersonal bliss with prepersonal ignorance.

Though Spirit is beyond ego, the non-egoic realm

has to be clearly differentiated into pre-egoic and trans-egoic; transcendence of ego implies the devaluation of ego levels rather than the elevation of the pre-egoic level. In the newborn child, the Self as the totality of the psycho-spiritual realm is not yet manifested; it is present in potential, but is not realised and remains therefore unconscious. In development, the personal ego transcends the prepersonal unconscious, and with the awakening of the ego as a self-conscious entity the relatively blissful ignorance of the unconscious is lost. In later developmental stages, individual consciousness re-awakens to the Self, but now in conscious and realised form.

Most people who are in need of psychotherapy do so because they are suffering from prepersonal fixations and they lack sufficient ego-strength to overcome those fixations. Psychotherapy first attempts to strengthen the ego in the process of ego transcendence rather than devaluing the ego.

As a major example of the pre/trans fallacy in psychological development Ken Wilber refers to Freud and Jung. Freud did accept a prepersonal 'id' and a personal ego but he reduced all sorts of spiritual experiences to a prepersonal 'fusion.' Jung correctly acknowledged the transpersonal realm but often confused this realm with the prepersonal, confusing the lower prepersonal collective unconscious with the higher transpersonal collective unconscious. As a result, the individual ends up in "a type of infantile psychological Garden of Eden."

Ken Wilber claims that many important theorists completely ignore the pre/trans fallacy view. His pre/trans fallacy, based on developmental and structural criteria, is not a model based on dogma, but is open to external and experimental verification.

Developmental and Structural Approach

As we have seen already in *The Atman Project,* the lower

levels do not embrace the higher levels as the higher cannot be explained by the lower. However, though the hierarchical levels are separate from each other, they are nevertheless interdependent and interpenetrating. The higher levels have capacities which are absent in the lower levels, e.g., psychology cannot be explained in terms of biology. The higher levels have correlations in the lower but can not be reduced to the lower. According to Ken Wilber, "the higher transcends but includes the lower—*not* vice versa. That is, all of the lower is 'in' the higher, but not all the higher is in the lower."[26]

As higher-order levels of consciousness emerge, they may repress the lower levels. These lower levels, which are threatening to the higher-order structure, are driven out of the consciousness, which itself is a distortion of the concept of self and blocks the higher-order integration. Psychotherapy aims at the re-establishment of this higher-order integration.

To his developmental model of consciousness Ken Wilber now adds the concept of 'self-system'. He distinguishes levels of consciousness from stages or phases of consciousness, which are often confused and one of the obstacles to a comprehensive paradigm. For Ken Wilber levels of consciousness as basic structures are essentially permanent and remain, whereas phases of consciousness as transition structures are temporary and pass. Each of the lower basic structures contributes and provides the data for the operation of the next level, without ceasing to be active. Transition or replacement stages serve only as stages and are outgrown; they emerge only to be replaced and not to be united.

Each basic structure is devoid of a self, but in the course of development a self-system emerges. In between the basic structures and the self-moral stages (like Maslow's self-needs as phase-temporary phenomena) lies the self-system.

In the course of its development the self-system, as a theoretical link between basic structures and moral selfstages, uses the basic structures as rungs in a ladder upon which it climbs. As such, the self-system, which includes the sense of identity, defence mechanisms and interpersonal relations, functions as the instrument of development and transcendence. Between levels the self is confronted with either an upward movement of increasing structural organisation and integration or a downward movement toward less organised and integrative structures.

At each stage of development, the lower rungs of the ladder are not destroyed, only one's exclusive identification with that rung is finished. The lower structures continue to operate, their capacities are preserved and the individual has still access to all the preceding and lower basic structures. However, a person at a more highly developed self-moral stage hardly responds to the lower levels.

So, in *Eye to Eye* Ken Wilber introduces a 'New Paradigm', which includes physical or exact science, social sciences and contemplative science; each has its own domain but also influences the others. Psychology, as a science of human behaviour, tends to reduce the mental to the physical level and to leave out the scientific admission of the inner reality of man, which can be studied by the introspective level of reason or meditation.

Transformations of Consciousness: *Conventional and Contemplative Perspectives on Development*

In *Transformations of Consciousness,* Ken Wilber deals with certain fundamental patterns in ontogenetic development. His evolutionary process, based on the full-spectrum model of human growth, includes stages of development investigated by conventional psychology, as well as by the world's great contemplative traditions. He connects the different stages of this developmental model with the possibility of qualitatively distinct corresponding psychopathologies and the correlative therapeutic interventions.

In attempting to integrate the conventional and contemplative schools of development Ken Wilber uses the "stage model" as a tool, and he links Sri Aurobindo's levels of consciousness with stages of development. But Ken Wilber maintains that the contemplative model lacks a certain knowledge of self-development, psycho- dynamics and object relations in the lower stages of development, which are extensively elaborated in conventional psychology. He suggests that conventional psychology has much to learn from contemplative traditions but also that the latter open themselves to the important insight of contemporary psychology. Ken Wilber regards it as inevitable that the realisation of optimal psychological well-being needs to be preceded by the realisation of becoming 'somebody' in order to become 'nobody.'

Ken Wilber describes nine basic levels or stages of human development and the particular pathologies that may arise at any of the levels and the therapeutic interventions related to each of these classes of pathology. In doing so he attempts to integrate the medical model into his structural, hierarchical spectrum model of conventional and contemplative human development.

The nine basic structures of consciousness development are divided into three each; the prepersonal, the personal and the transpersonal. In the presentation of each level Ken Wilber uses the same developmental procedures as discussed in his prior works and he constructs a "master template" from the structural comparisons of the contemplative traditions and the conventional developmental schools of psychology (see Table 1).

Table 1. Comparison and Correlation of Basic Structures with Pathologies and Treatment Modalities

	Sri Aurobindo's model according to Ken Wilber	**Wilber's model**	**Pathologies**	**Treatment modalities**
Pre-Personal Stages	1. Sensorimotor	Realm of sensation & perception	Psychosis'	Pharmacological & Physiological therapies
	2. Vital- emotional	Emotional & sexual level	Narcissistic-borderline disorders	Structure-building techniques, object-relation therapy
	3. Will-mind	Representational mind	Psychoneurosis	Uncovering techniques, Gestalt, Psychoanalysis
Personal Stages	4. Sense-mind	Rule / Role mind	Script-pathology	Transactional Analysis, cognitive therapies
	5. Reasoningmind	Formal/reflexive mind	Identity neurosis	Introspection, Socratic dialogue
	6. Higher-mind	Vision-logic	Existential pathology	Existential therapy
	7.Illumined- mind	Psychic; The beginning of transcendence	Psychic disorders	Psychosynthesis, Yoga therapy & Jungian therapy
Trans-personal Stages	8. Intuitive- mind	Subtle; the transcendent insight	Subtle pathology	Meditation
	9. Overmind	Causal; universal self	Causal pathology	Contemplation
	10. Supermind	Ultimate; the ground of all levels		

1. Ken Wilier starts the hierarchical developmental model with the sensory-physical realm, the level of matter, sensation and perception, Sri Aurobindo's physical-sensory level (the lower physical realm).
2. The phantasmic-emotional realm or the emotional-sexual level is related to Sri Aurobindo's lower vital level.
3. The Rep-mind or representational mind, which develops various stages of symbols and concepts, is similar to Sri Aurobindo's will-mind [mental will].
4. Rule/Role mind is able to adopt the role of others and rule various operations, Sri Aurobindo's sensemind.
5. Formal-reflexive mind indicates an introspective and self-reflexive mind, which is equated with Sri Aurobindo's reasoning mind.
6. Vision-logic, the integrative or creative synthetic mind, which has a higher-order synthesising capacity and what Sri Aurobindo calls the higher mind, "is the highest integrative structure in the personal realm."[27]
7. The psychic level indicates the development of the transpersonal realm and the transcendence of the mind's cognitive and perceptual capacities. 'This is Aurobindo's illumined mind."[28]
8. The Subtle level of transcendent insight Ken Wilber compares with Sri Aurobindo's intuitive mind.
9. The Causal level, Sri Aurobindo's overmind, "is said to be the unmanifest source or transcendent ground of all the lesser structures."[29] The ego-sense is abolished and replaced by a universal self.
10. The Ultimate, where consciousness re-awakens to the absolute Spirit, Ken Wilber compares with Sri Aurobindo's Supermind. It is not one level among others, but the condition of all other levels.

Pathology

Ken Wilber associates pathology with a failure to disidentify or detach from an exclusive involvement with a particular level in order to be integrated into the next higher basic level, i.e., fixation and negation, or a failure to differentiate or transcend a lower structure, or a differentiation from a component before it has been properly integrated (repression). In his outline of the Spectrum model—the prepersonal, personal and transpersonal ranges of development, he discusses the three corresponding stages of pathology resulting in an overall hierarchical model of pathology. A specific level of pathology will best respond to a specific type of psychotherapeutic intervention.

(a) *Prepersonal Pathologies:* Ken Wilber's model of prepersonal pathology is primarily based on the recent developments of psychoanalytic-developmental methods for treatment. There are three levels or stages of self-development in the prepersonal realm—the physica self, the emotional self and the mental self—and a developmental injury or trauma at a particular stage may cause a particular type of psychopathology.

1. When the physical self fails to differentiate from the physical environment then the infant remains lost in his or her undifferentiated state where the child is not able to distinguish the inside from the outside; this class of primitive pathology, where there is a severe distortion of the sense of reality, is known as psychosis.
2. When the emotional self starts to develop and the individual fails to differentiate one's emotional-psychological life from that of others and the self remains at the fusion stage, Ken Wilber relates to narcissistic personality disorders. If the self remains dissociated, he relates it to borderline disorders. In both syndromes the individual lacks a cohesive 'self-sense'.

3. Once the mental self begins to emerge and when the child begins to think, then this mental self becomes able to repress the previous emotional self (bodily impulses or drives), which expresses itself as neurosis. The difference between neurosis and borderline disorders is that in the former there is a conflict or repression within the self-structure, whereas in the latter there is a lack of or an underdeveloped selfstructure and the self is often overwhelmed by the environment.

(b) *Personal or Psychological Pathologies:* The intermediate or personal realm of development within the Spectrum of pathologies is characterised more by cognitive and existential conflicts as compared with psychodynamic prepersonal vulnerabilities.

4. When the rule/role mind emerges, the individual can imitate a role. Failure to find its place or role among others—Maslow's need for belongingness—Ken Wilber classifies as Cognitive Script Pathology.
5. With the development of the reflexive, introspective self-structure, the individual is no longer dependent on social roles and can rely on one's own individual principles of reason and conscience. Whatever goes wrong in the emergence of the self-reflective structure Ken Wilber calls the Identity neurosis.
6. The emergence of the existential mind has the centaur as its correlative stage of development. In this selfstructure body and mind are experienced as an integrated self. Failure to integrate the existential self (authenticity, self-actualisation, etc) may lead to existential pathology.
7. *Transpersonal or Spiritual Pathologies:* The transpersonal realm is also divided into three major levels of development and corresponding

pathology. Ken Wilber is frank enough to admit that some of the contemplative schools might disagree with his terminology of these higher stages or their possible pathologies. He invites the contemplative schools "to substitute more neutral terms."

8. The psychic disorders are related to the "lower level" of spiritual crises and pathologies which may occur spontaneously (e.g. *Kundalini* awakening) or invade the lower levels during periods of stress (e.g. psychotic-like episodes accompanied with spiritual insight, but through a self-structure that is neurotic, borderline or psychotic), or come up in the beginning of meditation practice. The beginner practitioner may be overwhelmed by: (a) psychic inflation when the spiritual insights are exclusively applied to the individual ego; (b) structural imbalance due to incorrect practice of the spiritual technique; (c) the fading of the initial spiritual experience; (d) split life goals; (e) pseudo-duhkha or psychic depression when the individual is overwhelmed by the painful nature of existence itself; (f) pranic disorders caused through misdirection of *Kundalini* energies in the early stages of its arousal; or (g) Yogic illness, when the higher psychic levels of consciousness overload the lower physical-emotional body.

9. Subtle disorders usually occur in the intermediate-to-advanced meditation practitioners. Ken Wilber describes three forms of subtle disorders: (a) Failure to integrate the Divine Presence as an image of one's own essential nature, (identity awareness with the Divine) after the practitioner is capable of it, he classifies as the Integration-Identity Failure, (b) In *pseudo-nirvana* the meditation practitioner mistakes the subtle forms of insight for final liberation, (c) In pseudo-

realisation, the subtle level equivalent of *pseudo-duhkha* on the psychic level, the individual fails to transcend the temporary and oppressive 'contents' of consciousness "and the soul is stranded on the shores of its own agony".

10. In the causal disorders the meditative practitioner fails to differentiate between the Formless or Unmanifest Realm and the world of Form or Manifest Realm. Ken Wilber describes two forms of this causal disorders: (a) Failure of the Formless consciousness to transcend the Manifest Realm, (b) Failure to integrate the subtle disjuncture between the Manifest and Unmanifest Realms.

In all these various forms of pathology, it is important to distinguish personality type or structure from the levels of personality organisation. According to Ken Wilber, "Almost all the commonly recognized personality *types* can occur at any level of personality *organisation;* healthy, neurotic, borderline, or psychotic. Even the more pathological character types—schizoid, paranoid, infantile—can occur within a neurotic structure."[30] For Ken Wilber, qualitatively different pathologies are associated with qualitatively different levels of self-organisation and self-development.

Psychotherapies

All these pathologies are best treated by different types of psychotherapy/ i.e. a specific-level of pathology will best respond to a specific type of psychotherapeutic intervention.

1. Severe forms of psychoses do not respond to psychotherapy and the only remedy which seems effective is pharmacological or physiological intervention.
2. For narcissistic or borderline disorders, in which there is not enough structure to differentiate self and object representations, or a lack of a

separated individuated self, object-relation therapy is helpful to strengthen the self through structure-building techniques. "These structure-building techniques, like optimal disillusionment or unification aim exactly at that differentiation-and-integration."[31]

3. In psychoneuroses uncovering techniques are used to bring back repressed unconscious aspects into consciousness where they can be re-integrated with the central self. These interpretative techniques include psychoanalysis and Gestalt therapy.
4. Ken Wilber divides script pathology into role and rule pathology. Role pathology is best treated by Transactional Analysis or family therapy, whereas the individual with rule pathology is more benefited by rational-emotive therapy or other similar cognitive therapies which help one encounter one's distorted and confused rules and beliefs.
5. In the identity neuroses, the individual is confronted with the emergence of an introspective self-sense through which one is able to apprehend one's internal life. "Introspection, in this context, refers to the techniques used in dealing with the difficulties or problems that arise from F-5 development [F relates to the Fulcrum of separation-individuation phase of development]; the formal-reflexive-introspective self and its turmoils."[32]
6. In existential pathologies, existential concerns overwhelm the self on the centauric level and block its functioning. Humanistic/existential therapies emphasise the concepts of intrinsic meaning and the autonomy of the self.

As described above, transpersonal or spiritual

pathologies are divided into the psychic, subtle and causal level. The various pathologies may occur at each level and are primarily treated by different forms of "spiritual" therapy.

7. For the "treatment" of psychic disorders Ken Wilber suggests that the techniques of contemplative discipline, Jungian therapy, prayer, and strengthening of the physical-emotional body are all applicable to this level of psychic pathology. In specific cases the meditative practitioner is advised to stop meditation immediately, and either consider another path "or ride it out sometimes under the care of a conventional psychiatrist"[33], or a yoga meditation teacher.
8. In subtle pathology, Ken Wilber advises the meditative person to intensify the path of subtle-level contemplation, and not to mistake subtle illuminations for the ultimate enlightenment. Psychotherapy can be used as an adjunct.
9. In causal pathology the final detachment or ultimate pathology, "a repeated movement' from manifest to unmanifest and back again—'burns' the root inclinations and desires for contracted and separated modes of self existence... the overcoming of this disjunction (a failure to integrate the manifest and unmanifest realms) or re-integration of emptiness-form are the 'supreme path'—wherein all phenomena are seen as already perfect expressions and seals of the naturally enlightened mind."[34]

Ken Wilber warns the reader that his hierarchical model of pathologies should be used cautiously, "there are no pure cases, the influence of cultural differences, genetic predispositions, genetic and traumatic arrests, and blended cases"[35] are all important factors in the process of pathology.

In all, it can be said that Ken Wilber in the *Transformations of Consciousness* attempts to describe the value of his spectrum model in the diagnosis and treatment of psychopathology. He outlines many forms of psychopathology which may occur at any developmental stage and he maintains that the three primitive forms of pathology—psychosis, narcissistic or borderline disorders, and neurosis—refer to three different levels of consciousness. A psychosis is a disorder on the physical emotional level, borderline problems are disorders on the emotional level (too much emotionality) and a neurosis is a disorder on the mental emotional level (repression of emotion). Unlike conventional psychiatrists, Ken Wilber discusses the pathological disorders which belong to the personal and transpersonal levels. It is important to ascertain at which level pathology finds its origin, physical, emotional, mental or spiritual, and treatment should take place at the corresponding level, i.e., use physical intervention for physical diseases and use spiritual methods for spiritual crises. However, treatment of other levels may be important as support or supplement. Ken Wilber is aware that illnesses do not originate in one separate level, what happens at one level influences, to a certain extent, all other levels.

Sex, Ecology, Spirituality: *The Spirit of Evolution*

In this book, the first of a three-volume set called the *Kosmos* Trilogy, Ken Wilber offers a broad orienting map of evolving men and their place in the larger Kosmos of matter, life, mind and spirit. From his previous works he elaborates on developmental, evolutionary themes in an extended version.

Consciousness is the most important instrument in evolution and Ken Wilber attempts to trace evolution within the context of perennial wisdom, in accordance with the insight and data of the various fields of contemporary scientific research. He links the evolution of consciousness with the fields of physical, biological and cultural evolution, as well as with anthropology, psychology, sociology, philosophy, mysticism, ecology and feminism.

Ken Wilber introduces several new topics in order to exemplify his previous ideas, and he expounds in detail his views on today's world of modernity and post-modernity which seems to him "slightly going mad". Nevertheless, this book, like his other works, does not offer a finished conclusion, it offers "a thousand hypotheses" or a metaphysics but with evidence. The first chapter of Book One in the cosmic Trilogy is based on orienting generalisations, i.e., "largely-agreed-upon orienting generalisations, from the various branches of knowledge", which after critical examination may produce profound conclusions.

Evolution and the Twenty Tenets as the principle of holistic systems theory.

In a unified holistic worldview, the real synthesis unites the domains of the physiosphere, biosphere and noosphere, and all of these domains again become an interrelated manifestation of Spirit. Human beings are complex individuals composed of the physical, biological, mental and spiritual levels, and cannot merely be interpreted in terms of the lower spheres such as the physiosphere or biosphere as they comprise only the physical and biological levels of a person. The major links in the continuous levels are termed body, mind and spirit, which correspond to the movement from nature to humanity to divinity. Each successive level represents "an increase in wholeness and integrative capacity."

Around the end of the 19th century modern science contributed to a worldview which separated the various spheres, and each sphere went its own way; facts from the physiosphere (natural sciences) were cut off from the values of the noosphere (human sciences). Nevertheless, new sciences discovered some self-organising and basic regularities which are applicable to all three spheres, and this unity of science, which Ken Wilber refers to as the evolutionary systems theory, claims to offer a coherent and unified worldview. In the holistic systems approach, everything in life is connected to everything else, and the whole consists of interlocking orders. The present crisis is due to a fractured worldview, a worldview that erroneously separates rather than integrates. The healing of this fractured worldview implies the recognition of the wholeness and interconnectedness of all life.

The systems theory is based on the notion of hierarchy, also referred to as holarchy, and like Ken Wilber's evolutionary model it ranks phenomena according to holistic capacities.

Reality is composed of several different but continuous grades or levels, from the lowest and least conscious to the highest and most conscious. These various levels of reality are composed of holons rather than things, processes, parts or wholes. A holon, a term borrowed from A. Koestler, is a relatively autonomous whole which is simultaneously a part of a greater whole, i.e., a phenomenon in the universe is neither a whole nor a part, but both simultaneously. Holons are hierarchically related to each other and holism between levels of the normal hierarchy represents an increase in wholeness or integrative capacity. The science of holarchy, as a multidimensional approach to the relation between each and all, studies the emergence of a series of increasing whole/parts. Each holon is composed of sub-holons which give rise to hierarchies of parts and wholes; "each deeper or higher holon embraces its junior predecessors and than *adds* its own new and more encompassing pattern or wholeness."[36]

This means that in a developmental sequence the whole at one stage becomes merely a part of a larger whole at the next stage. He deals with these holons in the physiosphere, (matter), the biosphere (life), noosphere, (mind), and the theosphere (the Divine). Ken Wilber is aware that any *hierarchical* model, [vertical, depth] a ranking of orders of events according to their holistic capacity, is opposed by the *heterarchical* model, [horizontal, extension], but he compares the hierarchical pattern of development between each level with transformation and the heterarchical pattern of development within each level with translation. The latter merely differentiates but, unlike the former, does not integrate.

He begins the dynamic systems theory with twenty orienting generalisations or tenets which represent patterns of existence or "tendencies of evolution". These common features are the most fundamental patterns of manifestation which are applicable to all surface development in all three domains of evolution—the physiosphere, biosphere and noosphere.

Each development involves a new transcendence, a new interiority, a greater degree of consciousness, a new integration and the possibility of new and higher pathologies. As mentioned before, Reality as a whole is composed of holons, but Ken Wilber uses 'Whole' not as a sum total of parts, but as the All, which is the sum total of whole/parts. Within this first tenet, Ken Wilber distinguishes Kosmos, the unending all which is composed of holons and includes the divine realm, from cosmos as the physical universe. A holon which has the capacity to preserve its own wholeness in the presence of environmental pressures Ken Wilber calls agency or 'self asserting tendency expressing wholeness', but as a part it must simultaneously adapt itself to other holons, a process which he calls 'communion or participating tendency'. Each holon possesses both agency and communion and they operate horizontally on any level. But a holon also has the capacity of self-transcendence or self-transformation, which results in a new whole, or the capacity of selfdissolution, which causes more fragmentation and less unity; these capacities operate vertically to higher or lower levels respectively. These four capacities taken together are in constant tension, i.e., the more a holon preserves its wholeness, the less it serves its parts in larger wholes.

Evolution involves a vertical self-transcendence to new forms of wholes and parts that integrates them both; not just a wider whole or a horizontal expansion but also a deeper whole or a vertical emergence. He relates changes in the horizontal dimension to translation and changes in the vertical dimension to transformation. Ken Wilber maintains that "the greater the vertical dimension of a holon, then the greater the depth of that holon; and the more holons on that level the wider its span."[37] He associates depth to the interior or qualitative dimensions in the hierarchy of a holon (whole), and span to the exterior or quantitative dimensions (part). Each subsequent level of growth brings about greater depth and less span in relation to a holon's predecessors, but greater span on its own level.

The self-transcendent capacities of holons enable new holons to emerge, and each new emergent holon transcends but includes its predecessors, i.e., whereas the deep basic structures are preserved, the surface transition structures are negated. The lower levels form the possibilities of the higher, and the higher form the probabilities of the lower. Though the higher transcends the lower it cannot ignore the lower level. However, each successive stage implies not only a greater integration but also the possibility of pathology; transcendence can end up in regression or differentiation with dissociation if the corresponding integration does not ensue. Holarchy goes pathological when arrogant holons do not embrace and transcend the preceding levels but repress, alienate and dissociate these holons upon which its own existence intimately depends.

Ken Wilber then makes some fundamental additions

to these twenty tenets which will not violate the systems theory. He connects the depth of a holon to consciousness and affirms that "the greater the depth of a holon, the greater its degree of consciousness."[38] The less depth, the more fundamental and less significant it is to the Kosmos and vice versa; the greater the depth, the less fundamental and more significant that holon is for the Kosmos. Many holistic theorists (New-Age paradigm) mistake great span (number of holons on any given level) for great depth (number of levels in any holarchy) and more fundamental for more significant; bigger or more fundamental is not a higher or deeper whole and this kind of growth only ends up in regression. Their holarchies are emphasising a horizontal, wider expansion and ignoring the vertical deeper expansion. However, greater depth involves both a vertical and horizontal expansion. Nevertheless, the realisation of the ultimate depth as the ultimate oneness with the Kosmos is not equal for all living beings. Though all beings are equally manifestations of Spirit, the realisation of ultimate depth, as the result of an evolutionary process of transcendence, depends on the holarchy of realisation. Growth is not a mere isolated affair (micro) but is inseparably related to the environment (macro). Though there are distinctions between individual and social growth, they are nevertheless interactive and the former is in relational exchange with the latter at all levels of its depth. And finally, evolution tends in the direction of increased differentiation/integration, autonomy, complexity, organisation and telos.

Ken Wilber is of the opinion that all these tenets of the systems theory are not a healing force for the fractured worldview, as they don't distinguish the individual and social dimensions on any level. But the individual and social levels are two aspects of the same level, and what is needed is "to construct a series of true holarchies of compound individuals, and then indicate at the same level of organization the type of environment (or social holon) in which the individual holon is a participant. [39] This needs to be done in the physiosphere and biosphere as well as the noosphere. At each stage of growth, a compound individual is related to a compound environment of the same level, which in turn is related to the cultural realm of that level.

The hierarchies of the holistic systems theory deal entirely with surfaces or exteriors (empiricism) and overlook almost entirely the interior, subjectivity and consciousness (introspection and interpretation). For the exterior, objective approaches the physical or empirical world is fundamental, it starts from material and empirical facts and deduces the existence of transcendental realities on the basis of empirical realities. For the interior subjective approaches, the primordial data are consciousness and intentionality, and the existence of transcendental reality is a deduction from interior, direct experiences. Although each approach is profoundly significant, transpersonal studies incorporates both these approaches.

The Four Quadrants Model

To do so Ken Wilber introduces the four major types of hierarchies in what he calls the 'four quadrants' model of development .in which he integrates the exterior and interior of the individual and social groups. In this four-quadrant model he distinguishes the interior (intention) and exterior (behaviour) of the individual, as well as the interior (cultural values and shared worldviews) and exterior (objective or material base of social systems) of the collective. In evolution the four different quadrants, as major aspects to each and every holon, are "intimately related and indeed dependent upon all the others, but none can be reduced to the others."[40]

Evolution occurs in all four quadrants and each quadrant is essential for completeness, because each holon has these four dimensions. Ken Wilber ties individual development to social and cultural evolution; cultural events have social correlates. Higher stages of consciousness development indicate wider patterns in all four quadrants, in self, in individual behaviour, in culture and in society.

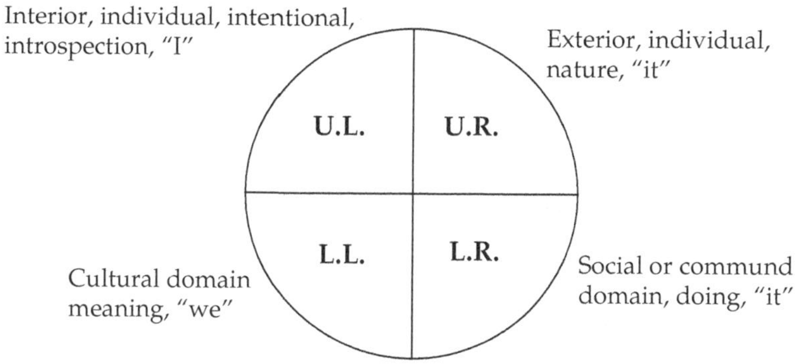

Figure 1. The Four Quadrants Model

Each quadrant has a different type of truth that cannot be reduced to the others. The upper right quadrant represents the exterior structure of the individual which deals with propositional truth (truth connected with objective, observable facts), whereas the upper left quadrant, the interior form of the individual, uses subjective truthfulness (truth connected with interpretation and meaning). The lower right quadrant represents the empirical or exterior forms of social systems and deals with objective social institutions or material social structures, and judges its validity through observable processes of the social action system which Ken Wilber refers to as "functional fit." The lower left quadrant is related to shared worldviews and values or the interiors of the social systems; its truth or validity is concerned with subjects in relation to mutual understanding such as goodness or righteousness also referred to as "cultural fit." Ultimately these four truths are the four facts of spirit as it radiates in the manifested world.

Each of these four validity claims has its own type of evidence and data: injunction (experiment), apprehension (collecting data), and confirmation/rejection (consensual justification). Assertions within each claim can be validated or rejected by the criterion of these three strands of genuine knowledge.

Each of these quadrants is formulated in a different language; the entire right half can be described in"it" terms, such as science, technology and empirical forms of social systems, as its exterior approaches can be studied empirically; the upper left is described in "I" language, such as self-consciousness and subjectivity, and the lower left in "we" language, such as ethics, common culture and intersubjective meaning, as its depth can be internally experienced (see Figure 1). For Ken Wilber, "any higher developments, in all four quadrants, have to occur through an individual's own effort (UL), evidenced in individual bodily transformations (UR), practiced in a microcommunity or sangha of the similarly depthed (LL) with its own microsocial structure (LR) ... but how they unfold will depend upon the mutual interaction and interplay between *all four quadrants*—intentional, behavioral, cultural and social—as all four continue to evolve in history, and *none* of that is predetermined in any strong sense."[41] The different left hand (ascending) and right hand (descending) approaches to consciousness must be integrated; the union of these two, the union of the one and the many, determines the approach to higher stages of consciousness development itself, and their union is the source and goal of genuine spirituality. These higher developments proceed in all four quadrants; in order for the realisation of Spirit to be complete all four quadrants ought to be taken into account as these four quadrants are all facets of Spirit.

What Ken Wilber calls 'flatland' or 'descending world' is the material world of flat and endless sensory forms without any deeper or higher potentials. It reduces the entire Kosmos to a bundle of 'its' where the 'I' and 'We' domains are almost entirely reduced to 'it' domains. It is a purely descending world without any ascending energy, like capitalism, consumerism, positivism, behaviourism or empiricism. The so-called 'flatland atomists' reduce all quadrants to the upperright quadrant, and they reduce all the higher order structures of this quadrant to atomic particles (gross reductionism). The 'flatland holists' reduce everything on the left half to a corresponding reality on the right half (subtle reductionism). The subtle reductionists recognise a surface hierarchy but leave out the depth dimension, such as value, consciousness, intuition, etc; they replace interior gradations of quality or degrees of interior depth by exterior gradations of quantity or functions of exterior span. Subtle reductionism is often holistic but this is only of the exterior variety, i.e., holistically interwoven 'its' lacking the holistic domains of the 'I' and 'We'.

In constructivism (cultural constructivism or interior holism) there is an attempt to reduce all quadrants to the lower left quadrant, i.e., reducing all knowledge claims to intersubjective constructions in the dynamic collective "We". They claim the absence of inter objective realities and objective truth, because the individual's ideas are built up according to one's interest. The reductionisms of the systems theory (exterior holism) attempt to reduce all reality to the lower-right quadrant, the dynamic collective 'It'; this means the reduction of all truths to functional fit, whereby the social system alone is the primary reality.

Both interior and exterior holism share their truths in the collective—one cultural and the other social, but the former occupies itself exclusively with subjectivism (We), whereas the latter deals mainly with objectivism (It).

According to Ken Wilber, the original holon is "a holon with four inseparable aspects (intentional, behavioral, cultural and social), each with its own validity claims (subjective truthfulness, objective truth, intersubjective justness, and interobjective functional fit)."[42] As long as the four quadrants themselves are not integrated, so long will this fractured worldview not contribute to a mutual harmony. "The healing impulse comes not from championing functional fit (Lower Right) but mutual understanding (Lower Left). And that depends first and foremost, we will see, on individual growth and transformation (Upper Left)."[43] He does not want the modernists or post-modernists to replace atomism by holism, but to integrate exterior 'it' with the depth of 'I' and the community of 'We', or integrate the biosphere and noosphere in a higher and deeper union.

The Path of Descent

Up to this point in Book One, Ken Wilber has discussed "the path of ascent" in the formative stages in the individual and collective evolution of the human species in the past and for the future. In Part Two, he describes "the path of descent"; the complementary movement in evolution, which is characterised by Spirit that delights in diversity, and which manifests itself in the emanation of the many out of the One. The Ascenders focus mainly on the uncreated Source and ignore creation, whereas the Descenders are more focused on the created world of manyness, seeing only creation.

Ken Wilber gives equal importance to the movement of ascent (Spirit transcendent to the world; Eros), and to the movement of descent (Spirit immanent in the world; Agape). In this improved version of his developmental process, all development (transcendence) is envelopment (immanence); the ascending force of the lower to the higher is accomplished by the higher force expressing itself in the lower (descent). "Reality is the integration of the Ascending [as the realisation of the other world] and Descending paths [as the creative Source of this world] that the Nondual awareness flashes."[44]

Systems theory is engaged in the relation with each and all, but leaves out the One, the Source of each and all. The horizontal dimension (surface structure/translation) reduces each to all, whereas the vertical dimension (deep structure /transformation) embraces all to One. In reconciling ascent with descent, the ascent towards the transcendent One culminates in descent towards the immanent Many. Reunion with the Kosmos involves a horizontal identification (descent) with Nature as well as a vertical movement (ascent) to the transcendent nondual One. This complementary movement of ascent and descent allows a wider identity and opening, in which natural phenomena are able to manifest Spirit which radiates through them. Without this unifying centre it is impossible to integrate the 'it', and 'we' spheres. By participating in the depth of the All embracing Each as a perfect manifestation of the One, one discovers the divine Source. Like Sri Aurobindo and Plotinus, Ken Wilber maintains that ascent is related to a change in perception in which "more and more of this world is perceived as Perfectly Divine until there is only the Perfectly Divine in all perception."[45]

He relates descent, Sri Aurobindo's delight of Existence, to compassion but unlike Sri Aurobindo's descent, Ken Wilber's descent, as we will see later on, misses the purifying function of the psychic in the process of transformation.

Modernism and Postmodernism

While examining in detail the shortcomings of modernism, Ken Wilber distinguishes two kinds of modernists: the eco camp as environmentalists and the ego camp as rationalists. Both camps are thoroughly caught in the modern descending path. The eco camp has reduced the higher levels (noosphere) to the lower levels (biosphere) without integrating the deeper possibilities. The eco camp faced the central problem of the relation between human subjectivity, the I, and the world and nature. In its attempt to return to nature, to become one with it rather than to control it, they emphasised the expression of ecstatic feelings in the unification with internal and external nature, thereby overlooking objectivity, autonomy and instrumentality. In their search forward to Nature, they went back to nature. The source of these spiritual feelings is not nature itself but transcendental Spirit, of which nature is an expression.

The descending ego camps were haunted by regression, a move downward to a previous lower level; they confused regression and higher order integration. Their way of embracing sensory nature ended up in pathological descent by validating pre-personal egoism. In their desire to control nature, the rational ego camp dissociated ego from nature and reduced the interior to the exterior without producing a global transformation. In its objectifying sciences of man, they focused on surfaces and external dimensions, overlooking internal phenomena such as value, meaning and purpose. The ascending ego camps were marked by repression, and no further ascent beyond ego; they ignored transpersonal illuminations, and confused transcendence and repression. Ken Wilber concludes that both camps had no place for the transcendent Spirit, as they assumed that nature itself is the ultimate reality.

While modernity has distinguished the four quadrants, postmodernism faces the task of the integration of the Big Three at the vision-logic level; the integration of the isolated individual with a meaningful social life and culture against the background of universal natural science. All these aspects are integral expressions of Spirit, none can be isolated from the other, and each has to be honored in its respective task. Going postmodern involves a change in consciousness and a rehash of man-made institutions.

Ken Wilber's Worldview

In a significant turn in his view of world's future Ken Wilber assumes a shift from the rational-industrial society to a vision-logic information-based society. This new information transformation brings with it a new worldview with new social institutions within a new cultural world space. But Ken Wilber is also of the opinion that this transformation is attended by greater problems, a huge nightmare may come with it. However, evolution does not mean a final extinction of humanity, though that is a genuine possibility; integration at the vision-logic level is possible as there are signs everywhere that this is taking place. With the emergence of vision-logic, the first stage going beyond rationality [mature Reason], the individual is able to integrate the noosphere with the biosphere and, on the cultural level, integrate culture and nature. Anyway, this higher integrative realm, forming a highly integrative personality, is still in the noosphere and not in the transpersonal domain. Even beyond the stage of vision-logic there are processes taking place which indicate the emerging glimpses of the Over-Soul. At present man is still not able to integrate the ascending and descending paths in the emergent World-Soul, but "the evolutionary understanding of nonduality has already been won by Schelling in the West and Aurobindo in the East ... their paths can be ours, collectively, now ... these roads are open to us, roads present but untravelled."[46] Ken Wilber assumes that an increasing number of individuals intuit the Over-Soul, the spiritual intuition of wholeness, but these individuals translate or interpret that intuition merely in terms of the upper-left quadrant (subjective introspection or "I"), thereby ignoring intersubjective (social service and cultural activities), and objective forms of Spirit (techno-economic infrastructures and social systems).

Others attempt to interpret these experiences merely in terms of the upper-right quadrant (objective observation or "It"), thereby ignoring the subjective interior dimensions of "I" and "we". The latter leaves out inner transformations as an aspect of the manifest All, whereas the former leaves out the objective reality as an aspect of the Selfs manifestation. According to Ken Wilber, "The idea seems to be that if I can just contact my higher Self, then everything else will take care of itself. But this fails miserably to see that Spirit manifests always and simultaneously *as* the four quadrants of the Kosmos."[47]

In the process of the integration of the Big Three—I, it, we—mind, nature, society and culture are taken up and integrated in Spirit, each sees itself not just as individual or collective fragments of the universe, but as vehicles of Spirit. "As Spirit/Consciousness evolves into the transpersonal domain, the Big Three appear as Buddha (the ultimate I), Dharma (the ultimate It), and Sangha (the ultimate We)... At the same time, the timeless and eternal nature of Spirit can nonetheless be intuited in (or through) any of the four quadrants."[48] As the only reality, Spirit must go out of itself in order to create the manifest world. "And so, Spirit knows itself objectively as nature; knows itself subjectively as mind; and knows itself absolutely as Spirit—the Source, the Summit and the Eros of the entire sequence."[49] These three broad movements can also be referred to as subconscious, self-conscious and superconscious, or prepersonal, personal and transpersonal.

Conclusion of Sex, Ecology, Spirituality

In this book, Ken Wilber explores some of the major presentday philosophical, psychological, ecological and spiritual trends. He points out the fractured general tendencies of such trends and articulates an integral worldview. His scholarship (based on the level of vision-logic with a higher order of synthesising capacity) creates a network of relationships and fits these together into a comprehensive whole. The *Kosmos Trilogy* asks the question: "How can we become more fully human and at the same time be saved from the fate of being merely human."[50] Ken Wilber offers the reader a broad orienting map of the place of men and women in relation to the Universe, Life and Spirit.

In Part One, describing the holonic Kosmos and the worldview of universal integralism, Ken Wilber traces evolution historically, from humanoids to postmodernism and psychologically, from pre-egoic levels of consciousness (infancy), through mental-egoic levels (personal) to trans-egoic levels (transpersonal). He opens the first chapter with orienting generalisations and attempts to unite the insights of all the various scientific disciplines into one concept: the hierarchy of holons. Evolution develops in an increasing complexity, differentiation and organisation, and has produced the physiosphere, biosphere and noosphere. The great wisdom traditions assume that human beings have different levels—body, mind and soul—but they don't correlate each of those levels with the four quadrants. Transpersonal studies should embrace and incorporate an all-quadrant view of human consciousness and development, covering all the levels in their behavioural, intentional, cultural and social manifestations. This multidimensional approach integrates consciousness (self), culture (ethics), and nature (environment). For Ken Wilber, individual growth requires the development of transpersonal stages, the realisation of these stages through practice, and the expression of them in all the four quadrants.

In Part Two he explores the complementary movement of the path of descent, the movement in which the One Self becomes the Many and creation becomes an expression of the One. In this major development Ken Wilber moves away from his earlier realisation of Spirit transcendent to Self and world, and he no longer denies earthly realities. Through his newly developed four quadrant model, he aims at a form of spirituality in which ascent and descent are integrated. Both paths are parts of one integral process with two distinct movements; when separated from each other they create a partial worldview. In Part Two, Ken Wilber also explains the concept of 'flatland', which prevents us from seeing the holistic Kosmos, as well as the fatal consequences of dividing the ascending and descending processes, and ways in which the two paths are united in the 'nondual Heart.'

The Eye of Spirit: *An Integral Vision of a World gone Slightly Mad*

In this work Ken Wilber presents his integral spiritual humanism and attempts to apply his integral orientation, inclusive and comprehensive, to the various fields of human knowledge, including the integration of science and spirituality. In a note to the reader Ken Wilber tries to explain the concept of integration and how to integrate the tradition of liberalism with a genuine spirituality. The liberals replace the individual's relationship to the Divine as the ultimate concern in life with the salvation of the individual's economic and political freedom. A spiritual liberalism integrates God and liberalism, a spirituality that rests on a liberal Spirit.

Ken Wilber relates the integral approach to the four quadrant model described in *Sex, Ecology, Spirituality.* Integral studies are related to an "all-level, all-quadrant" view of human consciousness, i.e., it covers not just all the quadrants, but also all the various levels within each quadrant. Ken Wilber explains this entire spectrum of levels in the four domains of human beings, from integral psychology to integral anthropology to integral philosophy to integral art.

He weaves earlier essays—*The Spectrum of Consciousness, Up from Eden, Eye to* Eye—together into new material. In the following chapters he gives commentaries and verifications of his earlier works and responds to the various criticisms he has received about his work in general and *Sex, Ecology, Spirituality* in particular.

In these chapters he outlines the major 'phases' of his works as Wilber—I, Wilber—II Wilber—III, and Wilber—IV.

In Wilber-I, *The Spectrum of Consciousness,* he fiercely expounds the Romantic viewpoints and refers to this early model as the "Romantic/Jungian/Wilber I" model. In this model the primal ground or perfect wholeness is present in the infantile pre-egoic structure, though in an unconscious form, i.e., the pre-egoic state is one with Ground but in an unconscious fashion. The self is totally one with the Ground in the pre-egoic and the transegoic stage, but the former union is unconscious and the latter is conscious. An infantile regression in the service of the ego, prior to transcendence of the ego, is the essential doorway to recontact the primal Ground. However, Atman is not lost in early evolution but in prior involution, and the Romantics, lacking a genuine understanding of involution, elevated prerational infantilism to transpersonal insight.

Wilber-II refers to the involution/evolution model of Sri Aurobindo and Plotinus. In *The Atman Project* and its sister volume, *Up from Eden,* Ken Wilber explores an integral psychology in which he unites East and West, from Buddha to Freud, and claims that "In the almost two decades since writing *Atman,* I have found its basic framework to be as sturdy and solid as ever."[51] Before they were published in book form both books were initially a validation of the Romantic version, but Ken Wilber discovered that this Romantic view was limited and he reworked the earlier drafts of both books. Human development does not proceed from unconscious Heaven (pre-egoic) to Conscious Hell (egoic), to conscious Heaven (transegoic), because the loss of consciousness with the Divine Ground, the loss of the unconscious Union, means that the individual world ceases to exist. The real course of manifest human development is from unconscious Hell to conscious Hell to conscious Heaven. The Romantics confuse pre with trans and elevate the prestates to the exaltation of the trans-states; the infantile state is basically prepersonal rather than the unconscious transpersonal. The loss of oneness from Spirit is called involution, the movement whereby Spirit unconsciously involves itself in the lower forms of its own manifestation. At each stage of involution, Spirit returning to itself, the individual remembers that he or she was once consciously united with the Divine itself. Infantile regression, as the core to the transpersonal domain, might occur only "if necessitated by a recontacting of Ground-as-prana or some earlier-fulcrum lost potentials, dissociations, pathologies, and so on (a regression in service of ego, prior to transcendence of ego)."[52] These developmental malformations at any of the self-fulcrums block subsequent higher development. Regression and recontacting of the infantile state is not a necessary prerequisite for higher spiritual development.

In *Up from Eden: a transpersonal view of human evolution*, he explores the idea that evolution itself is a spiritual unfolding, like Sri Aurobindo's vision. But unlike Sri Aurobindo, Ken Wilber claims to have combined that philosophical idea with anthropological data based on extensive empirical and anthropological evidence. However, this claim appears contradictory. In *The Eye of Spirit* Ken Wilber proclaims that "none of them [Teilhard de Chardin, Aurobindo and Hegel] had combined that philosophical notion with an actual hard look at anthropological data, and none of them had advanced any of the specific stages of this evolution based on any sort of extensive empirical and anthropological evidence. In this regard *Eden* was, I believe, a major advance."[53] But it seems rather strange to this author that Ken Wilber previously wrote in *Up from Eden*, "Aurobindo, of course, is one of the few geniuses and full mystics (East or West) who also had the opportunity and willingness to study the anthropological and paleontological records compiled so carefully by modem science, and he found those records to be not only compatible with his view but supportive of it."[54]

Cultural developmental stages accompany the evolution of cultural worldviews; what appears in individuals as a spectrum of consciousness (upper-left quadrant) appears in cultures as a spectrum of worldviews (lower-left quadrant). Ken Wilber assumes a correlation between the ontogenetic (history of the individual development of an organised being) and phylogenetic (history of the descent of families) formation of the human species. Ken Wilber alleges that he bridged the cross between the strength of Sri Aurobindo, Gebser and Habermas; Cultural evolution, in a sophisticated form, can be embraced as an explanatory principle in human history.

So we see that Wilber-II is more based on the ladder model in which spirituality develops gradually, step by step; the full process of human development can be seen as a spiritual process in which consciousness becomes clearer and enlarges until it unites with the spiritual level. In Wilber-I, the ego is seen as an 'enemy' of spiritual development but in Wilber- II the ego is no longer an obstacle but a stepping stone in the direction of spiritual development. Wilber-II replaces his old extrovert model of the Spectrum of consciousness by his new introvert model. The process of development indicates a progressive deepening and heightening of consciousness.

In Wilber-III, Ken Wilber realises that development is more complicated than he initially assumed and therefore he puts aside his homogeneous development (Wilber-II).

In *Eye to Eye,* Ken Wilber explores the full-spectrum approach to human consciousness and behaviour from a spectrum of the three valid modes of knowing; each of which discloses a different type of world; the world of sensibilia, intelligibilia, and transcendelia. To understand the Kosmos implies the inclusion of all three types of knowing. The nature of the Absolute can be disclosed only with the eye of contemplation and not with the eye of the flesh or the eye of the mind. Ken Wilber argues that metaphysics can be done only with the eye of contemplation. To be genuine, all future metaphysics must offer in addition to the sensory and mental experience, direct experiential data of the spiritual domain itself, through spiritual practice. These three strands of knowing are applicable to all levels in each quadrant, and with this integral vision science or nature touches the "it" of Spirit, consciousness or self touches the "I" of Spirit, and culture or ethics the "we" of Spirit.

In *Transformations of Consciousness* Ken Wilber adds a further differentiation of the various developmental levels to his model. He divides human consciousness—the upper left quadrant—into three main components: enduring-basic structures, temporary transition structures and the self or self-system. The self as a mediator between the basic and transitional structures has at each higher stage free access to the previous basic structures but not to the previous transitional structures.

A fulcrum of self-development, the stepping up of the self into a new level of consciousness, goes through the triple process of fusion, transcendence and integration. If a fulcrum gets disturbed it generates a specific level of psychopathology. The self, when identified with a basic structure, generates various transitional stages. These transitional structures, which include worldviews, are not integrated in the higher levels but are replaced. The exclusive identity with the lower level is dissolved, but the capacities of that lower structure are integrated into the higher structure. Though the development of basic structures is linear in which the lower cannot be bypassed, yet the self-sense can go sideways, regress or jump ahead, i.e., the self can be all over the developmental structures and is therefore not linear.

In his earlier works, Ken Wilber assumed that the individual has to negotiate all the lower levels first before spiritual stages can unfold, i.e., the lower stages cannot be bypassed. This does not mean that the individual can have spiritual experiences at any level or stage of growth, but the individual still has to grow to the point that he can integrate the depth of the spiritual experience, i.e., to actually live from those higher levels rather than temporarily having access to some of these higher levels of consciousness. "Spiritual experiences do not allow you to simply bypass the growth and development upon which enduring spiritual realization itself depends. Evolution can be accelerated, as Aurobindo said, but not fundamentally skipped over."[55]

Ken Wilber endeavours to refine this formulation by using his new Wilber-III model of enduring structures, developmental transitional lines and the self-sense which generates a transition structure, but is not a transition structure itself. Ken Wilber abandons his unilinear development and differentiates the self-sense from the lines of development which occur alongside each other and pass through the various stages. In his own words; "Ken Wilber- III explicitly distinguishes *the different developmental lines that unfold through those seventeen levels.* These different developmental lines include affective, cognitive, moral, interpersonal, object-relations, self-identity, and so on, *each of which develops in a quasi-independent fashion through the general levels or basic structures of consciousness.*"[56]

The various developmental lines involving both enduring and transitional structures often stand in a relation of "necessary but not sufficient", which means that "ethical development cannot race ahead of interpersonal development, which cannot race ahead of cognitive development, which itself rests on certain physiological maturational schedules (all juggled, of course, by the self)."[57]

The relatively independent lines of development are held together by the self-system. When the basic structure of awareness unfolds, the self-system may not be willing to follow the unfolding and remains on the lower level. In such cases the individual may have an increased spiritual development but he or she is not able to adapt or live authentically from that higher awareness unless the temporary higher *states* of consciousness are converted into enduring *levels* of consciousness through sustained practice.

Psychological and Spiritual Development

Ken Wilber meaningfully describes the different uses of the word "spiritual" in terms of lines or streams, and levels or waves, although he acknowledges that there are many more definitions of 'spirituality'.

According to Ken Wilber's interpretation of the word spiritual, spiritual development when defined as a separate developmental line with its own unfolding runs parallel with psychological development, whereas when defined as the highest reaches of all those lines (levels), its development occurs after psychological development is completed. Ken Wilber believes that both interpretations are acceptable, and spirituality does not exist only in the higher levels though he often refers to these higher domains as 'spiritual'.

In the development of the spectrum of consciousness, the nine or ten basic levels of consciousness represent the universal waves of developmental unfolding (the stage-like sequence common to all streams) through which the various developmental lines proceed, in other words, the different streams that move through those waves: the self or self system attempts to balance all the different streams with their waves of development.

Spiritual Level and Spiritual Line

In the first use of the term 'spiritual' as the highest wave of any stream, spiritual development cannot emerge stable unless the lower basic enduring structures or waves have been sufficiently secured. In this model spirituality exists only in the higher domains and can develop only after the lower domains are transcended. It needs a strong solidified ego before transcendence of the ego can take place. In the second use of the term 'spiritual' as a separate stream, its development can occur alongside the development of other transitional lines.

Most of the arguments about the relation of psychology and spirituality are due to the confusion of level or enduring wave with line or transitional stream. Nevertheless, Ken Wilber maintains that whether spirituality is seen as the highest wave or as a separate stream, the spiritual line itself still depends upon the movement from its prepersonal wave to its personal wave to its transpersonal wave, i.e., the spiritual stream runs through or moves from these three waves in a successive order to establish a stable adaptation rather than a temporary state.

Thus even if spirituality is viewed as a separate line, "it does show, on the long haul, a general unfolding through the expanding waves of consciousness [subconscious to conscious to superconscious waves], with developments in the spiritual stream depending upon previously established competences in that stream itself."[58] To express this complicated subject more simplistically, the higher stages of spiritual development must pass through the gateway of the integrative vision-logic level.

A global spirituality needs the deep integrative capacities of vision-logic, even though it seems that individual spiritual development can take place without this integral vision-logic level because it is a seemingly independent line of development.

When Sri Aurobindo's developmental model is viewed in terms of *waves*, then spiritual progress obeys "the logic of successive unfolding"; spiritual development proceeds when previous developments have been sufficiently conquered. In Ken Wilber's words, "Aurobindo's point is that meditation (or spiritual practice in general) can accelerate but not alter the form or sequence—of this developmental unfolding. As profound as Aurobindo's point is, let us refine it."[59]

Ken Wilber believes that both views are true on the condition that the terms spirituality and psychology are clearly specified. When psychology is classified as "mental and personal" and spirituality as "transpersonal" (the higher levels of the lines) then spiritual development can only proceed after psychological development has been secured. This is also Sri Aurobindo's view of successive unfolding in a linear manner. But this approach misses those different quasi-independent lines of development. These various developmental lines, psychological as well as spiritual, run parallel and do not unfold after each other in a linear way. Ken Wilber then treats Sri Aurobindo's surface, inner and higher development as three broadly distinct *lines;* each can develop quasi-independently. For Ken Wilber "this means that individuals (ontogenetically and phylogenetically) might make strides in psychic/ subtle development while still being relatively undeveloped in frontal structures (ego, rationality, conventional verbal, etc). This further points up why I believe these various streams are not stacked linearly on top of each other—and further, why progress in some lines might run ahead, or lag behind, others."[60] But as mentioned above, even if spirituality is defined as its own separate line these individual lines themselves do unfold in a linear sequence, as those lines rely upon the competences of the earlier structures and thus run from prepersonal to personal to transpersonal levels.

Wilber-IV, as represented in *Sex, Ecology, Spirituality,* A *Brief History of Everything* and *The Eye of Spirit,* relates the spectrum model to science, culture and society. The Wilber-III aspects are practically unchanged, but set in an 'all-quadrant, all-level' context. The individual subjective domain—consciousness, personality but also psychopathology—is always already embedded in objective, intersubjective and inter objective realities. The subjective domain is distributed across all quadrants with all their levels and lines. In the Wilber-IV model, the methodology of an integral approach to consciousness involves: (1) the three strands operative in all valid knowledge (injunction, apprehension, confirmation); (2) the four validity claims through which the three strands operate: propositional truth [upper-right], subjective truthfulness [upper-left], cultural meaning [lower-left], and functional fit [lower-right]; (3) the nine levels of development in each quadrant.

In Ken Wilber's previous works, he mainly described subjective individual development, but Wilber-IV describes not only the nine stages of development from Wilber-III, but they are now placed in the context of the other three quadrants, which causes a complex whole of thirty-six 'cells'. With the help of this model one can specify more clearly all the various forms of interaction between the four quadrants. Each quadrant does influence the other quadrants, but the attempt to reduce one of these quadrants to the other three quadrants Ken Wilber classifies as a form of reductionism. For him, all four quadrants are necessary for an integral theory of consciousness.

To recapitulate, Ken Wilber divides his body of work into four main periods: Wilber-I, the Romantic period, which is characterised by the pre/trans fallacy, confusing divine egoism with divine liberation; Wilber-II, the evolutionary and developmental period which replaced a 'recaptured goodness' model with a 'growth to goodness' view; Wilber-III subdivided development into levels and lines or 'waves' and 'streams'; development is not a ladder-like process but consists of numerous independent lines progressing through the levels; Wilber-IV sets development in the context of the 'four quadrants' model. Each period incorporates its predecessors, except Wilber-I, which has "some very good and some very confused ideas". *The Eye of Spirit* concludes with the transpersonal stages of consciousness.

Spirit

For Ken Wilber Spirit has two paradoxical aspects:

Spirit as the summit of being; as the highest level and goal of evolution (ascent or the transcendental nature of Spirit) and also as the essence of each and everything that exists, the Ground of the entire sequence (the immanent nature of Spirit).

Ken Wilber's nondualistic approach unites and integrates both aspects of Spirit. Spirit has evolved the instrument for its own self-realisation, and because of Spirit's involvement with this world, this world evolves with Spirit. But although Spirit occurs in the world of time, space and form, it is primordial, timeless and formless, and a certain amount of evolution is required to get in touch with this timeless/ formless Spirit, one's true Self. There is only Spirit, the each and the all are perfect manifestations of Spirit, and the separate self is in search of Spirit. Though Spirit is fully present at every moment, it is not yet realised. Spiritual practice does not aim at changing the state of consciousness, but directs the seeker into a stateless condition. In this ground of ever-present changeless awareness, the seeker sees the world with the eye of Spirit. When the separate selfsense has been annihilated, one will exist as a vehicle of Spirit.

The question immediately arises: does the ego exist in the higher stages of development? Ken Wilber consistently maintains two positions about this question. In the process of evolution, the ego's task will be diminished and finally abandoned to allow a place for superconsciousness. But transcendence of the ego does not mean a mere deformation or annihilation of the ego, "one still possesses an ego—it's just that one's identity is no longer exclusively bound to it."[61]

The existence of the egoic structure itself does not constitute our prison; it is only our exclusive identification with that structure which imprisons us. In the transegoic stage the ego is both negated and preserved. The ego is annihilated in the higher levels, when ego is referred to as an exclusive sense of identity with the individual body and mind. But the ego is maintained in the higher level when ego is referred to as that aspect of self-awareness or competency which deals with the gross conventional world. This means that one still possesses an ego in the higher levels but one's identity is no longer exclusively bound to it.

The Marriage of Sense and Soul: *Integrating Science and Religion*

In *The Marriage of Sense and Soul,* Ken Wilber uses his integral approach ('the all-level, all-quadrant' model) to integrate science and religion. Science, with its experimental and empirical method based on evidence, aims at the discovery of truth, but its truth is objective and does not offer meaning, value and depth. It is religion which offers the individual a fulfilling meaning to life, a wisdom which facts alone can never reveal. He relates religion to the common core of the world's great wisdom traditions, i.e., the Great Chain of Being, the interwoven levels of matter, body, mind, soul and spirit. Each level of reality has a specific branch of knowledge associated with it, for example, physics studies matter and mysticism studies the experience of Spirit.

Modernity in its process of differentiating art, morals and monological science went too far in its differentiating process, and ended up in dissociation, fragmentation and repression. Empirical science reduced the Great Chain of Being to systems of matter alone, and denied any real existence to art and morals. In the reconciliation of science and religion, Ken Wilber maintains that this integration is only possible in terms that are acceptable to both forces.

According to Ken Wilber, "In order to integrate religion and science, we need to integrate the Great Chain with the differentiation of modernity...this means that each of the levels in the traditional Great Chain needs to be carefully differentiated in the light of modernity."[62] In this integration, each of the levels, sensory, mental and spiritual is also divided according to the differentiation of modernity—art (I), morals (we) and science (it)—so you get the art, morals and science of the sensory realm, of the mental realm and of the spiritual realm.

Modernity discovered that the mind is not separated from the biomaterial brain, and transcendental events in consciousness have specific correlates in the brain. But the worldview of modernity reduced all interior dimensions of the 'I' and the 'we' to the exterior objective 'its' surfaces, thereby rejecting the Great Chain of Being. It used only the eye of the flesh to account for primary sensory reality without using the eye of mind and the eye of contemplation; the transcendental mind, measured by the eye of flesh, is reduced to a mere function of the organic body. In order to integrate science and religion a way has to be found in which the claims of the empirical as well as those of the transcendental realm are true.

Early postmodernism, in the forms of Romanticism and Idealism, revolted against the modernists' dissociations in its arguments for higher modes of knowledge, but their revolt failed due to the continuing denial of the interior domains by the scientific materialists. Later on, postmodern structuralism tried to unseat science itself and focused on the intrinsic role of interpretation in human understanding; there are no longer exterior surfaces which are related to objective truth but only interior depth processes, which are related to introspection and interpretation, and which can be seen by the eye of mind only. However, the emphasis on these issues was taken out of proportion and resulted in a denial of the reality of objective facts altogether.

The Poststructuralists, like the Idealists and Romantics, ended up with the dominance of the systems science, which denied any substantial reality of the I' and 'we' domains. Later, postmodernism, with all its extreme emphasis on interpretation and interior validation, became a new form of reason, but within a holistic chain of the exterior domains only, without genuine interior depth.

A true integration of science and religion includes the integration of art, morals and science; likewise, spirituality, by finding its own data and evidence with the eye of contemplation, must integrate the value spheres of the I, 'we' and 'it' domains.

According to Ken Wilber, "our task is not specifically to reintroduce spirituality and somehow attempt to show that modem science is becoming compatible with God.... Rather, it is the rehabilitation of the *interior in general* that opens the possibility of reconciling science and religion... Not Spirit, but *the within*, is the corpse we must first revive."[63]

Science, using the three essential aspects of the empirical method—injunction (the actual practice), apprehension (the domain brought forth by the injunction, i.e., the direct experience of data), and confirmation/rejection—is not wrong but partial. Science has to acknowledge the existence of subjective and intersubjective realms which are also responsible for generating knowledge. Although the existence of these interior domains cannot be investigated by empirical sensory science, these domains need not be denied and can be investigated in their own right. Science as genuine knowledge need not be restricted to sensory experience only ('narrow science'), but may also include a science of mental and spiritual experience ('broad science'). "Experiential evidence in each of these modes is actually quite public and shared, because each of them can be trained or educated with the help of a teacher."[64]

The three basic strands of knowing need not be used only in the narrow empiricism of sensory experience, but can also be used in the sensitive world of the deep structures of the interior realm—mental and spiritual experience.

Religion must also open its mythological truths and claims to direct verification/rejection by experiential data and evidence (direct spiritual experience). Applying the test of the three strands of valid knowledge allows a verifiable, repeatable injunction to generate the spiritual domain. Authentic spirituality is not based on sensory or mental experiences, but on direct spiritual transcendental or mystic experiences, data seen by the eye of contemplation; with the eye of contemplation Spirit or God can be seen. When the three strands of knowledge lose their grip on religion as a science of spiritual experience, then religion deteriorates to the eye of mind and becomes a set of dogmas and mental beliefs.

In order to gain access to the valid modes of knowing in the contemplative realm, the individual needs to engage the injunctive strands, i.e., perform the experiment through the practice of meditation or contemplation and verify the interior spiritual data with an experimental community of like-minded members.

As mentioned before, broad science applies the three strands of valid knowing not only to sensory experiences but also to mental and spiritual experiences; it assumes that the interiors of the 'I' and 'we' can be experientially explored by using the same three strands of valid knowing. This implies that broad science is applicable in all four quadrants representing intentional, behavioural, cultural and social aspects. Each of these aspects has correlates with all the others. The 'I' and 'we' need not be reduced to 'its, but are put on even terms with it, because the 'I', 'we' and 'it' can be equally accessed by using the three strands of broad science. According to Ken Wilber, "the four quadrants (or simply the Big Three) can thus be genuinely united, joined and integrated under the auspices of a deep science that is as operative in profound mystical experience as in geology, as applicable to moral aspirations as to biology—each domain, just as it is, is allowed its own form and structure and content—yet each is joined and united by the thread of direct experience and evidence."[65]

The method of the three strands of deep science is capable of integrating all four quadrants, even though each quadrant has its own validity or type of truth. When broad science is applied to the exterior upper-right quadrant, it generates objective truth (physics, neurology, behaviourism), to the interior upper-left quadrant, it generates subjective truth (introspective and depth psychology, art and aesthetics), to the lower-right quadrant, it generates inter objective truth (social systems science), and to the lower-left quadrant, it generates intersubjective truth (cultural sciences).

Ken Wilber maintains that although the Great Chain of Being claims to cover the whole of reality, it only covers the interior dimension of the individual. Because the Great Chain left out the other three dimensions of reality it could not catch up with the discoveries of science, cultural worldviews and social conditions, which are all interrelated with the interior upper-left hand quadrant. Sensory empirical science, as the exterior of Spirit, cannot see into the higher, interior domains of their own terms, but it can register their empirical correlates, because all interior events have exterior correlates. This provides a union of the transcendental and the empirical realm, as the higher level is not above but within the objective. Transpersonal research on the higher stages of individual growth must correlate its data with the corresponding changes in the other quadrants.

For Ken Wilber the four horizontal quadrants are present in each vertical level of the Great Chain of Being—body, mind, soul and Spirit. An integration of science and religion needs the integration of the Great Chain of Being with all the four quadrants. In this way, Ken Wilber's integral view, a harmonization of all levels with all quadrants, explores the various phenomena in each of the four quadrants and the correlation of each with the others.

In *The Marriage of Sense and Soul,* Ken Wilber elaborates on the co-relation and interaction of the inner worlds (soul) and the outer world (sense). He aims at a rehabilitation of the interior in general, which opens the possibility of reconciling science and religion.

One Taste: *The Journals of Ken Wilber*

In *One Taste,* Ken Wilber gives the reader a personal journal of his meditative practice and various mystical states based on his own experience. However, "these journals were not primarily meant to be a record of the details of my personal life, but rather a record of further attempts to convey the perennial philosophy."[66] The theme of the journal is based on the mutually inclusiveness of body, mind and soul, they are all "perfect expressions of the radiant Spirit that alone inhabits the universe ... There is only One Taste in the entire Kosmos, and that taste is Divine, whether it appears in the flesh, in the mind, in the soul."[67] In Ken Wilber's *Atman Project,* Consciousness, as a complete transcendence and release into Formless Consciousness, is a state of ultimate Unity. According to Ken Wilber; "Consciousness henceforth *operates* not on the world, but only as the entire World Process, integrating and interpenetrating all levels, realms and planes, high or low, sacred or profane."[68]. The dynamic aspect of God as a personal source of consciousness is dissolved into a static Formless impersonal consciousness.

Self-manifestation as a motivation for Atman's creation in the cosmic becoming is according to Sri Aurobindo not a sufficient motivation for Brahman/Atman to subject itself to the existence of human or worldly suffering. Atman does not undertake the cosmic process merely for the sake of returning from the human consciousness to Atman consciousness, its native state. Evolution does not take place only because of the latent principles and its urge to emerge, but also for a constant novelty of self-expression and self-finding, the ascension of a new humanity—in other words, a different and new evolutionary principle which creates a new evolutionary species. For Sri Aurobindo, evolution is not merely a process of awakening to Atman and overcoming the drama of self-suffering, but the realisation of a divine Life in a Gnostic society.

In *Transformations of Consciousness,* Ken Wilber still overlooks Sri Aurobindo's dynamic aspect of a bi-polar dimension in which there exists an interplay between Matter and Spirit. Sri Aurobindo does not want the sadhak (the spiritual practitioner of integral yoga) to escape into some formless Absolute. To the transcendent orientation or insight, he adds the universal and individual Divine, i.e., to bring the transcendental height into matter. Ken Wilber refers to the Formless source of the ascending arc of realisation as the "one constant" in the evolutionary equation and he emphasises the constant of the Formless source. However, this only amounts to a static realisation and he overlooks the dynamic aspects of the spiritual realisation.

Ken Wilber modifies his ideas about self-realisation in his first volume of the Kosmic Trilogy. On the subtle level, a unification takes place between the soul and God, whereas on the causal level, God and Soul are transcended in a pure Formless awareness. This pure formless Spirit, the goal and source of all manifestation, is experienced as the Godhead within. The realisation of this *Jivanmukta,* the state of freedom from duality, though the *summum bonum* of life, is not the end. To the state of Absolute unmanifest Formless Spirit, Ken Wilber adds the Absolute manifest world of Forms, as a perfect expression of Spirit. The unmanifest Formless and the world of manifest Form are experienced as a nondual consciousness. Ken Wilber's ultimate realisation is no longer a formless nondual experience in and on its own, but the realisation takes place only through the world of form which functions as the Source of the eternal search.

The manifest All as the Godhead evolves as All-Form, and the pure unmanifest does not evolve or involve but is the Source of all other levels and their ultimate Good. The Godhead is fully present in any manifest or unmanifest state, in the lower as well as the higher levels. However, there still seems to be a separation between the two, the Kosmos never finds the cosmos, "and since it will never find it [the Formless and the world of Form] it will never cease the search."[69]

In describing the formless Witness as 'One Taste' Ken Wilber refers to Ramana Maharshi's deep witnessing process of the I-I. In this pure Formless state there is only the pure nondual Consciousness, One Taste, one's true identity. According to Ken Wilber, "Once you find your formless identity as Buddha-mind, as Atman, as pure Spirit or Godhead, you will take that constant, nondual, ever-present consciousness and re-enter the lesser states, subtle mind and gross body, and reanimate them with radiance."[70] The lower realms with all their pain and suffering lose their primary importance and become vehicles of the Spirit. In the experience of One Taste "every single thing and event in the Kosmos, high or low, sacred or profane, has the same taste, the same flavor, and the flavor is Divine. All are gestures of God, which is to say, gestures of your own primordial Perfection, manifestations of your own radiant Emptiness, waves of your own nondual Consciousness."[71] This One Taste, which transcends and includes all possible states, is not a Witness but radical Spirit itself which is unqualifiable. In this pure Emptiness, though empty of any quality, the entire world of form is arising, described by Ken Wilber as, "Emptiness and Form are not-two. They are both One Taste in this moment. Emptiness and Consciousness are just two names for the same reality."[72]

One Taste, as the pure nondual Consciousness, represents a union of the One and Many, Emptiness and Form, i.e., the entire world of Form exists in the present

Formless awareness. By getting in touch with the formless Witness, the unqualified Godhead, the individual becomes one with the entire world of Form. It is interesting to read Ken Wilber's own experience of One Taste, "based on my own experience, I can testify to the existence of constant consciousness [in all the three states of waking, dreaming and deep dreamless sleep] and One Taste, both of them as prolonged and recurrent plateau experiences, sometimes lasting uninterruptedly 24 - 36 hours (although, in one case, constant consciousness persisted day and night for eleven days)."[73] If constant consciousness would not be noticed during the night Ken Wilber would take up several meditative or contemplative practices when he returned to the waking gross realm.

Ken Wilber describes One Taste not only in terms of Consciousness but also as a feeling of Being or feeling of existence. "The simple Feeling of Being is not an experience— it is a vast Openness in which all experiences come and go... The simple Feeling of Being, which is the simple feeling of existence, is the simple Feeling of One Taste."[74] In describing the feeling aspect of One Taste, Ken Wilber writes, "And once you taste One Taste, no matter how fleetingly at first, an entirely new motivation will arise from the depths of your very own being and become a constant atmosphere which your every impulse breathes, and that atmosphere is compassion. Once you taste One Taste, and see the fundamental problems of existence evaporate in the blazing sun of obviousness, you will never again be the same person, deep within your heart. And you will want—finally, profoundly, and most of all—that others, too, may be relieved of the burden of their sleep-walking dreams, relieved of the agony of the separate self, relieved of the inherent torture called time and the gruesome tragedy called space... Because of compassion, you will strive harder. Because of compassion, you will get straight. Because of compassion, you will work your fingers to the bone, push at the world until you literally bleed, toil till the tears stain your vision, struggle until life itself runs dry. And in the deepest, deepest center of your Heart, the World is already thanking you."[75]

In *One Taste* Ken Wilber also describes his integral approach to spirituality. For Ken Wilber religion serves not only to create meaning for the self which he relates to horizontal movement or translation, but religion also serves as a function for transcending the self, a type of vertical movement or a radical transformation. In the translative function, the self is given a new approach (in thought or feeling) to reality and the self learns to translate its world and its being in terms of the new approach. With transformation, the self itself is analysed, and the world is not only translated but transformed. Both functions are important and indispensable for spiritual development. Translation itself has an important and necessary function to fulfil in one's life, as without this function the seeker is bound to get lost in the process of *maya,* the illusion of the world. However, translation alone is not enough; later on in the maturation process this translative function, with its new approach, ceases to console and needs to be replaced by the transformative function with the transcendence of the self.

Ken Wilber also describes the translative function of religion in terms of legitimacy and the transformative function of religion in terms of authenticity. In the words of Ken Wilber, "This function of religion to provide a legitimacy for the self and its beliefs—no matter how temporary, relative, nontransformative, or illusory—has nonetheless been the single greatest and most important function of the world's religious traditions. The capacity of a religion to provide horizontal meaning, legitimacy, and sanction for the self and its beliefs—*that function of religion has historically been the single greatest 'social glue' that any culture has...* Where translative religion offers *legitimacy,* transformative religion offers *authenticity*. For those few individuals who are ready—that is, sick with the suffering of the separate self, and no longer able to embrace the legitimate worldview—then a transformative opening to true authenticity, true enlightenment, true liberation, calls more and more insistently... Transformative spirituality... settles instead into a glance that sees only a radiant infinity in the heart of all souls... It does not legitimate the world, it breaks the world; it does not console the world, it shatters it. And it does not render the self content, it renders it undone."[76]

An integral approach to spirituality combines the best of the translative and transformative functions of religion. Ken Wilber's evolutionary spirituality integrates liberal humanistic values with a transrational Spirit, i.e., "the joining of the Enlightenment of the West (or political freedom) with the Enlightenment of the East (or spiritual freedom)."[77]

Integral Psychology: *Consciousness, Spirit, Psychology, Therapy*

As Ken Wilber states, "My aim in this book, while focusing specifically on integral psychology, has also been an integral approach in general, attempting to take, not just the best of today's schools, but the best of premodern, modern, and postmodern insights, while jettisoning their extremist distortions. Obviously this type of approach can only begin with the most general of generalizations—outrageous generalizations, some would say—but if we are to start on this endeavor, we must start somewhere, and this type of approach is, I suppose, as good as any. But the major aim of this book is to act as just that: a beginning, not an end; the start of a discussion, not the finish."[78]

For Ken Wilber psychology studies human consciousness and its manifestations in behaviour. He meaningfully distinguishes the functions, structures, states, modes, development and behavioural aspects of consciousness. Different schools of psychology take one of these aspects as their subject matter, as if that aspect was the only aspect worth studying, but an integral psychology embraces every aspect of human consciousness.

While discussing each of these aspects, he describes in detail the difference between the basic levels, developmental lines and the self. The basic levels of existence—as levels of being and knowing—range from matter to spirit and infinitely shade into each other. As the highest level and the ground of all levels, Spirit is not the mere product of metaphysical speculation, but a direct experiential reality.

Structures, as levels of consciousness which can be either enduring (found in the basic level and remaining in existence) or transitional (found in the various developmental lines and tending to be replaced by subsequent stages), are stable patterns. A state is related to either natural states of consciousness such as the gross, subtle and causal, or altered states of consciousness. The natural states of consciousness are usually temporary states, but can become enduring structures when their potentials move from passing states to enduring states in the individual's development.

Having been accused of completely ignoring planes of existence, and referring to the levels of consciousness as the basic structure of knowing only in terms of epistemological components, Ken Wilber now explicitly includes the ontological aspects, the basic structures of being as planes or realms of existence. When basic levels refer to the subject, one speaks of levels of consciousness, and when these levels refer to objects one speaks of levels of reality. The basic levels are simultaneously levels of both knowing and being, and they are inextricably interwoven. Although they are both independent variables, they are also correlative structures, two sides of the same level, and Ken Wilber includes both of them in the basic structures or levels of the Great Chain of Being.

Lines of Development

As explained already in his previous works, through the basic levels flow about two dozen relatively independent developmental lines like the moral, interpersonal, cognitive, affective, ego, and spiritual lines, which mostly proceed from body (preconventional) to mind (conventional and postconventional) to spirit (post-postconventional), i.e., a largely universal, holarchical sequence.

Ken Wilber differentiates the actual levels—body, mind, subtle, causal and nondual, and the self at those levels— body-ego, ego, soul and self. In a similar way, although they have their root dispositions in specific realms, the ego, soul and self also have their own lines of development which can coexist together or develop in an uneven sequence.

The self includes the observing self (the "I" or proximate self), the observed self (the "me" or distal self) and the transcendental Self (the ultimate Witness); together they make up the overall self.

It is the proximate self which grows through a stage-like development by first identifying itself with a new level, then disidentifying and transcending it, and finally integrating it in order to move to the next higher level, but the overall self, containing different lines, does not follow a sequential development.

However, the proximate self as a developmental line also has constant functions, such as identification, will, defences, navigation, intersubjectivity, aesthetic apprehension, cognition, integration, etc. This functional self also undergoes its own development and is absolutely crucial in integral psychology.

In all, it can be said that for Ken Wilber an integral view of the major components of the evolution of consciousness are: "*the basic levels,* structures, or waves in the Great Nest (matter, body, mind, soul, spirit); *the developmental lines* or streams, (moral, aesthetic, religious, cognitive, affective, etc.) that move relatively independently through the great waves; *the states,* or temporary states of consciousness (such as peak experiences, dream states, and altered states); *the self,* which is the seat of identity, will, and defenses, and which has to navigate, balance, and integrate all the various levels, lines, and states that it encounters; and *the self-related lines,* which are the developmental lines most intimately connected with the self (such as the self's central identity, its morals, and its needs). In short: waves, streams, states, self, and self-streams."[79]

Ken Wilber's multidimensional developmental model sets all of these variables in the context of the four quadrants model.

The Integral Approach

Ken Wilber's integral approach investigates all the levels and lines in all of the quadrants. Exterior states are correlated to interior states, i.e., interior domains of intersubjective levels, lines and states have objective correlates which can be approached in scientific language, though they cannot be reduced to those correlates. Any state or level of consciousness can be investigated by adopting an "all-quadrant, all-level" approach.

States or levels of consciousness are profoundly moulded by objective facts (modern scientific discoveries), cultural backgrounds (intersubjective dimension, including ethics, values and collective worldviews) and social structures (interobjective dimension, including techno-economic production, social systems and social institutions). Consciousness is therefore not only a transcendental noumenon but deeply embedded in the context of and influenced by the four quadrants.

Integral Psychology

Ken Wilber's integral psychology attempts to include the best of modern research in the field of psychology, consciousness and therapy in the context of the truth of body, mind, soul and spirit without merely reducing them to empirical processes or objective systems. He suggests that a truly integral psychology "would involve the very best of premodemity (the Great Nest), modernity (the differentiation of the value spheres), and postmodemity (their integration across all levels in the Great Nest)—all-level, all-quadrant."[80]

An integral psychology involves levels, lines, states, ego, soul and spirit. The gross, subtle and causal lines and selves can exist alongside each other and develop independently; however, an enduring overall integral development includes a movement through the various levels in which none of the major levels of consciousness, frontal, intermediate, subtle and causal, can be bypassed.

Integral psychology honours the entire spectrum of consciousness, matter, body, mind, soul and spirit, in all the levels which modern research can confirm. According to Ken Wilber, "the job of an integral psychology (as a subset of integral studies) *is to coordinate and integrate the research findings in all the levels in all of the quadrants.* Integral psychology obviously focuses on the Upper-Left quadrant, but the whole point of the integral approach is that for a full understanding of this quadrant, it needs to be seen in the context of all the others."[81]

An integral psychology not only differentiates and integrates all four quadrants—organism, environment, consciousness and culture, but also the levels of consciousness unfolding themselves in all four quadrants. In the words of Ken Wilber, "For an integral psychology the basic levels of consciousness available to men and women need to be carefully differentiated into their various developmental lines. Through the levels or waves of the Great Nest (body, mind, soul, spirit) run numerous different developmental lines or streams (cognitive, moral, aesthetic, affective, needs, identities, perspectives, etc.). *It is the job of an integral psychology to track all of these various waves and streams as they unfold in any given individual.*"[82]

The all-level, all-quadrant model in integral psychology embraces the interrelatedness of all the four quadrants and investigates the developments of all the levels and lines in all of the quadrants. As described by Ken Wilber, "The integral psychology that I am presenting argues for an integrated approach to development in all of those quadrants —more precisely, an "all-level, all-quadrant" approach: following all of the levels and lines in all of the quadrants. This means following both the growth *in* each quadrant, and the growth in the capacity *of* the subject to grasp each quadrant (i.e., the growth in the subject's capacity to grasp its own subjective quadrant and the other quadrants as well). This means following the self's growth *in relation* to three environments or three worlds (the Big Three), namely, its relation to its own *subjective* world of inner drives, ideals, self-concepts, aesthetics, states of consciousness, etc.; its relation to the *intersubjective* world of symbolic interaction, dialectical discourse, mutual understanding, normative structures, etc.; and its relation to the *objective* world of material objects, states of affairs, scientific systems, cognitive objects, etc."[83]

A truly integral psychology needs to confront the rupture between the spiritual and material realms, and a constructive postmodern approach to an integral psychology embraces the insights of spiritual premodernity and scientific modernity without ignoring the weaknesses of either.

Pathology usually occurs as the self, on its way to a new and higher level, fails to differentiate and integrate the elements of that level. As each level of the Great Chain of Being has a qualitatively different make-up, so each pathology has likewise a different formation.

For Ken Wilber, pathologies faced by the self can occur at any self-stage, lower, intermediate or higher, where something of the differentiation-and-integration process goes wrong, i.e., the senior dimension does not transcend and include but transcends and represses, denies, distorts or dominates.

However, Ken Wilber is also aware that all kinds of pathologies are not just disruptions of the self, and he does not overlook the importance of psychosocial models of pathological development such as dysfunctional parenting or childrearing attitudes, and biologically influenced models of pathological development such as genetic factors or neuro- biological factors. The importance of both factors is indisputable, and developmental psychopathology needs to integrate all the discoveries of emerging research in these areas.

Actually for Ken Wilber, it requires all the four quadrants in order to understand pathologies in any of them, as "subjective events in individual consciousness (UL) are intimately interrelated with objective events and mechanisms in the organism (UR) ... All of those Upper-Right quadrant factors need to be carefully included in any understanding of individual psychopathology. This includes the partial truths of biological psychiatry... Likewise, we need to look specifically at the larger cultural currents (Lower Left) and social structures (Lower Right) that are inseparable from individual consciousness development. What good does it do to adjust and integrate the self in a culture that is itself sick?... Is that mental health?"[84]

Ken Wilber assumes that awareness in and of itself is the curable aspect of all the various levels of therapeutic treatment. Recontacting the alienated facets or fragmentations that produce pathology, meeting them with awareness and experiencing them fully, allows consciousness to release their distortions and reintegrate them again in the process of consciousness unfolding. Thus Ken Wilber observes that, "Every therapeutic school attempts, in its own way, to allow consciousness to encounter (or reencounter) facets of experience that were previously alienated, malformed, distorted, or ignored. This is *curative* for a basic reason: *by experiencing these facets fully,* consciousness can genuinely acknowledge these elements and thereby let go of them: see them as an object, and thus differentiate from them, de-embed from them, *transcend them*—and then integrate them into a more encompassing, compassionate embrace... Encountering (or reencountering) these disturbed or ignored facets allows them to be differentiated (transcended) and integrated (included) in the ongoing waves of ever-expanding consciousness."[85]

In Ken Wilber's view, each particular psychotherapeutic approach can not be used for all types of psychopathologies. He does not want to restrict the application of a given therapy only to one narrow wave of development but, "most forms of therapy increasingly lose their effectiveness when applied to more distant realms".

An integral psychotherapy works simultaneously with the surface, soul and spirit realms as they each unfold alongside each other. In this process of integral development, work on the lower realms cannot be bypassed in favour of work on the higher realms, as without a stable and strong frontal line development the higher realms cannot contribute to the integration of the lower and higher domains into a fullspectrum realisation.

An integral ongoing "all-level, all-quadrant" therapy aims at bringing awareness to the body, the shadow, the persona, the ego, the existential self, the soul and spirit; the return journey (within) to the past in order to recontact the early distorted scripts can be used as a means to unearth the future, a journey to the real depth of the Self beyond surface layers of the proximate self.

But Ken Wilber's integral therapy is not only individual but also cultural, social and spiritual, because an integral therapy would "attempt to address as many facets of the quadrants as is pragmatically feasible in any given case... The idea is to simultaneously exercise all the major capacities and dimensions of the human bodymind physical, emotional, mental, social, cultural, spiritual."86

A general overview of Ken Wilber's *Integral Psychology* shows us a rather complex image of man and gives us his definite formulation of his general psychological model. His integral psychology tries to integrate the insights of the premodern, modern, and postmodern development. Integral psychology admits the existence of the inner dimension of the individual which can be developed and can transcend the borders of the personal. For Ken Wilber, this inner dimension is embedded in the body, culture, and society; he does not reduce any one of them to the others, yet he is aware of their influence upon each other. Culture and society do influence the individual, but he does not deny the existence of a relatively autonomous and responsible individual self.

A Brief History of Everything*: An integral vision for business, politics, science and spirituality*

In his latest work, Ken Wilber gives a brief overview of an integrative vision he calls a 'Theory of Everything'. In the first four chapters he introduces his vision and in the last three chapters he outlines its relevance in the real world. Ken Wilber uses the term integral in the context of unity-in-diversity, i.e., sharing commonalities along with differences. He distinguishes horizontal from vertical integration: the former involves the integration of the four quadrants at any given level, whereas in the latter there is a movement to a higher level of integration altogether.

The integral level of the vertical integration depends on the highest level of development; the ultimate integral level is the nondual Kosmos itself.

In his genuine *A Theory of Everything,* Ken Wilber uses the Human Consciousness Project (a psychological correlate of the Human Genome Project) as a crucial part of the psychological research work of "a cross-cultural mapping of all of the states, structures, memes, types, levels, stages and waves of human consciousness."[87] In this overall map, as a psychological component of a history of everything, which will be supplemented with the findings from the physical, biological, cultural and spiritual dimensions, Ken Wilber uses, as an example, the 'Spiral Dynamics' model, based on the ideas of Clare Graves and refined by Don Beck and Christopher Cowan. Their books contain a developmental model which is applicable to group dynamics in the society. Spiral Dynamics proceeds through eight stages, waves or memes ("a meme is a basic stage of development that can be expressed in any activity"). Beck and Cowan use various memes and colours that are related to these different waves or memes and they are available to each and every individual in potential form. The first six levels, as subsistence levels, are characterised by 'first-tier thinking', whereas the last two levels, as being levels, are marked by 'second-tier thinking'.

Ken Wilber gives a brief description of all the eight waves, beginning with Beige, the level of basic survival; then comes Purple, the level of magic and animistic thinking, followed by Red, the level of egocentrism and impulsiveness; afterwards Blue appears, the level of mythic fundamentalism and rigid social hierarchies; then comes Orange, the level of scientific materialism, individualism and the modernists, followed by Green, the level of pluralistic relativism, egalitarianism and postmodernism. Ken Wilber places early vision- logic in the Green colour, i.e., early vision-logic differentiates formal systems into multiple concepts. With the completion of the Green wave, human consciousness can move into second-tier thinking, the integrative stages of development where the individual becomes aware that each level is crucially important for the complete functioning of the overall Spiral. The middle and late vision-logic levels are able to integrate the differentiations of Green to varying degrees. The individual on the second tier thinking can think vertically as well as horizontally, and is able to think in terms of the overall Spiral rather than in terms of any one level. Yellow, the level of integration, integrates differences and pluralities into independent flows. Finally, there is Turquoise, the holistic level where the Universal holistic system unites feeling with knowledge and which uses the entire Spiral. Spiritual dynamics, however, does not include the higher transpersonal waves and the different (altered) states of consciousness. Ken Wilber adds three higher levels, the psychic, subtle and causal, i.e., a 'third-tier' level. For Ken Wilber, the third-tier waves are more integral, "as the integral level depends upon the highest level that we recognize".

Ken Wilber relates the Spiral Dynamics to the all-quadrant, all-level model. The Upper-Left quadrant (the interior of the individual) contains a full spectrum of levels or waves of development, different streams, different states of consciousness and different types of consciousness, as already explained in *Integral Psychology.* But this individual subjective consciousness is intimately related with the objective organism and brain (Upper-Right quadrant), with the interobjective patterns of consciousness, i.e., social systems and environment (Lower-Right quadrant) and with the intersubjective patterns of consciousness, i.e., cultural settings and communal world views (Lower-Left quadrant). As discussed in the sections on *Sex, Ecology, Spirituality* and *Integral Psychology* above, each of these quadrants has its own waves (from matter to body to mind to soul to spirit), streams (including moral, spiritual, cognitive, aesthetic, somatic, interpersonal, etc.), states (waking, dreaming, sleeping, altered, meditative) and types (personality types, gender types). "The self as the navigator of the great River of Life acts to bind the multiple waves, states, streams and realms into something of a unified organization."[88]

Ken Wilber maintains that Sri Aurobindo investigates only the Upper-Left quadrant. Later on, we will see whether or not this criticism is sufficiently grounded.

Using the results of the research work of Clare Grave, Don Beck and Christopher Cowan, Ken Wilber assumes that approximately only 1 to 2 per cent of the population is at an integral second-tier stance in which an integral transformation may occur and where truly integral solutions become available. Pluralistic relativism, with its strong subjectivism, easily falls prey to narcissism, which, in turn, destroys a Theory of Everything. With this culture of Narcissism, Ken Wilber introduces the pathology of the Green level, i.e., *Boomeritus*. Boomeritus refers to the baby boom generation and their extraordinary vitality, creativity and idealism, but also their self-absorption and narcissism. According to Ken Wilber, "Boomeritus is that strange mixture of very high cognitive capacity (the green meme and noble pluralism) infected with rather low emotional narcissism".[89] For Ken Wilber boomeritus is one of the greatest barriers to an integral unfolding because "it appears that boomeritus intensifies a *fixation* to the green meme, making it almost impossible to let go of. Because narcissism finds such a happy home in pluralism, both get stuck with each other".[90]

Ken Wilber does not overlook the strengths of the people at the Green level, which include an extraordinary vitality, creativity and enrichment of human potentials. The Greens use early vision-logic in order to grasp different systems and pluralistic concepts that exist in different cultures. "Green has been responsible for basic initiatives in civil rights and environmental protection. It has developed strong and often convincing critiques of the philosophies, metaphysics and social practices of the conventional religious (blue) and scientific (orange) memes, with their often exclusionary, patriarchal, sexist and colonialistic agendas. On the other hand, as effective as these critiques of pre-green stages have been, green has attempted to turn its guns on all post-green stages as well, with the most unfortunate results. This has made it very difficult, and often impossible, for green to move forward into more holistic, integral constructions."[91]

Individuals on the green wave, having detached themselves from rational and dogmatic religious thinking, imagine themselves to be the creators of a new paradigm but in their attempt they reject each and every form of universal thinking and universal truth. *A Theory of Everything* includes postmodernistic influences and Ken Wilber affirms that the individual is not a fully autonomous being but is influenced by culture and society. Nevertheless, he also affirms the existence of an individual self, and he does not want to reduce this individual self to culture and society, where one no longer has responsibility, depth and quality. Ken Wilber acknowledges a universal truth in which there is autonomy and responsibility for the individual.

Development passes through three stages; the selfish preconventional stage, the sociocentric care stage and the post conventional worldcentric stage, which is the beginning of the possibility of developing a truly integral embrace. In this developmental process each higher stage includes an increase in sociocentric consciousness and universal care and a successive decrease in narcissism. The moment the fixation and attachment of the green wave is removed, second-tier consciousness can move forward and replace the pluralistic relativism with a universal integralism.

Ken Wilber is aware that ultimately it is the spiritual practice and not the theoretical knowledge that is the guide for the seeker's spiritual journey to the inner realms of being. His theory of everything may be an essential aid as an orientation in the exploration of the field but it is not sufficient to replace the actual practice of spiritual discipline. For Ken Wilber the transformation from the green wave into mature second-tier consciousness needs to be supplemented by an integral transformative practice, a practice based on an all-level, all-quadrant model which involves exercising physical, emotional, mental and spiritual levels in self (I)' culture ('we') and nature (science, 'it'). If these exercises are done only in the 'I, it ends up in boomeritus; extended in culture, the individual gets involved in community service where relationships are used for improving one's own growth and the growth of others; getting involved in nature honours nature and promotes one's capacity to care. For Ken Wilber this integral practice is "the most powerful way to trigger transformation to the next wave".

A genuine theory of everything does not claim to be a fixed or final theory; according to Ken Wilber, his Theory of Everything "is destined only to pass into yet further, better visions". Everybody's theory explains some aspects of truth and all of these aspects need to be refined and included in a new theory of everything. Unfortunately, Ken Wilber devotes only a few pages to elaborate on his integral practice. Many of his readers had complained that they were overwhelmed by all the exercises from each quadrant level. They had the feeling that they were failing in their own practice in comparison with the all-level, all-quadrant model. Ken Wilber attempts to redress the situation, as follows: "The idea of integral transformative practice is simple enough, namely, exercise physical, emotional, mental and spiritual levels in self, culture and nature... My intent, rather, was simply to suggest that individuals might like to supplement their present practice with a few others from areas they were perhaps neglecting—to complement, not condemn, their present practices... My intent was to *invite* people to expand their options, and *not* to condemn any practices that they were already doing".[92]

Conclusion 'A Theory of Everything'

For Ken Wilber reality, as the Great Chain of Being, has several levels ranging from matter to God. This Great Chain of Being can be labelled as body, mind, soul and Spirit, which are levels of consciousness as well as levels of reality. However, materialistic science rejects the idea of the inner dimension of man, soul and Spirit, and Ken Wilber attempts to find a way to rehabilitate the spiritual dimension within Western culture and metaphysics and to provide an academic basis for spiritual experiences and practice. His integral approach takes up as many visions of other researchers as possible in order to formulate a theory of everything. Such a theory is not based only on natural sciences but includes all facets of human experience. The inner dimension of man seems to be of a different reality when compared to the outer dimension and these two different realities cannot be reduced to one separate reality. In Ken Wilber's integral theory of consciousness, he uses the four-quadrant model, which distinguishes not only an individual outer dimension (UR) and an inner dimension (UL), each consisting of at least nine levels which are reflected in all the quadrants, but also an interobjective social (LR) and intersubjective cultural dimension (LL). He does not ignore the outer dimension, and in his later works the body is no longer at the lowest rung of the ladder, but is a reality which runs parallel to the whole inner dimension. Nevertheless, this inner dimension cannot be reduced to physical processes of the brain, though it leaves its mark upon it. Each phenomenon of consciousness, including the- higher mystical states of consciousness, leads to an identifiable pattern in the brain, which can be studied by exact science. Ken Wilber integrates all discoveries of contemporary neurobiology, minus its reductionism. He is of the opinion that Sri Aurobindo did not pay sufficient attention to this insight. He claims that his integral approach is applicable to any aspect of human life, and is able to relate a number of disciplines to each other in a complete and coherent vision. Ken Wilber's writings are by no means finished, almost every year he writes a new book in which he elaborates on his latest developmental vision about science and spirituality.

NOTES

1. Ken Wilber, *The Spectrum of Consciousness,* p. 53.
2. Ibid., p.118 - 119.
3. Ibid., p.272.
4. Ibid., p.20.
5. Ken Wilber, *Journal of Transpersonal Psychology,* Vol.7, No.2, 1975.
6. Ken Wilber, *The Spectrum of Consciousness,* p.152.
7. Ibid., p.279.
8. Ibid., p.288.
9. Ibid., p.241.
10. Ibid., p.295.
11. Ibid., p.29.
12. Ken Wilber, *The Atman Project,* p.101
13. Ibid., p.103.
14. Ken Wilber, *Journal of Transpersonal Psychology,* Vol.ll, 1979, p.2.
15. Ken Wilber, *The Atman Project,* p. 160-161.
16. Ibid., p.173.
17. Ibid., p.40.
18. Ken Wilber, *Up from Eden,* p.187.
19. Ibid., p.286.
20. ibid., p.255.
21. Ibid., p.320.
22. Ibid., p.323.
23. Ken Wilber, *Eye to Eye,* p.9.
24. Ibid., p.10.
25. Ibid., p.153.
26. Ibid., p.129.

27. Ken Wilber, *Transfortnations of Consciousness*, p.72.
28. Ibid., p.72.
29. Ibid., p.73.
30. Ibid., p.108.
31. Ibid., p.130.
32. Ibid., p.134.
33. Ibid., p.138.
34. Ibid., p.144.
35. Ibid., p.107.
36. Ken Wilber, *Sex, Ecology, Spirituality*, p.49.
37. Ibid., p.56.
38. Ibid., p.57.
39. Ibid., p.83.
40. Ibid., p.120.
41. Ibid., p.314.
42. Ibid., p.139.
43. Ibid., p.143.
44. Ibid., p.348.
45. Ibid., p.361.
46. Ibid., p.522.
47. Ibid., p.496.
48. Ibid., p.6O6.
49. Ken Wilber, *A Theory of Everything*, p.303.
50. Ibid., p.x.
51. Ken Wilber, *The Eye of Spirit*, p.51.
52. Ibid., p.164.
53. Ibid., p.69-70.
54. Ken Wilber, *Up from Eden*, p.313.
55. Ken Wilber, *A Theory of Everything*, p.153.
56. Ken Wilber, *The Eye of Spirit*, p.212.
57. Ibid., p.246.
58. Ken Wilber, *The Atman Project*, p.143.
59. Ken Wilber, *The Eye of Spirit*, p.225.

60. Ibid., p.245.
61. Ibid., p.340.
62. Ken Wilber, *The Marriage of Sense and Soul,* p.14.
63. Ibid., p.142.
64. Ibid., p.153.
65. Ibid., p.177.
66. Ken Wilber, *One Taste,* p. VII.
67. Ibid., p. VIII.
68. Ken Wilber, *The Atman Project,* p.74.
69. Ken Wilber, *Sex, Ecology, Spirituality,* p.316.
70. Ken Wilber, *One Taste,* p.70.
71. Ibid., p.82.
72. Ibid., p.126.
73. Ibid., p.318.
74. Ibid., p.302.
75. Ibid., p.323.
76. Ibid., p.29-30.
77. Ibid., p.79.
78. Ken Wilber, *Integral Psychology,* p.193.
79. Ibid., p.89.
80. Ibid., p.87.
81. Ibid., p.67.
82. Ibid., p.191.
83. Ibid., p.283.
84. Ibid., p.112.
85. Ibid., p.99.
86. Ibid., p.113.
87. Ken Wilber, *A Theory of Everything,* p. 7.
88. Ibid., p. 54.
89. Ibid., p. 27.
90. Ibid., p. 28.
91. Ibid, pp. 14-15.
92. Ken Wilber, *The Collective Works,* Volume 8, Introduction.

Chapter Six

Sri Aurobindo's Metaphysical Vision

A BRIEF EVALUATION OF SRI AUROBINDO'S WRITINGS

Before elaborating on Sri Aurobindo's integral sadhana and its difficulties, it is essential to explore the metaphysical foundation of the integral Yoga, which forms the basis of his integral sadhana. In the following two chapters the author brings out some of the salient points of Sri Aurobindo's metaphysical vision. To get a more complete insight into this vision, he briefly discusses Sri Aurobindo's main works as used in this comparative study, as well as the aim of integral Yoga, the process of integral transformation and the constitution of the various parts of the being.

The author copiously uses quotations of Sri Aurobindo's writings and often repeats his very words wherever possible without using the quotation marks. He is aware that some of the material in the following chapters has already been discussed in detail in *The Concept of Personality in Sri Aurobindo's Integral Yoga Psychology and A. Maslow's Humanistic/Transpersonal Psychology* and *The Quest for the Inner Man*, but for the sake of clarity these topics are essential here.

In *The Life Divine,* Sri Aurobindo sets forth his thesis regarding life, man, the world and God. In this *magnum opus* he outlines the possibility of a new life for the individual and the human race in which a new supramental consciousness would manifest and impel life on earth, bringing about a radical transformation in its character. *The Life Divine* describes the manifestation of the divinity in man, as well as the reconstruction of an individual's entire physical, social, economical, political and cultural environment by the transforming power of the Divine. *The Life Divine* is based on an evolutionary model with the Supermind as the evolutionary destiny of humanity. In the divine life, a greater value will be placed on spiritual unity than on mental analysis, vital action or physical materialism. Individual and collective ego and desires will be replaced by a vision of the truly individuated person and gnostic community. The ultimate goal or highest spiritual destiny of man is to establish the Kingdom of God in a material world. This increased fulfilment of the limitless possibilities inherent in life is the outflowering of the Divine in the individual and in collective humanity.

Sri Aurobindo gives hope for a positive future in his vision of a divine life, albeit not without formidable difficulties. The new ingredients in Sri Aurobindo's metaphysics of life-transformation and world-transformation are his conception of the interrelated processes of evolution and involution, the principle of integration at every stage of the forward movement of consciousness and, lastly, the creative role of the Supermind. Sri Aurobindo views the adventure of consciousness as an upward movement (evolution), a downward movement (involution), and an inward movement (integration and transformation). A divine life here is the inevitable outcome of Nature's evolutionary endeavour. Sri Aurobindo works out in detail how this foundation of the Life Divine on a terrestrial base is to be promoted and ultimately accomplished.

In this difficult process of spiritual evolution towards unity and harmony, it is not only the discovery of the individual soul, the universal Self and the awareness of the Divine being which are crucial steps of self-achievement; matter, life, and mind also have to receive the transforming touch of the Spirit. The lower instrumentation is a responsive field of experimentation where the first decisive advances towards the Supermind may be made. If the inner urge towards spiritualisation is strong enough to pierce the barrier between mind and Supermind, then man need not be written off as a failure; otherwise the future will lie, perhaps, with another race.

In *The Synthesis of Yoga,* Sri Aurobindo presents his metaphysical treatise of *The Life. Divine* from the viewpoint of yogic practice; in this work, he postulates the method and foundation of his integral Yoga. In the four parts of the synthesis, he elaborates on the theory and practice of the *Yoga of works,* the *Yoga of knowledge,* the *Yoga of devotion* and his *Yoga of self-perfection.* In his synthesis of spiritual discipline, all these various paths draw on the divine Power and when harmonised they can become the means for an integral Yoga. In one of the *Arya* Journals, he observes that, "Truth of philosophy is of a merely theoretical value unless it can be lived, and we have therefore tried in the *Synthesis of Yoga* to arrive at a synthetic view of the principles and methods of the various lines of spiritual self-discipline and a way in which they can lead to an integral divine life in human existence. But this is an individual selfdevelopment, and therefore it was necessary to show too how our ideal can work out in the social life of mankind.

In *the Psychology of Social Development* [The Human Cycle] we have indicated how these truths affect the evolution of human society. In *the Ideal of Human Unity,* we have taken the present trend of mankind towards a closer unification and tried to appreciate its tendencies and show what is wanting to them in order that real humanity may be achieved."[1]

Yoga is the effort towards self-perfection by reuniting God and Nature in a perfected human life and for Sri Aurobindo, "the true and full object and utility of Yoga can only be accomplished when the conscious Yoga in man becomes, like the subconscious Yoga in Nature, outwardly conterminous with life itself."[2]

In ordinary Yoga, one main power of being or one group of its powers is made the means or path, but in Sri Aurobindo's synthesis of Yoga all powers are combined and included as a transmuting instrumentation so that man develops in totality and not just in part. Another aspect which has been overlooked by the various yoga's is the development of humanity, and ultimately service of the Divine, rather than the mere desire for individual salvation. Personal realisation in this world is a means for effecting a total transformation of individual and universal man. Sri Aurobindo's Yoga does not merely aim at reaching the highest possible spiritual levels, but also at bringing down the supramental-Force to our earthlife. In *The Synthesis of Yoga,* the essence and methods of the earlier Yogas are taken up in the inclusive and integral Yoga of self-perfection.

The Life Divine and *The Synthesis of Yoga* are based on the sound foundation of scriptural texts, but also on the basis of enlightenment gained through Sri Aurobindo's own intuitive mystic vision and spiritual experiences. Both works were written, not as a mere system of thought to expound the theoretical aspects of his philosophy, but as a practical guide to integral living. They show proper paths to tread in order to reach the adventure of self-discovery and self-exceeding.

It is *The Life Divine* and *The Synthesis of Yoga* that are most often referred to by some of the interpreters or commentators of the transpersonal movement. In these works, it seems that Sri Aurobindo is primarily concerned with existential questions, but unlike the humanist existentialists, Sri Aurobindo is not concerned only with humanity and he gives full attention to the means of going beyond the limitations of present humanity in order to live a divine life.

In *The Human Cycle,* he attempts to apply his integral yogic vision to sociology, and this *psychology of social development* is essentially teleological, i.e., social evolution is the development of the integral relation between the individual, the community and mankind in which each seeks its own fulfilment and realises the purpose of the Divine. These relations of the individual, the community and mankind are viewed against a metaphysical background and the rationale of social evolution in its spiritual basis.

For Sri Aurobindo spiritual life, as the fulfilment of God's intention, has an individual but also a collective dimension. Collectivity, like the individual, is an expression of the manifesting Godhead; both aim to manifest God. The one actualises the possibility of the Divine's self-revelation in each individual centre, whereas the other works to elicit the potentialities in the collective. Though the destiny of the individual is also the destiny of man in society, yet the process of the development of the collectivity is slower than in the case of the individual.

For Sri Aurobindo, human societies like individuals, pass through certain psychological stages on their way to a predetermined evolutionary achievement. Sri Aurobindo uses Karl Lamprecht's model of social developmental stages and agrees that "human society progresses through certain distinct psychological stages which he [Lamprecht] terms respectively symbolic, typal and conventional, individualist and subjective. This development forms, then, a sort of psychological cycle through which a nation or a civilisation is bound to proceed."[3] Though Sri Aurobindo believes in these psychological facts of history, he does not agree that every cultural unit, society or nation must necessarily pass through such uniform patterns. Human progress is not circular but spiral; the cycle moves forward even if it completes a round. According to Sri Aurobindo, "Obviously, such classifications are likely to err by rigidity and to substitute a mental straight line for the coils and zigzags of Nature. The psychology of man and his societies is too complex, too synthetical of many-sided and intermixed tendencies to satisfy any such rigorous and formal analysis. Nor does this theory of a psychological cycle tell us what is the inner meaning of its successive phases or the necessity of their succession or the term and end towards which they are driving."[4]

Nevertheles, Sri Aurobindo uses Lamprecht's psychological theory for the purpose of his own views. He begins *The Human Cycle* at the fourth stage of the evolution of Nature, where man becomes self-conscious. Sri Aurobindo suggests that the historical evolution starts with an infrarational stage in which mankind acts principally out of customary responses to desire, need and circumstance which are crystallised in social, economic and political institutions. As man proceeds and moves towards a rational stage his or her 'intelligent will' becomes a judge of one's thoughts, feelings and actions. In the course of time, development gives rise to a subjective trend which seeks inspiration of a higher source than of enlightened will and reason. This growing subjectivity of the human mind may culminate in a suprarational stage, the age of the spirit. These stages are discernible in the evolution of the individual man as well as of the collectivity; they are not exclusive of the rest and each contains some elements of the others in varying degrees.

The infrarational stage has three noticeable periods in its growth, described as the symbolic, typal and conventional stages. In the first, evolution is predominantly religious and spiritual and men express their perceptions of the world largely in myth, art and poetry. The typal stage is predominantly psychological and ethical; everything else is subordinated to the psychological and ethical ideas. In the conventional stage form prevails, and conventional functions such as class and caste become fixed according to external standards instead of individual merit.

The age of reason is at first necessarily individualistic and increasingly democratic; the second phase is more socialistic. In this age, progress and freedom play a dominant role.

The subjective age, which emerged in the present century, is characterised by a step towards self-knowledge. Man begins to live from within and is discovering one's self-developing soul, yet man often mistakes one's ego for the Self. It is only when there is a full awareness of the necessity for realising a Self, which relates the good of each to the rest of the world, that the age of subjectivism will fulfil its function.

Sri Aurobindo envisages a stage beyond these stages, which he called the coming of a spiritual age of human society, the establishment of a new order in a spiritualised society. In such a society man is not subjected to a religious order but each individual inwardly and outwardly lives a divine life.

In *The Human Cycle,* Sri Aurobindo analyses the problem of the individual and the society from an inner psychological point'of view, whereas in *The Ideal of Human Unity* he elaborates the same general theme but from a more outward, political viewpoint.

As for the individual and society, so for the entire human race, there is one Spirit, the divine Reality, which manifests itself singly in the individual and pluraly in humanity. In *The Ideal of Human Unity,* Sri Aurobindo describes the attempts that have been made to arrive at a unification and integration of humanity. These attempts—

humanitarianism, socialism, democracy but also scientific, political and economic developments—failed because they lacked sincerity in approach and they only served the externals of a world order. For Sri Aurobindo, these mechanical unifications in the external field were a necessary preparation, but at present there is a need for a spiritual religion of humanity. While exploring the inevitability of a lasting united humanity, through the idea of a religion of humanity, he maintains that such suprarational union cannot be achieved by means of social, economical, political or any other external machinery of society, but needs first a spiritual aspiration, an awakening in mankind which creates a psychological oneness before a true outward union can be established. Each and every man must surrender both inwardly and outwardly to the force of spiritual consciousness. He envisages a gradual spiritualisation of society, a progressive movement towards the divine life in the entire universe.

The spiritual religion of humanity is able to bring about a real transformation in human consciousness; at first this change has to be accomplished in the individual and thereafter in a larger number of individuals. In this way a higher spiritual consciousness can descend in the social mind. For Sri Aurobindo, the spiritual religion of humanity plays an important social role in human history by transforming every aspect of human life; when it gets more deeply rooted in mankind, the spiritual age can come into existence replacing the old repetitive human cycle of social development. The necessary spiritual transformation for the creation of the ideal human unity or perfect society comprises not only individual self-perfection but also the perfection of one's fellow human beings.'

The most important book from the standpoint of the practice of sadhana, the *Letters on Yoga,* comprises his correspondence with the practitioners of integral Yoga, where he elaborates on their psycho-spiritual difficulties and doubts, and their requests for help and guidance.

In these letters, he attempts to give various sadhaks some psycho-spiritual, often strict and difficult guidelines for behaviour and some understanding of the psychological difficulties of their spiritual journey. His answers to these questions were not the usual logical-intellectual interpretations, but came from his higher spiritual experiences and his supreme understanding of human nature. The seekers on the journey placed their difficulties in the day-to-day course of the sadhana before Sri Aurobindo, and he wrote to them explaining and clarifying their developments and guided them to speed up their progress. In his endless compassion and ever-ready support, he led the seekers along the steep path of integral sadhana.

He gave importance to the correspondence because it was an effective instrument for his central purpose—the evolution of mankind: "there are a large number of Sadhaks whom it has helped to awaken from lethargy and begin to tread the way of spiritual experience, some who have been absolutely hopeless for years who have undergone a conversion and- entered from darkness into an opening of light... for the majority of those who wrote, there has been a real progress."[5] Though each individual has his own line of spiritual development, and what is valid for one seeker need not be so for others, yet certain fundamental truths are common to all types of sadhana.

His language in the letters is less formal than the expository prose of *The Life Divine* and *The Synthesis of Yoga,* and gives a more immediate impression of the psycho-spiritual experiences the seeker is bound to come across.

Aim Integral Yoga

Yoga as a means of uniting the individual, the universal and the transcendent reality, proceeds through a systematic awakening of man's inner potential. Sri Aurobindo means by this "a methodised effort towards self-perfection by the expression of the potentialities latent in the being and a union of the human individual with the universal and transcendent Existence we see partially expressed in man and in the Cosmos."[6]

The union with the Infinite and the Eternal is a direct move- ment of the consciousness and the being of man, through a series of self-purifications and self-enlargement. The whole meaning of the process of Yoga is related to a change of consciousness, which takes the seeker from the surface into the depth and heights of one's consciousness; it shows man the secret of the Divine and, brings to the seeker the intricate presence of the Immanent, the Cosmic and the Transcendent Reality. To rise to a higher consciousness means not only a change of consciousness but also a change of life. Sri Aurobindo describes the aim of integral Yoga: "to open the consciousness to the Divine and to live in the inner consciousness more and more while acting from it on the external life, to bring the inmost psychic into the front and by the power of the psychic to purify and change the being so that it may become ready for transformation and be in union with the Divine Knowledge, Will and Love. Secondly, to develop the Yogic consciousness, i.e., to universalise the being in all planes, become aware of the cosmic being and cosmic forces and be in union with the Divine on all the planes up to the overmind. Thirdly, to come into contact with the transcendent Divine beyond the overmind through the supramental consciousness, supramentalise the consciousness and the nature and make oneself an instrument for the realisation of the dynamic Divine Truth and its transforming descent into the earth-nature."[7]

Sri Aurobindo elaborates on his concept of Yoga as integral on the basis of two insights: first, he synthesises the Yoga of action, devotion and knowledge into his system of Yoga, and secondly, his yoga aims at the full development of body, mind and soul. Integral Yoga implies the binding together of all these various parts by the power of the

Self or the in-dwelling Divine. Moreover, the individual induces all humanity to go with him or her on the same path. This synthesis of yoga cannot be arrived at by a simple combination of the various systems of yoga or a successive practice of the various systems.

Integral Yoga "takes up the essence and many processes of the old Yogas—its newness is in its aim, standpoint and the totality of its method.... There is nothing that distinguishes it from the old Yogas except the aim underlying its comprehensiveness."[8]

Sri Aurobindo's Yoga is a yoga of transformation, and unlike the traditional systems of Yoga not a mere yoga of realisation and liberation from life. This transformation results in a new species radically different from the present human species. On a collective scale, it results in a spiritualised society (gnostic society) of 'spiritual' individuals.

According to Sri Aurobindo, "No synthesis of Yoga can be satisfying which does not, in its aim, reunite God and Nature in a liberated and perfected human life or, in its method, not only permit but favour the harmony of our inner and outer activities and experiences in the divine consummation of both. For man is precisely that term and symbol of a higher Existence descended into the material world in which it is possible for the lower to transfigure itself and put on the nature of the higher and the higher to reveal itself in the forms of the lower."[9]

Integral Yoga aims at the transformation of life by bringing down into it the Light and Power of the divine Truth and its dynamic certitudes. It does not aim at a world-shunning asceticism but at a change of life and existence. The descent of the new consciousness attained by the ascent is the seal of integral sadhana.

For Sri Aurobindo, "the principle of this yoga is not

perfection of the human nature as it is but a psychic and spiritual transformation of all the parts of the being through the action of an inner consciousness and then of a higher consciousness which works on them, throws out their old movements or changes them into the image of its own and so transmutes lower into higher nature."[10]

The aim of the practitioner of integral Yoga must be the possession of God, to be perfect as God in His being, and the attempt to bring all mankind to the same divine perfection. This implies replacement of egoism by divine consciousness and the bringing of the kingdom of heaven on earth, i.e., effectuating God in the world, but also realising God as transcendent of the Universe. This self-perfection is not actually a self-annulment or a withdrawal from the universe, but an attempt to effect a perfection in the universe. "The world is a movement of God in His own being; we are the centres and knots of divine consciousness which sum up and support the processes of His movement. ... The world is a formula, a rhythm, a symbol-system expressing God to Himself in His own consciousness—it has no material existence but exists only in His consciousness and self-expression; we, like God, are in our inward being that which is expressed, but in our outward being, terms of that formula. Out of imperfection we have to construct perfection ... out of matter to reveal Spirit. To work out this end for ourselves and for humanity is the object of our Yogic practice."[11]

It is clear that the aim of integral Yoga is not only freedom from the bondage of human nature but perfect control over it, with a view to transforming, spiritualising and divinising it.

INTEGRAL TRANSFORMATION

Integration

In passing from one level to another or in climbing to higher spiritual levels, the lower faculty is compelled to take up as much as it can assimilate of the higher, enlarging itself and arriving at a more complete self-accommodation to higher faculties.

Sri Aurobindo, like Ken Wilber, does not want to renounce or reject what has already been given to the individual in the lower strata in the process of the Divine's Self-manifestation. Integration takes up what has already been evolved into each higher grade as it is reached. In the words of Sri Aurobindo, "Not to abandon the lower to itself, but to transfigure it in the light of the higher to which we have attained is the true divinity of nature."[12]

The curve of evolving consciousness brings out what was held from the beginning by the original Consciousness in all things. It would not be possible for the lower to evolve into the higher unless potentialities of the higher were already inherent within the lower. The lower levels of development contain within themselves the essential principle of that which exceeds them, "the lower term of being in which we now live contains in itself the principle and intention of that which exceeds it and it is by its own self-exceeding and transformation into that that it can find and develop into a complete form its own real essence."[13]

For Sri Aurobindo integration is related to the transformation of the different, often conflicting parts of the being brought about by the control and the working of a higher principle into an organic whole, so that they can move in perfect union with the divine Will. Integration implies the reconciliation of the disparate parts of the being, the conscious and the unconscious parts, but also the concealed subliminal and superconscious parts of the being. True integration is not a superficial association between various parts and cannot be done by the mental and vital being but only from within by the soul, as it is the soul which functions as the centraliser of truth and can harmonise it with the truth of the other parts. An integral spiritualised consciousness links the highest, the Superconscious, to the lowest, the inconscient; it reveals the hidden true significance of the lower, and enables them to overcome their separateness from the Divine Reality.

The lower domains as instruments

Mind, life and body are instruments and not prisons for the working of the Divine Force, and once the seeker opens to this Force he or she can be a perfect instrument of her Power. However, for Sri Aurobindo the present functioning of the lower instrumentation is characterised by a separation in consciousness from the Divine Truth. But for an integral transformation, the lower instrumentation of mind, life and body must be capable of divinity in their potential working, and in the end the higher must be able to remould the lower realms themselves into a perfect image of its eternal Truth. *The discords of the lower need not merely be resolved into a harmonious whole or dominated by the higher, but need to be purified, eliminated and transformed,* so that the spiritual life of man can create in him or herself the perfect Man, and use the lower instrumentation as a perfect vessel of divine self-expression. "The lower faculty is compelled to take up as much as it can assimilate of what the higher had already given and to attempt to re-establish it by its own methods. By the attempt it is itself enlarged in its scope and arrives eventually at a more supple and a more ample self-accommodation to the higher faculties. Without this succession we should be obliged to remain under the exclusive domination of a part of our nature while the rest remained either depressed and unduly subjected or separate in its field and therefore poor in its development."[14]

Transformation

Transformation expresses certain spiritual concepts and spiritual facts of integral Yoga. In a spiritual sense, a realisation makes the experience more real and dynamic, and implies "the making real to ourselves and in ourselves of the Self, the transcendent and universal Divine". For Sri Aurobindo, a spiritual realisation may bring an opening or heightening or widening of the consciousness but by itself does not necessarily transform the being as a whole. One can realise the Divine everywhere, the summit experience in spiritual life, yet remain untransformed in one's nature. It is, therefore, only one means towards the Divine transformation along with self-perfection and spiritual emancipation from Nature.

In transformation, there is a process of heightening, widening and integration of the range of consciousness; an ascent to a new level and a taking up of the lower levels. This transformation takes up and remakes into a new power of awareness the inner existence as well as the outer being and world-being. In the words of Sri Aurobindo, "If the control of that highest spiritual being is to be brought into our waking life, there must be a conscious heightening and widening into immense ranges of new being, new consciousness, new potentialities of action, a taking up—as integral as possible, of our present being, consciousness, activities and a transmutation of them into divine values which would effect a transfiguration of our human existence. For wherever a radical transition has to be made, there is always this triple movement—ascent, widening of field and base, integration—in Nature's method of self-transcendence."[15]

In this process of transformation, when the lower consciousness is transformed by the light of the higher spiritual consciousness, the seeker does not merely receive the influences from the higher descending Forces but one also needs to live deeper within and ascend into higher and wider levels, i.e., a bringing down of the static and dynamic divine consciousness in every part of the being. There must be a descent of the Power not only into the mind, but into all the parts of the being down to the physical and below in the subcouscient, before a real transformation can take place.

If the lower parts of the being are to be truly transformed they must be made to consent to their own transformation, but this is difficult to bring about because they cling to their own habits, impulses; reactions, pleasures and sufferings. The moment the sadhak receives a call to exceed and transform him or herself into a greater being and wider nature, one is often encountered by resistance and revolt. The lower instrumentation of an individual is too much under the influence of ignorance and the inferior movements of its natural inclinations, and that's why it cannot function as a proper instrumentation. The development, enlargement and removal of the limitations of the lower instrument, raised to its fullest powers and its subsequent transformation, allows a richer preparation for the supramental action.

Sri Aurobindo uses the concept of transformation in a special sense: "a change of consciousness radical and complete and of a certain specific kind which is so conceived as to bring about a strong and assured step forward in the spiritual evolution of the being of a greater and higher kind and of a larger sweep and completeness than what took place when a mentalised being first appeared in a vital and material animal world."[16] In this radical change and conversion of the natural parts into their spiritual equivalents the whole of human nature may be sublimated and transfigured into the divine Supernature. Such a transformation of human nature can only be achieved when the essence of the being is permeated in the spiritual principle, in which all movements become a harmonised process of the Spirit. According to Sri Aurobindo's concept of it, transformation enables the sadhak to live in the Divine not only in the absorbed ecstasy of trance, but to live the Life Divine on earth at all times, in all the parts and elements of the being—physically, vitally, mentally and spiritually.

During the process of transformation, before the lower gradation of being can come to a point at which the higher can manifest in it, the lower needs to surrender itself first to the pressure from some superior planes where the new power is dominant. It has to be purified, reorganised, reformed, liberated and perfected in order to become a faultless instrument. In this way, the lower parts of the being are exalted and get a greater fullness and significance in the reality of their power and performance; they become "manifestations of the truth of being ... they would themselves be conscious motive-powers of the Spirit and although not yet in the full force of their entirely realised spiritual substance, they would not be subjected to a lesser instrumentation fragmented, diluted, diminished, obscured by the substance of the Nescience."[17]

The impurities and inadequacies of an unstable instrumentation, due to the discord between the various activities of mind in itself, as well as between the activities of the vital and physical being, creates various kinds of limitations. It is for this reason that the characteristic limitations of the instruments must be purified of 'defects', but the power of the instruments of our normal nature also needs to be heightened and enlarged for the greater action of the divine Force.

Purification

The passage from the human to the divine involves two stages one of preparation in which the instruments must become pure and another of the soul's manifestation in and illumination of the life through its pure and fit instruments. For an active perfection of the lower domains, a process of purification of the working of all the members of the lower instrument is inevitable. Sri Aurobindo assumes that "Mind, heart, the soul of vital desire, the life in the body are the seats of impurity; it is they that must be set right if the working of the spirit is to be a perfect working."[18] Obstructions and impurities of the lower instrumentation prevent the higher from acting and using the lower as a clear mirror in which the divine reality can be reflected.

The True being itself, the spirit in man, needs no purification; it is pure in itself and is not affected by the faults of its instrumentation of mind, heart and body, the seats of impurity. This instrumentation must be rectified if the working of the spirit is not to be obstructed by its present concession to the pleasure seeking of the lower nature. Sri Aurobindo describes purification as, "a release... it is a throwing away of limiting, binding, obscuring imperfections and confusions; purification from desire brings the freedom of the psychic Prana [the pure activity which gives the sadhak a psycho-spiritual base], purification from wrong emotions and troubling reactions the freedom of the heart, purification from the obscuring limited thought of the sense-mind the freedom of the intelligence, purification from mere intellectuality the freedom of the gnosis."[19]

This purity has an integral character, as the complete purification of one instrument depends on the complete purification of all the other members. In the words of Sri Aurobindo, "the purification of each member of our being profits by the clarifying of every other, the progressive tranquillisation of the emotional heart helping for instance the purification of the understanding while equally a purified understanding imposes calm and light on the turbid and darkened workings of the yet impure emotions ... yet love itself needs to be clarified by divine knowledge."[20]

The integral purification is, therefore, a great source of difficulties and disappointments, as when the sadhak thinks that his or her intelligence is purified it is still subject to clouding by the emotions of the heart and will. But sadhaks need not despair, as one important instrument, sufficiently purified, can be used as a means for the purification of others, "one step firmly taken makes easier all the others and gets rid of a host of difficulties." Even if the higher spiritual influences are accepted by the lower instrumentation there is still the danger of seeking to capture the descending Powers for egoistic advantages and degrade these spiritual influences into an aggrandised lower instrumentation for desire. Vital craving in the form of desire carries into its pursuit a sense of limitation, dissatisfaction, and early disappointment. To get rid of desire is, therefore, indispensable for the purification of the lower instruments.

To turn the vital being from a 'troublesome power' into an obedient instrument of an unattached mind, and to turn the will into an unattached structure are the first steps in purification. Even here, the will of the transcendent Spirit, the divine *Shakti* (the principle of spiritual force in divine nature) or *Tapas* (spiritual effort by concentrating of the will to conquer the lower nature), may get jostled with one's ego for various reasons; when the individual soul moves away from the universal and transcendental truth. The will of the transcendent Spirit gets mixed up with an alien personal energy, which interferes with the divine principle.

Any method recommended in any yogic system, which is suitable to the nature and temperament of the sadhak, can be pursued for some time as a means of quieting one's mental agitations. But in integral yoga nothing tangible is gained until the psychic being is brought to the fore and gains control of the processes initiated. The sadhak's identification with the psychic being gives him or her a secure poise from which he or she can observe and deal with even the least movements of one's nature, its secret forces and the subtle interrelations of its parts. In psychic consciousness; we feel each impure movement in our nature not as something sinful which has to be severed but as a play of energy. It is the psychic being which makes it possible for the seeker to open the human nature to the Divine if they submit to the psychic influence.

For Sri Aurobindo, "It is only the inmost psychic being unveiled and emerging in its full power that can lead the pilgrim sacrifice unscathed through these ambushes and pitfalls; at each moment it catches, exposes, repels the mind's and life's falsehoods."[21] As useful aids during this difficult passage Sri Aurobindo advises "the method of detachment from the insistence of all mental and vital and physical claims and calls and impulsions, a concentration in the heart, austerity, selfpurification and rejection of the old mind-movements and lifemovements, rejection of the ego of desire, rejection of false needs and false habits, but the most central way is to found all such or other methods on a self-offering and surrender of ourselves and of our parts of nature to the Divine Being."[22]

The systematic purification of the whole being can also be brought about through the triple method of Yoga—knowledge, love and work—in a growing attitude of self-surrender, a growing vision of the psychic being, and an implicit faith in the divine guidance.

It should be clear by now that for Sri Aurobindo this total purification of the complex instrumentality in all the parts of the being is not, ultimately, the narrower moral purification of the ethical nature. As described by Sri Aurobindo, "purification must not be understood in any limited sense of a selection of certain outward kinetic movements, their regulation, the inhibition of other action or a liberation of certain forms of character or particular mental and moral capacities. These things are secondary signs of our derivative being, not essential powers and first forces."[23]

In integral sadhana, the sadhak has to gain a more deep-rooted psychological insight regarding the primary forces of one's nature, and to strike at their roots rather them changing or curing symptoms of impurity.

Liberation

Sri Aurobindo describes liberation as "that inner change which is essential to perfection and indispensable to spiritual freedom ... it implies always two things, a rejection and an assumption, a negative and a positive side; the negative movement of freedom is a liberation from the principle bonds, the master-knots of the lower soul-nature, the positive side an opening or growth into the higher spiritual existence."[24]

The knots of the mind and the heart come to the seeker in the form of ego and desire, and the liberation from ego and desire together form the central spiritual freedom. The ego, as the fulcrum of ignorance and bondage, supports falsehood of a separate existence rather than dwelling upon the idea of oneness and unity. An intellectual knowledge of the spiritual truth of oneness or the elimination of the active sense of the ego is not a true spiritual liberation. For Sri Aurobindo a spiritual liberation from the ego means the replacement of the ego by a oneness in the transcendental Divine and identification with the universal Being. This transcendent existence or this universal Spirit is a truth which the purified intelligence can apprehend, but it can only be realised and lived in Spirit. According to Sri Aurobindo a spiritual liberation from, the ego "is a lifting up and surrender of the whole being to him [the Divine], by which not only do we become one with him in our spiritual existence, but dwell too in him and he in us, so that the whole nature is full of his presence and changed into the divine nature; we become one spirit and consciousness and life and substance with the Divine and at the same time we live and move in and have a various joy of that oneness."[25]

The *integral* liberation comes when "the soul is liberated both from attachment to the lower action of nature and from all repugnance to the cosmic action of the Divine.... The liberation of the Nature becomes one with the liberation of the spirit, and there is founded in the integral freedom the integral perfection."[26]

A complete liberation from the ego and desire creates a superiority over the qualitative modes of the inferior nature when the play of the 'infinite' is no longer subject to the limited play of concorded discords. The liberation of the individual soul is the primary necessity and the pivot on which all else turns. There is a tendency of this single liberated soul to extend the same divine self-consciousness to other individual souls of our terrestrial humanity.

Liberation is, therefore, not only the freedom of an unbroken contact of the individual being in all its parts with the Divine; an integral liberation also includes the acquisition of the divine nature, the most complete and final release of all.

Perfection

Purification and liberation are indispensable antecedents of perfection; when the self is purified and liberated into its self- existent being then spiritual perfection becomes possible. Human perfection usually aims at things outward, like social action and a rational cooperation with our fellow men and our environment. It is concerned with a good, rich and happy way of life. It is also the manifestation of a more subjective ideal, it endeavours to raise intelligence and will to a nobler, ethical and finer emotional instrumentation. This human perfection must include self-mastery and a mastery of the surroundings; man's urge to self-perfection is to be self-ruler no longer subjected to the unfettered instinctual stimuli-response system.

Integral Yoga takes up this aim but places it in a wider spiritual context, opening it to the divine degrees of the Spirit, and Sri Aurobindo distinguishes, therefore, this human perfection from integral spiritual perfection. Perfection as used in integral Yoga refers to a growth out of a 'lower' non-divine into a 'higher' divine nature.

Sri Aurobindo describes perfection in this way: "for the integral Yoga perfection will mean a divine spirit and a divine nature which will admit of a divine relation and action in the world; it will mean also in its entirety a divinising of the whole nature, a rejection of all its wrong knots of being and action, but no rejection of any part of our being or of any field of our action."[27]

Sri Aurobindo does not want to limit the description of the individual's and the world's undivine perfection solely to moral evil or suffering, on the contrary, he wants the sadhak to consider the general principle of imperfection, i.e., the principle 'of division and ignorance. However, imperfection is only a first condition and opportunity for the achievement of a greater perfection in the manifestation of the hidden divinity, and "our imperfect status is a starting-point and opportunity for. the achievement of another higher, wider and greater will that shall be divine and perfect not only by the secret spirit within it but in its manifest and most outward form of existence."[28] As such, imperfection becomes a necessary term in the manifestation of. the divine nature. The soul s dissatisfaction with imperfection and its divine aspiration for the elimination of all imperfections from one's nature is a law of the being, but also a law against which the sadhak revolts.

To be an active master rather than being in mental control of one's nature, the sadhak's natural mental, vital and physical personality must rise above the mechanical determinism of Nature. Mind, life and body act upon each other in discord, in a mixed harmony in their various activities. Perfection can be attained only when the present nature is dealt with radically. Its temporary, immediate determination of utility, enjoyment, maintenance, need, possession, etc., must be transformed into a larger harmony of action in order to arrive at some principle of a higher utility and freer instrumentation. In Sri Aurobindo's words, "the body is given us as one instrument necessary to the totality of our work and it is to be used, not neglected, hurt, suppressed or abolished. If it is imperfect, recalcitrant, obstinate, so are also the other members, the vital being, heart and mind and reason. It has like them to be changed and perfected and to undergo a transformation. As we must get ourselves a new life, new heart, new mind, so we have in a certain sense to build for ourselves a new body."[29] The sadhak should also abandon one's separate individuality and universalise oneself in order to work out his or her purpose.

Sri Aurobindo describes three requirements by which this perfection can be arrived at: (1) growing into a perfect equality, a sign that the sadhak has passed beyond the egoistic determination of one's nature; (2) raising all the active parts of the human nature to their higher capacities so that they become capable of being divinised into true instruments of the perfect divine action. To divinise the perfect nature, the seeker has to replace his or her limited human energy by the divine Power, which requires the sadhak's surrender to and faith in the divine guidance; (3) the ascent of the mental being into the supramental being, beyond mental limitations.

This "*Yoga-siddhi,* the perfection that comes from the practice of Yoga, can be best attained by the combined working of four great instruments. There is, first, the knowledge of the truth, principles, powers and processes that govern the realisation ... Next comes the force of our personal effort [a watchful introspection and a constant practice and vigilant will of self-modification and self-transformation] ... and the direct influence of the Teacher. Last comes the instrumentality of Time."[30] The aim of these external instruments is to awaken the sadhak's soul to the Divine within. When the normal instruments are perfected, then they are no longer disturbed by undue interference from each other, and when this perfection rises in its capacity for action, then the instruments will be ready for transformation in which they will discover a luminous spiritual truth of the whole perfected nature. The whole object of an integral Yoga of self-perfection is "to grow into the truth and power of the Spirit and by the direct action of that power to be made a fit channel of its self expression— a living of man in the Divine and a divine living of the Spirit in humanity."[31]

Difficulties in the process of perfection like ego-claims, grief, revolt, impatience can be overcome by a complete self-surrender to God. "This complete self-surrender must be the chief mainstay of the Sadhaka because it is the only way, apart from complete quiescence and indifference to all action—and that has to be avoided—by which the absolute calm and peace can come. The persistence of trouble, the length of time taken for this purification and perfection, itself must not be allowed to become a reason for discouragement and impatience ... recurrence of trouble serves to bring out the presence of the defect, put the Sadhaka upon his guard and bring about a more enlightened and consistent action of the will to get rid of it. When the trouble is too strong to be kept out, it must be allowed to pass and its return discouraged.... Thus persisting it will be found that these things lose their force more and more, become more and more external and brief in their recurrence, until finally calm becomes the law of the being. This rule persists so long as the mental Buddhi [the thinking mind] is the chief instrument; but when the supramental light takes possession of mind and heart, then there can be no trouble, grief or disturbance."[32]

An integral purity which enables a perfect reflection of the divine being in oneself and the perfect outpouring of this truth in us, is the condition of an integral liberation which in turn prepares the integral perfection of humanity, a perfection founded on a certain free universality of being, of love and joy, of knowledge and will in unegoistic action. It is this integrality which is aimed at in integral Yoga. The cultivation of these three constituent elements of Yoga makes the nature a pure and perfect instrument for divine work.

Triple transformation

Another way to understand Sri Aurobindo's views on integral transformation is to place this process in the context of the triple transformation: the psychic transformation, the spiritual transformation and the supramental or the perfect integral transformation.

The transition beyond the human into the Divine, a transformation effected by sadhana, needs to be based on a total and integral change of consciousness. A descent of the whole higher consciousness into the mind may change the mind but need not change the vital nature; a higher power in the vital may enlarge the vital movements but leaves the physical consciousness unchanged; the descent of Light may change the inner being while the outer remains an imperfect instrument. There must be a descent of Light and Power not only in the mind but also into all the parts of the being down to the physical and below in the subconscient before a real transformation can take place.

Sri Aurobindo distinguishes two successive movements of consciousness; an inward movement in which the seeker discovers an inner being which is much larger in its potentialities than our external being, and an upward movement beyond our present mental level into a static cosmic movement. However, for Sri Aurobindo transformation can be complete only when the psychic movement inward to the inner being, and the opening upward to the higher existence are supported by the action of the supramental Consciousness and Force. The descending force of the Divine, which works through the Supermind, transforms the mental, vital and physical status of the person; but so long as there is a hiatus between the Divine and earth existence there can be no radical change of the surface existence. This hiatus between mind and

Supermind can be bridged through the process of triple transformation. As Sri Aurobindo says, " the gulf between Mind and Supermind has to be bridged.... This can be done only by the triple- transformation: there must first be the psychic change, the conversion of our whole present nature into a soul-instrumentation; on that or along with that there must be the spiritual change, the descent of-a higher Light, Knowledge, Power, Force, Bliss, Purity into the whole being, even into the lowest recesses of the life and body, even into the darkness of our subconscience; last, there must supervene the supramental transmutation—there must take place as a crowning movement the ascent into the Supermind and the transforming descent of the supramental Consciousness into our entire being and nature."[33]

Psychic Transformation

As has already been indicated, to overcome the various psychological difficulties and problems in the process of purification and liberation the sadhak is advised to go inward and discover one's true Person, the psychic being. Each time there is a purification of the outer nature it becomes more possible for the inner being to reveal itself, and once the psychic being is in front the sadhana becomes natural. Psychicisation, the first step in the process of the triple transformation, leads to a psychic change of the lower nature bringing right vision into the mind, right feeling into the vital and right movement into the physical.

This psychic change purifies the egoistic mental, vital and physical movements; each of these movements is spiritualised so that the mind, the vital and the physical become manifesting instruments of a greater oneness. In this change the mixed and limited members of our being are no longer dependent on mental preferences, vital passions or physical cravings but on the recognition of the soul's potentialities.

Sri Aurobindo describes psychic transformation as, "a

modification of the substance of the consciousness especially in the vital-emotional part, and as such a modification prolonged or repeated till it became permanent would mean a great step in what I call the psychic transformation of the being. It is just these modifications in the inner substance that make transformation possible."[34]

If the psychic being comes to the front, then a deeper mutation enables the descent of the spiritual force to become more effective; for the preliminary soul-change in the totality of the conscious being emancipates mind, life and body from the limitations of their own imperfections and impurities.

To experience the soul's complete emergence needs the direct contact of the surface being with the spiritual Reality. To achieve this contact, the soul may use the thinking mind as an instrument and put a psychic impression on the intellect and intuitive intelligence, i.e., at first the mind of the higher mental thinker, then the mind of the sage. As a result, the mind becomes pure, tranquil and impersonal; in its search the highest thinking mind becomes aware of an impersonal Reality, a supreme Good, Truth, Beauty and Bliss. But this direct contact of the soul with the spiritual Reality can also be brought about through the consecration of the heart, when the approach is made through the spiritual Reality of love. The nascent spiritual man appears in the emotional nature first as the devotee and might later develop into the saint. A larger change, however, needs a consecration of the pragmatic will, which is possible by a gradual elimination of the ego-will and its motive power of desire.

Sri Aurobindo emphasises a combination of thesse different approaches made by the soul to get in touch with the spiritual Reality, as explained by him: "A combination of all these three approaches, the approach of the mind, the approach of the will, the approach of the heart, creates a spiritual or psychic condition of the surface being and nature in which there is a larger and more complex openness to the psychic light within us, and to the Reality now felt above and enveloping and penetrating us."[35]

The psychic being, with its spontaneous self-giving, lights up thoughts, emotional movements, and vital and physical habits. It substitutes right movements for wrong ones and makes them pure instruments for the innermost psychic.

The psychic's characteristic power is "to turn everything towards the Divine, to bring a fire of purification, aspiration, devotion, true light of discernment, feeling, will, an action which transforms by degrees the whole nature. Quietude, peace and silence in the heart and therefore in the vital part of the being are necessary to reach the psychic."[36]

Although psychic transformation is a necessary condition for the total transformation of our existence and brings all kinds of inner changes, it has certain limitations. In the first place, it can open up the hidden divine ranges of our being, but it needs a spiritual transformation from above to possess our self in its universality and transcendence. By itself, the psychic being might be content to be united with the cosmic consciousness and become purely passive, remote from mastery and action in the world, i.e., it may lose its individuality in its source and experience this as its ultimate mission. Another limitation is related to the action of the psychic being when it comes up to the surface. In its action the psychic being gets mixed with the surface disabilities which it has to use to express itself and for this reason it cannot remain distinct in its purity. The inferior instrumentation reflects a modified manifestation of things as the psychic intimations get jumbled with mental ideas, vital desires and habitual physical tendencies. Under these conditions the true psychic light gets diminished in the mind into a mere idea, the psychic feeling in the heart into a mere sentiment and the psychic will to action into a blind vital enthusiasm. Moreover, the psychic being does not emerge full-grown, it evolves and moves through a slow development; its power to impress the outer instruments is imperfect because in its push for action it has to rely on these instruments and by the obscurity of our consciousness it is separated from its inner reality.

For a spiritual change the psychic or, more widely speaking, the psycho-spiritual transformation is essential but not sufficient. The old Yogas have been mainly confined to the psycho-spiritual occult range of experiences, a kind of static liberation without any dynamic descent. In integral Yoga, when the lower field has been sufficiently prepared by a certain amount of psycho-spiritual experience, the sadhak's consciousness is drawn upward to ranges belonging to the higher spiritual consciousness, not merely to receive from there, but to live there and bring it down to change the lower consciousness altogether. Without the inner psycho-spiritual experience nothing lasting can be done, but there must also be a realisation of the Divine in the outer consciousness. If the sadhak does not go beyond the psychic transformation, then there is only an inner change while the outer nature continues to be moved by the mechanical effects of past energies and may remain incoherent.

Spiritual Transformation

The psychic development prepares the lower nature to receive the higher spiritual consciousness with a complete receptivity and right attitude. To explore spiritual experiences before purification may create a dangerous situation; an ambition or any other vital motive mixed up with the spiritual seeking often leads to the growth of an exaggerated egoism. Sri Aurobindo advises the sadhak not to plunge blindly into spiritual experiences in sadhana without a fairly long period of preparation and purification. When the soul is in front, the sadhak gets the right guidance from within, which makes the descent of the higher consciousness safe and easy.

While psychicisation, as a change from within, unifies the depth of the being with the surface, spiritualisation, as a change that descends from above, unites the manifested existence with Knowledge, Power, Bliss and Purity into the whole being. These two movements indicate two necessities in sadhana and are complementary to each other; the psychic change must be completed by an ascension to the higher ranges of consciousness, as this brings us in contact with cosmic consciousness, a greater sensory perception of the world and its objects, which is at present hidden from us. When sadhaks are in contact with the cosmic consciousness and universalise themselves, they must recast their individual minds in the illuminative self-existing truth of a cosmic mentality, their individual lives enlarged into the dynamic movement of universal life and allow an opening of their bodies to the forces of universal Nature. These ascents, which are powerfully illuminating and liberating, often take place in trance, but are also possible during a concentration of the waking consciousness.

This new consciousness brings to the sadhak spiritual awareness of the Infinite, which is able to remove barriers and break down the limitations of the lower nature. According to Sri Aurobindo, "It is the aim of the sadhana that the consciousness should rise out of the body and take its station above... Thus liberated one opens to all that is above this station, above the ordinary mind, receives there all that descends from the heights, observes from there all that is below. Thus it is possible to witness in all freedom and to control all that is below and to be a recipient or a channel for all that comes down and presses into the body, which it will prepare to be an instrument of a higher manifestation, remoulded into a higher consciousness and nature."[37] The spiritual transformation culminates in an ascent of consciousness which establishes itself on a higher plane and from where it governs the mind, life and body, but it achieves also an increasing descent of the powers of the higher consciousness, which becomes more and more the whole normal consciousness. But the descent of the higher Force, descending from centre to centre till it has occupied the whole being often comes down in an extremely intense way and its influence is often resisted by the lower instruments. For Sri Aurobindo, "What is needed [in such cases] is the establishment of the calm and wide consciousness at the base of the whole Nature, so that when the lower nature ap- pears it will not be as an attack or struggle but as if a Master of forces were there seeing the defects of the present machinery and doing step by step what is necessary to remedy and change it."[38]

Spiritual transformation, like psychic transformation, has its limitations. According to Sri Aurobindo, "If the psychic mutation has not taken place, if there has been a premature pulling down of the higher Forces, their contact may be too strong for the flawed and impure material of Nature ... or the descending influence may withdraw or be split because the nature cannot contain or keep it. Again, if it is Power that descends, the egoistic mind or vital may try to seize on it for its own use and a magnified ego or a hunting after powers and self-aggrandising masteries may be the untoward result."[39]

The spiritual consciousness, like the inner consciousness, is diminished in its working when it is dependent on mere human instrumentation of the mind and may even lead to vital errors. In the words of Sri Aurobindo, "the numerous mistakes of reception or the imperfections of the vessel may impede the transformation ... at any moment the work may be stayed, because the nature is able to receive or assimilate no more,—for it has reached the present limits of its capacity,— or because the mind may be ready but the vital, when faced with a choice between the old life and the new, refuses, or if the vital accepts, the body may prove too weak, unfit or flawed for the necessary change of its consciousness and its dynamic transformation."[40]

The spiritual mind can unite the individual mind with the cosmic mind on its highest plane and make possible an action of universality, even if it cannot transform the whole human nature (the Inconscient) into the Supernature. "The Power has to come at intervals and work meanwhile behind the veil or hold itself back through long periods of obscure assimilation or preparation of the recalcitrant parts of Nature; the Light has to work in darkness or semi-darkness on the regions in us that are still in the Night.... A light and power of the Overmind working in its own full right and in its own sphere is one thing, the same light working in the obscurity of the physical consciousness and under its conditions is something quite different and far inferior in its knowledge and force and results."[41]

The psychic transformation, having risen into the spiritual change, has to be completed, integrated and uplifted by the supramental transformation.

Supramental or Integral Transformation

All powers of consciousness suffer a diminution of their dynamic capacities when they descend and work in the obscurity of the lower domains. They are, therefore, not able to bring about an integral transformation, the complete divine dynamisation of nature, a total and radical transmutation of even the darkest and most inconscient parts of the mind, life and body. However, these instruments of the Spirit are not condemned to function forever on the irretrievable basis of division and darkness, but are meant to recover their essential unity and be converted into the divine counterparts of light and purity; a union of the sadhak's instrumental being no less than of his or her soul and spirit must change one's imperfect nature into the very likeness of Divine Nature.

Sri Aurobindo defines the integral or supramental transformation as follows: "A supramental change of the whole substance of the being and therefore necessarily of all its characters, powers, movements takes place when the involved Supermind in Nature emerges to meet and join with the supramental light and power descending from Supernature. The individual must be the instrument and first field of the transformation; but an isolated individual transformation is not enough and may not be wholly feasible. Even when achieved, the individual change will have a permanent and cosmic significance only if the individual becomes a centre for the establishment of the supramental Consciousness-Force as an overtly operative power in the terrestrial working of Nature. ... There must be an emergent supramental Consciousness-Force liberated and active within the terrestrial whole and an organised supramental instrumentation of the Spirit in the life and the body. ... On this basis the principle of a divine life in terrestrial Nature would be manifested."[42] An isolated individual transformation is, therefore, not enough; the emergent Consciousness-Force must be active within the terrestrial whole so as to make the manifestation of the Divine in the earth-consciousness possible.

This integral transformation includes the double movement of an ascent towards divine knowledge, power and delight and a descent of the supramental Consciousness-Force in human nature. In the words of Sri Aurobindo, "There must be an ascension of the whole being, an ascension of spirit chained here and trammelled by its instruments and its environment to sheer Spirit free above, an ascension of soul towards some blissful Super-soul, an ascension of mind towards some luminous Supermind, an ascension of life towards some vast Super-life, an ascension of our very physicality to join its origin in some pure and plastic spirit-substance.... At the same time, there must be a descent too to affirm below what we have gained above: on each height we conquer we have to turn to bring down its power and its illumination into the lower mortal movement."[43]

A real integral transformation, therefore, needs not only a direct and unveiled intervention from above, but also a total submission and surrender of the lower consciousness and a cessation of its insistence on its own separate law of action.

The double movement of ascent and descent results in the union with God, where the false opposition and gulf between the lower and the higher existence, the finite and the Infinite is broken down; this is the divine fulfilment of the individual in the complete harmony of the cosmic consciousness and the realisation in the cosmic being of the transcendent *Sachchidananda*.

"At each stage, the higher parts of the nature may be provisionally but incompletely organised in the new consciousness while the lower are in a state of flux or formation, partly moving in the old way though influenced and beginning to change, partly belonging to the new kind but still imperfectly achieved and not yet firm in the change."[44] In this integral transformation the divine Force can come in freely and use the mechanical instruments as perfect conscious parts of its own manifestation; the lower instruments are not merely changed into passive channels for higher supramental activities but are themselves supramentalised, i.e., the supramentalisation of the physical, vital and mental parts of the being. This process of change does not take away anything from the external truth of the lower realm; it only removes its limitations with the help of the supramental Truth.

For Sri Aurobindo, "its governing presence [of the supramental principle] in the lowest forms assures us, because of the unity of all existence, that there is a possibility of their awakening, a possibility even of their perfect manifestation here in spite of every veil, in spite of all the mass of our apparent disabilities, in spite of the incapacity or unwillingness of our mind and life and body. And what is possible, must one day be, for that is the law of the omnipotent Spirit."[45] The integral transformation of human nature and life will be the ultimate perfection of man.

For the completion of this integral transformation, a passage from the obscure harmony of a blind automatism of Nature to the luminous authentic motion of the self-existent truth of Spirit, "a long, difficult stage of constant effort, energism, austerity of the personal will, *tapasya,* has ordinarily to be traversed before a more decisive stage can be reached."[46] The difficult result of this integral transformation can become possible only through a total reversal of our consciousness, a shifting of the position of the consciousness from the outer to the inner self, a habitual action from this inner self and an opening of the individual to the cosmic consciousness. Next, the sadhak has to open towards the participation in an action of Supernature, i.e., "the surrender of the whole being to the light and power that come from the Supernature, is a second condition which has to be accomplished slowly and with difficulty by the being itself before the supramental transformation can become at all possible."[47]

Sri Aurobindo assumes that the sadhak is already quite advanced in the psychic and spiritual transformation before the beginning of an integral transformation can take place. Sadhaks must first acquire an inner Yogic consciousness (the subliminal consciousness) in which their ordinary views of things and motives of life are replaced. Going still deeper they discover their veiled psychic entity, which psychicisises all their inner and outer parts and turns them into a conscious instrumentation of the soul. Then the being is spiritualised by a descent of a divine Light, Force, Purity, Freedom and Wideness.

The three steps of transformation, as described

above, should not be considered as strictly successive; the spiritual transformation may begin before the psychic transformation has reached its culmination, or the integral transformation may intervene in the midst of the psychic or spiritual transformation in order to speed up its pace and shorten the way.

The supramental plateaus of consciousness are far beyond the grasp of mental description or the possibility of translating such a process into a mental scheme. It is not possible for the untransformed mind to translate the radically different height of the supramental Consciousness-Force into human language. Sri Aurobindo does not ask everybody to become supramental; in the first step of transformation he asks sadhaks to turn their attention to psychic love and use the vital not for its own sake but as an expression of the soul's realisation. The difficult supramental change must be regarded as the end of a far-off perspective; it must not be turned into a first aim or an immediate objective. Yoga is a rapid conscious evolution of the being but, howsoever rapid, all evolution must proceed by stages. For Sri Aurobindo, "a hasty and ignorant mind, a too eager force easily forgets this necessity; they rush forward to make the Supermind an immediate aim and expect to pull it down with a pitchfork from its highest heights in the Infinite. This is not only an absurd expectation but full of danger."[48]

Transformation is not the central object of the traditional Yogas but, rather than a spiritual escape from life or a departure into some kind of celestial transcendence, the object of Sri Aurobindo's integral Yoga is a full descent of a new consciousness into the whole nature of man, which is essential to transform life.

Sri Aurobindo has formulated the idea behind the philosophy of integral transformation as follows: "An integral transformation is the integral aim of the Being in Nature; this is the inherent sense of her universal urge of self-transcendence. It is for this reason that the process of Nature is not confined to a heightening of herself into a new principle; the new height brings with it a widening and establishes a larger field of life in which the power of the new principle may have sufficient play and room for its emergence ... it includes a taking up of that which is lower into the higher values. ... Our mental, physical, vital existence need not be destroyed by our self-exceeding, nor are they lessened and impaired by being spiritualised; they can and do become much richer, greater, more powerful and more perfect; in their divine change they break into possibilities which in their unspiritualised condition could not be practicable or imaginable."[49]

NOTES

1. *The Arya*, 4th Volume, No.12, Reprinted 1990.
2. *The Synthesis of Yoga*, p. 4.
3. *The Human Cycle*, p.2.
4. Ibid., p.2.
5. *On Himself*, p. 180.
6. *The Synthesis of Yoga*, p. 2.
7. *Letters on Yoga*, p. 509.
8. Ibid., p. 99.
9. *The Synthesis of Yoga*, p. 4.
10. *Letters on Yoga*, p. 848.
11. *The Hour of God*, p. 50-51.
12. *The Life Divine*, p. 36.
13. Ibid., p. 486
14. Ibid., p. 68.

15. Ibid., p. 737.
16. *Letters on Yoga, p. 98.*
17. *The Life Divine,* p. 1012.
18. *The Synthesis of Yoga,* p. 616.
19. Ibid., p. 647.
20. Ibid.,p. 295.
21. Ibid., p. 157.
22. *The Life Divine,* p. 907.
23. *The Synthesis of Yoga,* p. 618.
24. Ibid., p. 647.
25. Ibid., p. 651.
26. Ibid., p. 663.
27. Ibid., p. 664.
28. *The Life Divine,* p. 397.
29. *The Synthesis of Yoga,* p. 702.
30. Ibid., p. 47.
31. Ibid., p. 592.
32. Ibid., p. 695.
33. *The Life Divine,* p. 891.
34. *Letters on Yoga,* p. 1113.
35. *The Life Divine,* p. 904.
36. *Letters on Yoga,* p. 1197.
37. Ibid., p. 1128.
38. Ibid., p. 1677.
39. *The Life Divine,* p. 914.

40. Ibid., p. 915.
41. Ibid., p. 915-916.
42. Ibid., p. 962 - 963.
43. *The Synthesis of Yoga,* p. 123.
44. *The Life Divine,* p. 956.
45. *The Synthesis of Yoga,* p. 454.
46. *The Life Divine,* p. 929.
47. Ibid., p. 929.
48. *The Synthesis of Yoga,* p. 268.
49. *The Life Divine,* p. 727 - 728.

Chapter Seven

The Psycho-spiritual Nature of Man

For Sri Aurobindo, man is the nucleus of the divine transformation, and man's main task is to transform the inconscient into the conscient and the superconscient.

The psycho-spiritual constitution of man is described by Sri Aurobindo not only in terms of the various layers of consciousness, but also in terms of the different parts of the being. There is a broad overlap between them, as it is through the various parts of the being that the seeker becomes aware of the various layers of the vertical consciousness.

When Sri Aurobindo refers to the many different levels of consciousness, he places them under three systems that are active simultaneously:

(a) a surface system, made up of the physical, vital and mental levels of consciousness which constitute the outer being;

(b) a vertical system, an ascending and descending series of super-imposed levels, extending from below the surface mind (the inconscient and the subconscient) to far above the reasoning mind (the higher mind, illumined mind, intuitive mind, overmind and supermind) up to Sachchidananda;

(c) a concentric or depth system behind the surface being in each of its levels, consisting of the inner or subtle physical, inner vital, inner mental being, and the inmost or psychic being.

THE PSYCHO-SPIRITUAL CONSTITUTION OF MAN IN TERMS OF THE VARIOUS LAYERS OF CONSCIOUSNESS

For Sri Aurobindo "there is a state of being experienced in Yoga in which we become a double consciousness, one on the surface, small, active, ignorant, the other within, calm, vast, equal, observing the surface being with an immovable detachment or indulgence or, it may be, acting upon its agitation to quiet, enlarge, transform it. So too we can rise to a consciousness above and observe the various parts of our being, inner and outer, mental, vital and physical and the subconscient below all, and act upon one or other or the whole from that higher status. It is possible also to go down from that height or from any height into any of these lower states and take its limited light or its obscurity as our place of working while the rest that we are is either temporarily put away or put behind or else kept as a field of reference from which we can get support, sanction or light and influence or as a status into which we can ascend or recede and from it observe the inferior movements."[1]

The Surface or Waking Consciousness

Man's outer or surface consciousness is composed of the mental, the vital, and the physical consciousness. The mental consciousness is related to the cognitive elements and functions, whereas the vital or Life-Nature is made up of feelings, emotions, desires and instincts. The physical consciousness or body consciousness has its own obscure limited and automatic awareness which one perceives as nervous and sensational modes of consciousness. The surface consciousness functions as an instrument of expression of the inner consciousness and the psychic; but at the same tune it receives influences from the inconscient and the subconscient below from, the subliminal behind and tvom the superconscient above as well as from the surrounding environment.

The Inner or Subliminal Consciousness

Sri Aurobindo distinguishes that which lies *below* the level of surface consciousness—the subconscient, from that which lies *behind* the surface consciousness—the subliminal.

"The real subconscious is a nether diminished consciousness close to the Inconscient; the subconscient, which we call subliminal is, on the contrary, a consciousness larger than our surface existence. But both belong to the inner realm of our being of which our surface is unaware, so both are jumbled together in our common conception and parlance."[2]

It can be said that there is near the surface consciousness an obscure subconscious element, but behind it is the depth of the subliminal, the totality of our concealed inner being. According to Sri Aurobindo, "the subliminal, with the subconscious as an annex of itself is the seer of inner things and of supraphysical experiences; the surface subconscious is only a transcriber. ... Our waking state is unaware of its connection with the subliminal being, although it receives from it,—but without any knowledge of the place of origin,— the inspirations, intuitions, ideas, will-suggestions, sense suggestions, urges to action that rise from below or from behind our limited surface existence. ... The subliminal has the right of entry into the mental and vital and subtle-physical planes of the universal consciousness, it is not confined to the material plane and the physical world."[3]

The subliminal consists of mind, life and senses like the surface being, but unlike the surface subconscious they extend to wider domains, have wider powers and are free from our limitations. The subliminal works constantly behind our normal waking self and is to a certain extent responsible for our movements and actions. The subliminal opens itself to the universal consciousness and is aware of the workings of a universal Mind, universal Life and universal subtle Matter-force. When the existing veil between the surface and the subliminal self is lifted, a free and conscious flow of energies from the inner to the outer self is made possible.

According to Sri Aurobindo the subliminal self "exceeds the physical mind and physical organs although it is aware of them and their works and is, indeed, in a large degree their cause or creator. It is only subconscious in the sense of not bringing all or most of itself to the surface, it works always behind the veil. ... This description is no doubt truest of the deeper parts of the subliminal; in other layers of it nearer to our surface there is a more ignorant action and those who, penetrating within, pause in the zones of lesser coherence or in the No-man's-land between the subliminal and the surface, may fall into much delusion and confusion."[4]

For Sri Aurobindo this surface subconscious cannot be explored by the sadhak's surface mental consciousness, but needs to be investigated and controlled by the subliminal consciousness and the Superconscient.

If the inner consciousness does not manifest, the outer will never get transformed but, once the inner consciousness remains stable and one lives in it, the exterior parts can be dealt with more thoroughly and become a proper instrumentation for the activities of the psychic being.

The Subliminal Consciousness and the Environmental Consciousness

The subliminal consciousness is separated from the environing cosmic consciousness through a limitation of subtler sheaths of our being, just as the surface consciousness is separated from universal Nature by the gross physical sheath. According to Sri Aurobindo, "The subliminal has besides a formation of consciousness which projects itself beyond all these sheaths and forms a circumconscient, an environing part of itself, through which it receives the contacts of the world and can become aware of them and deal with them before they enter. The subliminal is able to widen indefinitely this circumconscient envelope and more and more enlarge its selfprojection into the cosmic existence around it. A point comes where it can break through the separation altogether, unite, identify itself with cosmic being, feel itself universal, one with all existence. In this freedom of entry into cosmic self and cosmic nature there is a great liberation of the individual being; it puts on a cosmic consciousness, becomes the universal individual."[5]

The environmental consciousness thus serves as a medium of transition between the individual and the universal inner consciousness. Whereas the inner physical consciousness can be thought of as "connected with" the body, and the higher consciousness as "above" the body, so the environmental consciousness "surrounds" the body (aura) and through it the individual comes into contact with cosmic forces and with other beings. The universal forces of benediction do not pour directly into the individual; they first have to enter one's environmental consciousness. According to Sri Aurobindo, "The subliminal extends itself into an enveloping consciousness through which it receives the shock of currents and wave-circuits pouring upon us from the universal Mind, universal Life, universal subtler Matter-forces."[6] The environmental consciousness, in which are determined our unseen connections with the world around us, is not wholly our own realised self, but our self plus the external world-nature.

Experiences rejected from the surface consciousness either sink into the subconscious or settle into the environmental consciousness, from where they try to return even after long intervals. After subconscious movements have been expelled by the conscious self these rejected movements do not re-enter the subconscious or get abolished, but move into the individual's circumconscient where they no longer belong to the individual self. It is through this subtle circumconscient medium that waves of universal forces, such as desire, passion, sex, suggestions, etc., come in and take possession of the external being. However, according to Sri Aurobindo, "If the wall that separates this inner existence from the outer self were penetrated, we could know and deal with the sources of our present mind-energies and life-action and could control instead of undergoing their results."[7] But this can only be done when the individual has acquired a high degree of self- mastery.

The Subconscient

The environmental consciousness must not be confused with the subconscient. What is stored in the subconscient (impressions and memories) rise up from there into the conscious parts of the being. In the environmental consciousness things are not stored up and fixed, they move about there.

For Sri Aurobindo there are different planes of the subconscient:

(a) He distinguishes the subconscient from the submental although both appear to the individual as inconscient. The submental, which is below and inferior to mind, is void of mentality and less in possession of itself. The subconscient proper lies below even the physical and vital consciousness, it is the Inconscient vibrating on the borders of consciousness. According to Sri Aurobindo, "when we stand back from it [the mind], when we can separate our mind from its sensations, we perceive that this is a nervous and sensational and automatically dynamic mode of consciousness, a gradation of awareness different from the mind: it has its own separate reactions to contacts and is sensitive to them in its own power of feeling; it does not depend for that on the mind's perception and response."[8]

(b) The inconscient is not really inconscient at all, but a dwelling place of a secret consciousness, a suppressed or concealed consciousness in which there is everything but nothing is expressed. The incoscient uses matter as its field and this inconscient we see at work in matter, for it creates the material universe. For Sri Aurobindo, "Inconscience is a phenomenal state; consciousness is an inherent and eternal state of being, inconscience is its temporal, temporary and apparent condition when it forms itself by its own energy into Matter and material objects. Its consciousness involves itself in inanimate Matter and it seems there an inconscience. ... So it seems, but so it cannot be; there is something hidden from us which we have to discover. It is the consciousness behind the Energy, the conscious Being behind the action that we have to discover."[9] We may say, therefore that the inconscient is the most involved state of consciousness below the subconcient; it is an instrument of a secret consciousness which has created the miracle of the universe, and from this seemingly inconscient Matter emerge, successively, life and mind. The essential purpose of a growing evolution here is the emergence of consciousness in an apparently inconscient universe.

(c) The subconscient proper, lying below the normal and waking consciousness, below the level of mind and conscious life is the obscure consciousness that operates in the purely physical and vital parts of the being. The mind has no control over the subconscious area, and Sri Aurobindo describes

> this region as "the extreme border of our secret inner existence where it meets the Inconscient, it is a degree of our being in which the Inconscient struggles into a half consciousness. ... Or, from another viewpoint, this nether part of us may be described as the antechamber of the Inconscient through which its formations rise into our waking or our subliminal being."[10]

In integral Yoga the subconscient is that emerged part of our being in which there is no waking consciousness and coherent thought, will, feeling or organised reaction, but it does receive obscurely the impressions of all things and stores them up in itself. Sri Aurobindo observes that "The subconscient is the main support of all habitual movements, especially the physical and lower vital movements. When something is thrown out of the vital or physical, it very usually goes down in the subconscient and remains there as if in seed and comes up again when it can."[11]

This obscure mind—full of fixed notions and habitual reactions formed by our past—or obscure vital full of habitual desires and nervous reactions, or a most obscure physical which governs the condition of the body, surge up from time to time into the waking consciousness and are largely responsible for our chronic illnesses, and for the rigidity of our character structure.

The Superconscient

This is a level of consciousness beyond our present level of human consciousness, with which the normal individual being has no contact and which seems to it unconscious. In the superconscient are included the higher planes of mental being as well as the native heights of the supramental being. The superconscient is One with the self and the soul of the world and not governed by any phenomenal diversity, it is in possession of the truth and the delight of things. Sri Aurobindo describes the superconscient as follows: "If the subliminal and subconscient may be compared to a sea which throws up the waves of our surface mental existence, the superconscience may be compared to an ether which constitutes, contains, overroofs, inhabits and determines the movements of the sea and its waves. It is there in this higher ether that we are inherently and intrinsically conscious of our self and spirit... it is through that ether of superconscience that we can pass to a supreme status, knowledge, experience. Of this superconscient existence through which we can arrive at the highest status of our real, our supreme Self, we are normally even more ignorant than of the rest of our being; yet it is into the knowledge of it that our being emerging out of the involution in Inconscience is struggling to evolve."[12]

It is not possible to reach the summit or source of this supramental consciousness all at once, and moreover it is difficult for the intellect to grasp what is meant by the supramental consciousness, as it can only be understood after a certain approximation in experience.

THE PSYCHO-SPIRITUAL CONSTITUTION OF MAN IN TERMS OF THE DIFFERENT PARTS OF BEING

Man is not made up of one part, there are many parts, each having a personality of its own and each acting on its own behalf and in its own way. Man known to us is not the real man or the complete man, in one's true perspective. The confused or inadequate knowledge that we have of ourselves is due to the double aspect of our being, the outer and inner aspects. According to Sri Aurobindo, "Men do not know themselves and have not learned to distinguish the different parts of their being; for these are usually lumped together by them as mind, because it is through a mentalised perception and understanding that they know and feel them, therefore they do not understand their own states and actions, or, if at all, then only on the surface. It is part of the foundation of yoga to become conscious of the great complexity of our nature, see the different forces that move it and get over it a control of directing knowledge. We are composed of many parts each of which contributes something to the total movement of our consciousness, our thought, will, sensation, feeling, action, but we do not see the origination or the course of these impulsions; we are aware only of their confused results on the surface upon which we can at best impose nothing better than a precarious shifting order."[13]

It is through the practice of Yoga that the seeker discovers the extraordinary complexity of one's own being and finds "that every part of us—intellect, will, sense-mind, nervous or desire self, the heart, the body—has each, as it were, its own complex individuality and natural formation independent of the rest; it neither agrees with itself nor with the others nor with the representative ego which is the shadow cast by some central and centralising self on our superficial ignorance. We find that we are composed not of one but many personalities and each has its own demands and differing nature. Our being is a roughly constituted chaos into which we have to introduce the principle of divine order."[14]

In the outer surface nature, all parts are present together and it needs a strong power of introspection, self-analysis and close observation to find out the composition of our nature and the relation and interaction of these parts with each other. In the words of Sri Aurobindo, "A time must come for every seeker of complete self-knowledge when he is thus aware of living in two worlds, two consciousnesses at the same time, two parts of the same existence. At present he lives in the outer self, but he will go more and more inward, till the position is reversed and he lives within in this new inner consciousness, inner self and feels the outer as something on the surface formed as an instrumental personality for the inner's self-expression in the material world. Then from within a Power works on the outer to make it a conscious plastic instrument so that finally the inner and the outer become fused into one."[15]

Sri Aurobindo's dynamic view of the multi-layered structure of the psycho-spiritual make-up of the being needs a more detailed elaboration in order to avoid confusion regarding the different parts in the organisation of the being.

The Outer Surface Being

The different parts of the surface being each have a separate function and are distinct from one another, yet all of these external aspects interact with each other.

This surface being is composed of three parts:

1. The physical being.
2. The vital being.
3. The mental being.

The Physical Being

The body is just not unconscious matter, but a vehicle or expression- of consciousness made up of physical energy substance. The physical being is therefore not merely the gross body, but possesses a distinct consciousness of its own which is different from that of the mind and the vital, although interpenetrated by them. In Sri Aurobindo's words, "Each plane of our being-mental, vital, physical has its own consciousness, separate though interconnected and interacting; but to our outer mind and sense, in our wakmg experience, they are all confused together. The body, for instance, has its own consciousness and acts from it, even without any mental will of our own ... and our surface mind knows very little about this body-consciousness. ...It is part of the yoga to become aware of this separate consciousness of the body, to see and feel its movements and the forces that act upon it from inside or outside and to learn how to control and direct it even in its most and (to us) subconscient processes."[16]

The physical being consists of three parts:

(a) the body or material physical, the most visible part of the physical being, is mostly influenced by the subconscient rather than by the mind or the vital. It is automatic and mechanical in its functioning, has its own physical instincts and is subject to illness, decay and finally death. Regarding this gross material part, "it is hot necessary to specify its place, for that is obvious, but it must be remembered that this too has a consciousness of its own, the obscure consciousness proper to the limbs, cells, tissues, glands, organs."[17]

(b) the vital-physical (nervous being) refers to that part of the physical which is interfused with the vital consciousness. It functions as the instrument of the smaller sensations and desires of the outer gross physical material life, and its irrational actions are completely determined by its habitual instincts and impulses.

(c) the mental-physical is that aspect of the physical being which partakes of the characteristics of the mental consciousness. The mind in the physical being is fixed on physical objects and happenings. For Sri Aurobindo the mental-physical, when left to itself, functions like a machine, repeating customary past thoughts and old movements. The mental-physical part of the being has no direct experience of the existence of supraphysical things, it can only respond, with great difficulty, to the higher forces.

The physical being is mainly occupied with the corporeal life and habits of life, mind and the body. This is the normal type of personality, where all the other tendencies latent within the individual are subordinated to the maintenance of body and life. It blindly obeys the mind and the vital. The physical being, clouded by obscurity and limitations, determines the greater part of our waking self. It can be freed from these limitations through a constant union with the psychic centre of the being.

The Vital Being

The vital consists mainly of desires, impulses, and emotions of possession and enjoyment. It is often narrow and limited and subject to dualities such as pleasure and pain. If is under the strong influence of the ego and if uncontrolled, when it is enslaved by desires and passion, it brings disorder and disaster. Sri Aurobindo distinguishes four parts of the vital being;

(a) the central-vital consists of the stronger vital longings and reactions, e.g., ambition, pride, fear and passions of various kinds.

(b) the physical or lower vital does not act according to reason and is entirely concerned with insignificant desires and feelings such as food-desire, sex-desire, anger, disliking, etc. It supports all kinds of inferior movements of action and all kinds of external egoistic activities.

(c) the mental-vital gives a mental expression by thought, speech or otherwise to the emotions, desires, passions and other movements of the vital being. It expresses vital tendencies without subjecting them to the intellect. Through this mental-vital various vital passions, impulses and desires arise which distort the thinking mind.

(d) the higher vital or most mentalised part of the vital nature the larger dynamic movement of the conscious life-force is concerned with creation, with giving and self-giving, is capable of great love, sympathy, altruism, and is responsive to the greater objects of Nature.

The vital being is mostly related with self-affirmation, life-enlargement, and the claims of the ego, power and excitement. The nature of the predominantly vital individual is more active, stronger, and more chaotic than that of the physical man, but it is also more creative and energetic. Though this part is obscure and full of perversions it is an indispensable mediator between the inner being and the outer life and only a vigorous vital mind and mental will can govern the kinetic vital energies. The vital is essential for the divine or spiritual action, without it there can be no complete realisation in sadhana and in life. It is for this reason that the vital and its life-power must not be rejected and condemned in its very nature. Nevertheless, Sri Aurobindo insists on the dangers of the unregenerated outer vital which is full of desires and lower-passions, and the necessity of mastery and purification of them. He emphasises the subordination and subjection of the vital to the psychic and spiritual influences. According to Sri Aurobindo, "when people speak of a vital man, they mean one under the domination of vital force not controlled by the mind or the spirit. The vital can be a good instrument, but it is a bad master. The vital has not to be killed or destroyed, but purified and transformed by the psychic and spiritual control."[18] By the practice of sadhana the vital must receive from the self above its equality to all things and from the psychic within its general love.

The Mental Being

The vital has to be clearly distinguished from the mental; on the surface they are intermingled, but in themselves they are quite separate forces. The term 'mental being' refers to that part of the human being which deals with the cognitive functions and processes, and all the mental movements that are part of the individual's intelligence.

Sri Aurobindo divides the mental being into three parts:

(a) The physical mind, which binds us to the brain instrument and identifies us with the bodily consciousness, seems to us determined by the body because it is preoccupied with the physical workings, which it uses for its conscious superficial action in the material world. The physical mind, as the lowest sub-plane of the intelligence, attaches most''importance to objective things and outer life, and the subjective or inner existence is subordinated, to the greater claims of the exterior reality. It perceives the physical as factual and real, and whatever is not physical or objective is regarded as unreal. Other subjective beings are accepted only in so far as they can become objects of our external consciousness. However, the physical mind, preoccupied with worldly pleasures and material affluence, is less obstinate and can be more easily opened to the inner forces, because it is less dependent on the subconscious than the material and vital physical. Despite this, the physical mental being is limited in its functioning and without the influence of a widened consciousness the physical mind remains outward-oriented.

(b) The vital mind, as a mediator between the vital and mental, has its utility in ordinary life and human actions, but it often limits and falsifies the mental truth according to its own desires, passions and cravings. The vital mind, though energetic and creative, does not think or reason and if it uses any thought it does so not for the sake of reason but for the service of life-power; it imposes the dictates of these powers on the faculty of reason. The vital mind, as an instrument of desire, attaches immense importance to the satisfaction and fulfilment of the vital nature and life force. It is mostly concerned with defence mechanisms and practical needs, but also craves for the actualisation of unrealised possibilities. The vital mind is not satisfied with the physical and objective only, but seeks too a subjective, a purely emotive satisfaction and pleasure; it always enlarges desire and creates a dissatisfaction in order to look for something more than what life seems able to give it.

(c) The mental mind as a reflective mentality is the source of the pure thinker in us; it sees the world not in terms of life and body but of mind. Its preoccupation is with knowledge, the search for truth and the effort to know itself and the world. It inquires into everything, affirms and questions the evidence of the senses, follows the conclusions of reason, but unbuilds these mental constructions again to arrive at different, often opposite conclusions. The philosopher, scientist, intellectual creator, the idealist, and the dreamer are the present mental beings at the highest attained summit. Though the pure mental mind is the highest reach of the intellect acting for itself, for its own purpose, yet it cannot arrive at a final certainty, certitude or absolute conviction as it proceeds from a fundamental ignorance and has no hold on assured truth; there is still the veil created by ignorance between the mental and supramental action. The thinking or reasoning mind has therefore its own defects and limitations; it knows first by analysing, only thereafter it synthesises. It can control lower nature but cannot change it. Yet the thinking mind is a higher faculty than the vital mind. It has the capacity to discriminate between good and evil, virtue and vice; but in the performance of these functions it is often influenced by the physical or vital mind. Only by a strong will and severe self-discipline is the former able to rule the latter.

It is difficult for the human mind to harmonise these three parts of the mental being. According to Sri Aurobindo, "the ordinary man lives mainly in the habitual, [thought-mind or physical mind] and experiences a great difficulty in using at all or entering into the movement of the pure ideative mentality. [pure reasoning mind] The creative pragmatic mind [vital mind] is commonly too much occupied with its own motion to move freely and disinterestedly in the atmosphere of pure ideative order. ... The pure ideative mentality tends to construct abstract systems of truth, intellectual sections and ideative edifices, and either misses the pragmatic movement necessary to life and lives only or mainly in ideas, or cannot act with sufficient power and directness in the life field, and is in danger of being divorced from or weak in the world of the practical and habitual mentality."[19] Mind, therefore, can create a considerable mentalised harmony, but it cannot integrate the whole being and nature. These mental harmonisations can be steps on the way but are not final.

Human beings are complex entities. The material body, as the individual's foundation, supports a conscious life principle and a mental functioning; it is often difficult to distinguish these from each other, yet they remain separate entities in a dual experience. Not only can these various parts of the being be at war with each other, but each one is also divided against itself—each different part of the being has its different movements and all these discordant movements obstruct and influence each other. In integral Yoga the seeker aims to become aware of the separate yet interconnected consciousness of each plane, and to feel its movements and the forces that act upon it from inside or outside.

For Sri Aurobindo the outer being is only a means of

expression and not one's real self. The seeker is advised not to identify with it, for then the individual can change it so as to express the true inner personality of the Light.

The Inner or Subliminal Being

The outer being is by no means complete in itself, and the individual's total existence is much larger than one s apparent surface nature. This external being which we suppose to be ourselves is a confused mixture of mind formations, life movements and physical functions. When the individual goes behind, into the hidden planes of one's being, one discovers a large inner or subliminal existence.

According to Sri Aurobindo, "We find that the contradictions and the struggles of our surface consciousness are largely due to the contrary or mutually discordant tendencies of our mental vital and physical parts opposing and unreconciled with each other and these again to the discord of many different inner possibilities of our being and even of different personalities on each level in us which are behind the intermixed disposition and differing tendencies of our surface nature. But while on the surface their action is mixed together, confused and conflicting ... we find in this inner or subliminal being the means of directly distinguishing between what rises from within and what comes to us from outside, from others or from universal Nature, and it becomes possible to exercise a control, a choice, a power of willed reception, rejection and selection, a clear power of self-building and harmonisation which we do not posses or can operate very imperfectly in our composed surface personality but which is the prerogative of our inner Person."[20]

However, there is often a struggle between the inner and outer parts, the latter remaining attached to the things of the ordinary life while the former wants the Divine.

The inner being, unlike the outer being, receives and

responds to the physical and universal world directly, through the subtle senses of its more subtle inner bodies. It has the power to enter into direct contact with another consciousness or with other objects, and is able to achieve immediate knowledge of the occult. By entering into the subliminal or identifying oneself with it the seeker is able to observe the springs of one's thoughts and feelings, and the sources and motives of one's actions.

Like the outer being, the inner being is also comprised of three levels:

(a) the inner or subtle physical "is closest to the physical, and most like it. But yet the conditions are different. For instance, the subtle physical has a freedom/ plasticity, intensity, power, colour, wide and manifold play of which, as yet, we have no possibility on earth."[21] By identifying oneself with the inner physical being the individual can observe, the operative energies that build up the surface personality. This subtle physical is capable of clairvoyant faculties and telepathic communication.

(b) the inner vital, unlike the surface vital, is wide, vast and strong, without limitations. It is the reservoir of pranic energy which is in constant contact with the universal energy outside. When purified it can be an instrumental force for all the divine realisations as it is without ego and knows itself to be a projection and instrument of the Divine.

(c) the inner mind can directly know things by intuition and inspiration. The inner mental is much more comprehensive than the outer mental, it exceeds the physical mind and physical organs although it is aware of them.

The subliminal is connected with the small outer

personality by certain centres of consciousness. These channels of communication are also known as the various chakras. By opening these channels, the inner being can enter into the outer being. Only a little of the inner being reaches outer life, but according to Sri Aurobindo; "that little is the best part of ourselves and responsible for our art, poetry, philosophy, ideals, religious aspirations, efforts at knowledge and perfection."[22] So our surface being, though largely influenced by the subconscient, is also influenced to a significant extent by the subliminal from which it receives its inspirations, intuitions, etc.

The movement of going and living within brings a rush of new experiences, a larger capacity, greater vision and an enlargement richer than any delight gained in the vital and mental existence. An awaking of the inner being is characterised by the development of a state of neutral equanimity, an absence of attachments, and this quietude slowly penetrates the deeper layers of the being, where it prepares the outer life for a first change. The subliminal creates a larger, wider awareness and is able to open, penetrate and illuminate the submental and the subconscient.

The Inmost or Psychic Being

The individual's external consciousness is rarely aware of one's inner being because it is veiled from it. But once the inner being is awake it opens inwardly to the soul and above to the Self. Within this inner being of man is revealed the central being, the transcendent and Universal Atman. Sri Aurobindo distinguishes two aspects of the central being, the upper and the lower.

The upper part, the *Jivatman* is that aspect of man whtch does not change or evolve as it stands above the personal evolution, it transcends time as well as the individual expressions of life and mind. The central being as Jivatman puts forward a representative power on each plane of the individual nature: on the mental plane, the true mental being *(Manomaya Purusha)*, on the vital plane, the true vital being *(Pranamaya Purusha)*, and on the physical plane, the true physical being *(Annamaya Purusha)*. The true representative of the inner being is the psychic being *(Chaitya Purusha)* which is mostly concealed behind the mental, vital and physical plane.

This lower part of the central being, the *psychic being*, represents the true individuality in the process of evolution. The psychic being, as the centre of the individual self, is almost a deputy of the Jivatman, expressing itself in each individual life and existence and supporting it.

This evolving psychic being, in the projection of the Spirit, individualises what is eternal in potentiality. "The psychic is not universalised like the Jivatman, but is the individual soul supporting from its place behind the heart-centre the mental, vital, physical, psychic evolution of the being in Nature."[23] The difference between the self or Atman and the psychic being is that the former is felt as universal and the other as individual, and one psychic being can be in sympathy with the other but cannot unite, as pointed out by Sri Aurobindo, "the psychic being cannot take up more than one body. There is only one psychic being for each human being."[24]

At its origin the psychic being is only a spark of the divine consciousness, it is not fully master of itself and it is only through successive lives that it builds up a conscious life. In other words, the psychic being is the soul consciousness developing its manifestation from life to life, with the mind, vital and body as its instruments.

Sri Aurobindo differentiates the psychic being from the vital being. The *psychic entity*, (the soul) in its manifestation, takes two forms:

(a) The surface desire-soul, a superficial psychological element which is involved in vital cravings, desires, emotions, and happiness. It is centred on the individual's egoistic existence and this external form therefore creates the basis for one's egoistic self. In most men the soul is covered by the action of the external nature and many people mistake the vital being for the soul, because it is the vital which animates and moves the body. Thus Sri Aurobindo observes that, "All or most of the works of life are at present or seem to be actuated or vitiated by this soul of desire; even those that are ethical or religious, even those that wear the guise of altruism, philanthropy, self-sacrifice, self-denial, are shot through and through with the threads of its making. This soul of desire is a separative soul of ego and all its instincts are for a separative self-affirmation; it pushes always, openly or under more or less shining masks, for its own growth, for possession, for enjoyment, for conquest and empire."[25]

(b) The true soul, a pure power of love, light and joy, "is the psychic personality in us that flowers as the saint, the sage, the seer; when it reaches its full strength, it turns the being towards the Knowledge of Self and the Divine, towards the supreme Truth, the Supreme Good, the supreme Beauty, Love and Bliss, and opens us to the touch of spiritual sympathy, universality, oneness. ... If the secret psychic Person can come forward into the front and, replacing the desire-soul, govern overtly and entirely and not only partially and from behind the veil this outer nature of mind, life and body, then these can be cast into soul images of what is true, right and beautiful and in the end the whole nature can be turned towards the real aim of life, the supreme victory, the ascent into spiritual existence."[26]

The psychic being in its one-pointed orientation towards the Divine does not create rigidity, as the intellect does (its power is related to a spiritual feeling rather than to knowledge), or bigotry of impulses, as the one-pointed vital forces do. "Its action is like a searchlight showing up all that has to be changed in the nature"; it sees the Divine essence everywhere. Sri Aurobindo describes the character of the psychic being as: "In the first long stage of its growth and immature existence it has leaned on earthly love, affection, tenderness, goodwill, compassion, benevolence ... on all that can help to refine and purify the grossness and commonness of human nature; but it knows how mixed are these human movements at their best and at their worst how fallen and stamped with the mark of ego and self-deceptive sentimental, falsehood.... It may still admit the human forms of movements, but on the condition that they are turned towards the One alone ... It lifts the being towards a transcendent Ecstasy ... but it calls down also this transcendent Love and Beatitude to deliver and transform this world of hatred and strife and division and darkness and jarring Ignorance. It opens to a universal Divine Love, a vast compassion, an intense and immense will for the good of all... It is not attracted or misled by mental imitations or any vital misuse of these great deep-seated Truths of existence; it exposes them with its detecting search-ray and calls down the entire truth of divine Love to heal these malformations."[27]

This psychic being as one's own individual soul-being makes it possible for the individual to open and uplift the whole lower nature to the Divine and suffuse it with a spiritual consciousness; but it can also contribute to a quieting and purification of the mental, vital and physical consciousness if they submit to the psychic influence. If the psychic is in front it becomes easy to remain conscious of the things that have to be changed and purified in the external nature so that they become fit instruments of the Divine.

It is always the psychic being that is the real cause of and greatest help in the seeker's turning towards the spiritual life, but for a full opening of the psychic being the sadhak has to get rid of the mixture of vital motives with one's sadhana. Thus Sri Aurobindo observes, "Purity, simple sincerity and the capacity of an unegoistic unmixed self-offering without pretension or demand are the condition of an entire opening of the psychic being."[28]

The psychic personality is connected with *Prakriti* (Nature) and therefore not purely metaphysical but empirico-metaphysical. In itself it carries all divine possibilities, but in its actions the psychic being is affected by the limitations of the mental, vital and physical. The soul is therefore not the overt guide and master of one's thoughts and actions; it has to rely on the outer instruments and its expression is not always pure since it is mixed with the activities of the outer being. It is only by the heart's aspiration to the divine that the psychic being gets free from these limitations.

The Higher domains of Being

Like an opening of the heart centre within to the psychic being there is also an opening of the mind centre above towards a higher divine spiritual consciousness. The psychic and the spiritual belong to different planes; the psychic is involved in the external manifestation and is able to create a spiritual aspiration, whereas the spiritual is concentrated in the Divine above the external manifestation. The spiritual realm is independent of the psychic but gives the latter more strength and width. Usually, consciousness is imprisoned in the mental, emotional and sensational centres, but when the individual opens up the surface being begins to ascend in order to join itself to this higher consciousness, a vast consciousness full of freedom, peace and light. This is described by Sri Aurobindo thus: "We are not merely embodied minds; there is a spiritual being, a spiritual plane of Nature. Into that we have to heighten our force of consciousness.... Our imperfect mental instrumentation is not the last word of our possibilities; for there are in us, dormant or invisibly and imperfectly active, other principles beyond mind and closer to the spiritual nature, there are more direct powers and luminous instruments, there are greater ranges of dynamic action than those that belong to our present physical, vital and mental existence." 29

The spiritual mind is distinct from the ordinary mind; the latter is not a power of knowledge, it sees as if through distorting spectacles and its knowledge is coloured by its instruments. The spiritual mind is open to all knowledge from above, it does not think with the brain as it has vaster means of awareness than thought. It is marked by oneness and through this pure consciousness the seeker enters into the awareness of the Spirit and is able to see all things in their essential reality.

The spiritual planes above the mind are the meeting place of the ascending and descending forces; they range from what Sri Aurobindo terms the Higher Mind, the Illumined Mind and the Intuitive Mind up to the Overmind and the Supermind.

In the elaboration of the higher grades of the mind, Sri Aurobindo points out, "in themselves these grades are grades of energy-substance of the Spirit: for it must not be supposed, because we distinguish them according to their leading character, means and potency of knowledge, that they are merely a method or way of knowing or a faculty or power of cognition; they are domains of being, grades of the substance and energy of the spiritual being, fields of existence which are each a level of the universal Consciousness-Force constituting and organising itself into a higher status."[30]

The 'Higher Mind' as "a luminous thought mind" functions as an instrument of truth-cognition in its cognitive aspects, as it seems to be in possession of Truth. This thought is not an acquired knowledge but a self-revelation of eternal Wisdom.

The cognitive aspects of the Higher Mind are described by Sri Aurobindo as: "This higher consciousness is a Knowledge formulating itself on a basis of self-existent all-awareness and manifesting some part of its integrality, a harmony of its significances put into thought-form. It can freely express itself in single ideas, but its most characteristic movement is a mass ideation, a system or totality of truth-seeing at a single view; the relations of idea with idea, of truth with truth are not established by logic but pre-exist and emerge already self-seen in the integral whole."[31]

In its conative aspects it is marked by the effectuation of the Truth, laying a foundation of change and preparing the whole being for a superior truth of existence. Sri Aurobindo describes the conative aspects of the Higher Mind as: "this greater more brilliant Mind works always on the rest of the being, the mental will, the heart and its feelings, the life, the body, through the power of thought, through the ideaforce. The idea is put into the heart or the life as a force to be accepted and worked out; the heart and life become conscious of the idea and respond to its dynamisms and their substance begins to modify itself in that sense, so that the feelings and actions become the vibrations of this higher wisdom; the will and the life impulses are similarly charged with its power and its urge of self-effectuation."[32] By the realisation of the Higher Mind, the seeker becomes less bound to the automatism of the lower vital nature; the latter is now mastered by a greater enlightened thought, sight and will which is in touch with the Infinite.

In the 'Illumined Mind' the seeker proceeds from the power of Truth-thought to the power of Truth-sight. In the Illumined Mind thought is only a subordinate movement expressive of sight. The Illumined mind, turning the spiritual thinker into a mystic seer, illumines and transforms the thinking mind, but also the vital and physical being with its direct inner vision, inspiration and spiritual sight. According to Sri Aurobindo, "A consciousness that proceeds by sight, the consciousness of the seer, is a greater power for knowledge than the consciousness of the thinker. ... As the Higher-Mind brings a greater consciousness into the being through the spiritual idea and its power of truth, so the Illumined Mind brings in a still greater consciousness through a Truth-sight and Truth-light and its seeing and seizing power. It can effect a more powerful and dynamic integration; it illumines the thought-mind with a direct inner vision and inspiration, brings a spiritual sight into the heart and a spiritual light and energy into its feeling and emotion, imparts to the life-force a spiritual urge. ... In the transformation by the Higher Mind the spiritual sage and thinker would find his total and dynamic fulfilment; in the transformation by the Illumined Mind there would be a similar fulfilment for the seer, the illumined mystic, those in whom the soul lives in vision and in a direct sense and experience."[33]

As a power of Truth-vision, the 'Intuitive Mind' can take up into itself the intuitive functionings of all the parts of one's nature and recast them into its own higher mode, thereby achieving a more intense infegration of the being than was yet possible. Intuition can perform all the functions of reason and intelligence but by a superior process, grasping the object directly.

Sri Aurobindo distinguishes various forms of intuition; a power of revelatory truth-seeing, a power of truth-hearing, a power of truth-touch, and a power of true discrimination of the exact relation of truth to truth. But in the present stage of evolution the action of intuition in the individual is imperfect in kind as well as intermittent in action; it is clouded and altered to the needs of the heart or intellect.

As Sri Aurobindo further observes, "Intuition sees

the truth of things by a direct inner contact, not like the ordinary mental intelligence by seeking and reaching out for indirect contacts through the senses etc. But the limitation of the Intuition as compared with the supermind is that it sees things by flashes, point by point, not as a whole. Also in coming into the mind it gets mixed with the mental movement and forms a kind of intuitive mind activity which is not the pure truth, but something in between the higher Truth and the mental seeking. It can lead the consciousness through a sort of transitional stage and that is practically its function." [34] Intuition, being frequently interrupted by the mental movement, is therefore not in a position to give the individual an integral experience of the ultimate truth.

Intuition, as an edge or ray of a superior light, comes as a play of lightning flashes but is still blocked by our primary mind-substance. The next step of the ascent leads us to the Overmind. Sri Aurobindo describes the Overmind as a superconscient cosmic Mind which is in direct contact with the supramental Truth-consciousness. The preceding stages are not cosmic in nature but in the Overmind the consciousness expands to become a palpable principle and manifestation of cosmic Truth. To the vertical ascent is added a vast horizontal expansion of consciousness and in this boundless largeness the separate ego-sense disappears entirely. Egocentric movements may still continue, but the centralising ego-sense is entirely subordinated and only occurs as a ripple in the cosmic wideness. The power of the Overmind releases the mind from its close partitions so that the cosmic consciousness can open itself in the seeker, who then becomes aware of the cosmic spirit and the play of cosmic forces.

Sri Aurobindo explains the difference between the global Overmind Consciousness and the individual's imperfect synthetic mental .consciousness: "To the Overmind, for example, all religions would be true as developments of the one eternal religion, all philosophies would be valid each in its own field as a statement of its own universe-view from its own angle, all political theories with their practice would be the legitimate working out of an Idea Force with its right to application and practical development in the play of the energies of Nature. In our separate consciousness these things exist as opposites; each claims to be the truth and taxes the others with error and falsehood ... at best, each must claim to be superior, admit all others only as inferior truth-expressions. An overmental Intelligence would refuse to entertain this conception; it would allow all to live as necessary to the whole or put each in its place in the whole or assign to each its field of realisation or of endeavour."[35]

Though the Overmind is full of light and power, it is here that the separation of the Truth begins and where there is no longer the perfectly unifying knowledge, i.e., the Overmind takes various aspects of the Divine and separates them into different entities. It admits aspects of the One Truth but separates them, which originates tension in the limited surface mind. The Overmind can unite the individual mind with the cosmic mind, but it cannot lead beyond itself; it cannot dynamise the Transcendent, for it is only the Supermind that has the direct power of manifestation of the Transcendence. .

The 'Supermind' is difficult to describe in our ordinary mental language, for it is a different consciousness altogether and acts in a different way. Whatever may be said of it is likely to be misunderstood and only by growing into it can the seeker know what it is. As a general description, the Supermind may be characterised as a Truth-consciousness free from ignorance, in which the sense of integrality is never lost.

Supermind is situated between *Sachchidananda* and the lower creation, and is described by Sri Aurobindo as "a spiritual consciousness acting as a self-luminous knowledge, will, sense, aesthesis, energy, self-creative and unveiling power of its own delight and being.... Supermind lends itself to the action of the inferior instruments; it is always there indeed at the core as a secret support of their operations. In matter it is an automatic action and effectuation of the hidden idea in things; in life its most seizable form is instinct, an instinctive, subconscious or partly subconscious knowledge and operation; in mind it reveals itself as intuition, a swift, direct and self-effective illumination of intelligence, will, sense and aesthesis. But these are merely irradiations of the supermind which accommodate themselves to the limited functioning of the obscurer instruments: its own characteristic nature is a gnosis superconscient to mind, life and body. Supermind or gnosis is the characteristic, illumined, significant action of spirit in its own native reality."[36]

The Supramental vision is marked by an original unity in which there is no division. It differentiates but does not divide, it maintains the many in unity but it always acts on the truth of the indivisible unity. The Self is in each, each is in the Self and each is the Self; but the Self here is not the hard core of the ego in ignorance but the divine Self. All existence in all its variety and the whole cosmos is contained in the Supermind, but it also transcends the cosmos. In its transcendental vision the Supermind sees the universe in its right relation to the eternal reality of which it is one expression, and in its universal vision it sees all that is individual in terms of the universal as well as in its own individual terms; yet it also knows each in its inmost essence, of which everything else is a resultant expression.

CONCLUSION

Man with his many personalities consists of a multi-layered dynamic structure. The gradation of the various planes as a whole appears to be a great connected complex movement, and it is often difficult to distinguish them from each other. Mind identifies itself with the movements of the various parts, but when the seeker draws back one discovers that each part has a consciousness of its own. Each different part of the being has its own movements and all sorts of discordant movements obstruct and influence each other. Nevertheless, the various parts of the being are interdependent and the development of each of them depends on the development of all the other parts. The higher, from which the lower is derived and to which it is destined to be converted, precipitate their influences on the lower and the lower react to the higher, manifesting within themselves something that corresponds to the higher power and its action.

Through the practice of sadhana the seeker can become aware of the complexity of our present human nature, the confused interactions of the various parts on each other and the precise nature of the conversion each part must undergo in order to move from the mentalised vital animal to the fullness of one's submerged hints of Godhead.

It must be remembered, however, that while this classification is helpful for psychological self-knowledge, discipline and practice, it should not be erected into too rigid a formula. As these things run very much into one another, a synthetical sense of these powers is as necessary as the analytical.

Man in his or her real nature is a Spirit using the various parts of the outer being for an individual and communal experience of self-manifestation in the universe. This Spirit, in its infinite existence, limits itself in apparent being for individual experience, i.e., it assumes in the universal and individual nature the complexity of the infinite in the finite. The Supermind, mind, life and the body are the four instruments which the Spirit is using for its manifestation in the workings of Nature.

The first object of the sadhana aims at the expansion of the sadhak's self-awareness. As a *preliminary* step the seeker begins to acquire more and more control over the movements of all the faculties, through the practice of self-observation. At this time the seeker becomes aware of the need for self-purification—moral and psychological purity—to ensure further growth. This double operation of self-observation and self-purification is dealt with on all the levels of being.

According to Sri Aurobindo, "the transition to the higher principle means not only a difficult conversion of his whole mind and reason and intelligence, but in a certain sense a reversal of all their methods. ... In fact, the change is only possible if there is first a spiritual development on our present level of consciousness and it can only be undertaken securely when the mind has become aware of the greater self within, enamoured of the Infinite and confident of the presence and guidance of the Divine and his Shakti."[37]

Sri Aurobindo advises the sadhak to replace one's mental structure with the intuitive guidance of the Divine Grace, which is behind all one's activities. With this change in attitude the sadhak calls down the Divine Force and enables it to act on his or her activities. The constant aspiration to acquire higher levels of being, in order to establish some harmony in the chaos of the various parts of the being, needs a constant rejection of everything which is unwilling to undergo the process of transformation.

Nevertheless, to acknowledge the presence of Grace and to rely on its spiritual Force, which is supporting the seeker, does not grant that it will become operative. If the chaos in the various parts of the being is allowed an inner freedom to experiment, then could it be that a premature change increases the outer chaos rather than creating something more integral, even though the force of the Divine Grace is beyond this chaos and ultimately arranges everything? Does this chaos need some psychological structure and social order first, with all its limitations, before it can attempt any higher organisation in the various parts of the being, so as to avoid a possible catastrophe?

The results of Sri Aurobindo's psychological interrogations may not be very concrete in their conclusions, but their methods imply a broader base for understanding the various planes and parts of the being and human life; it includes the discovery of the inmost and highest self of man. Sri Aurobindo's metaphysical language is not always expressed in psychological terms, but this does not mean that the complexity of being has no psychological significance.

NOTES

1. *The Life Divine*, p.345-346
2. Ibid., p.223
3. Ibid., p.426-427
4. Ibid., p.560
5. Ibid., p.541
6. Ibid., p.735.
7. Ibid., p.736.
8. Ibid., p.559.
9. *Essays Divine and Human*, p.314-315.
10. *The Life Divine*, p.422-423.
11. *Letters on Yoga*, p.357.
12. *The Life Divine*, p.561-562.
13. *Letters on Yoga*, p.233.
14. *The Synthesis of Yoga*, p.69.
15. *Letters on Yoga*, p.1025-1026.
16. Ibid., p.347.

17. Ibid., p.348.
18. Ibid., p.346.
19. *The Synthesis of Yoga,* p.812.
20. *The Life Divine,* p.533-534.
21. *Letters on Yoga,* p.255.
22. Ibid., p.1165.
23. *Leiters on Yoga,* p.277.
24. Ibid., p.442.
25. *The Synthesis of Yoga,* p.164.
26. *The Life Divine,* p.226-227.
27. *The Synthesis of Yoga* p.146-147.
28. *Letters on Yoga,* p.1099.
29. *The Life Divine,* p.731-732.
30. Ibid., p.938.
31. Ibid., p.940.
32. Ibid., p.941.
33. Ibid., p.945-946.
34. *Letters on Yoga,* p.264.
35. *The Life Divine,* p.283-284.
36. *The Synthesis of Yoga,* p.599
37. Ibid., p.770.

Chapter Eight

Sadhana in Integral Yoga and Its Difficulties

INTRODUCTION

Sadhana as a vision and a path for the perfection of man prescribes methods and techniques for the alleviation of human suffering at various levels. Hindu philosophy, understood as a sadhana, starts with the practical need of explaining the human problem of suffering and ends with the spiritualisation and liberation of man. In other words, how to deal with and free man from the notion of suffering inherent in the human condition. According to T. Wilson, "*Sadhana* connotes the successful achieving of a desired end. The notions of activity, movement, change, process, struggle, and power are inherent in the concept. *Sadhana* is the instrument for the attainment of perfection *(siddhi)*. *Sadhana* is the healing of the division between theory and practice. The means by which the end is attained is not specified by the term; hence *sadhana* can be used in the context of science, of industry, of jurisprudence, of warfare, of persuasion, of instruction, of prayer and even of magic. No matter how siddhi is reached, the means to siddhi is sadhana."[1]

For T. Wilson, sadhana as a system of thought and way of life aims at the perfection of man through knowledge, morality, faith and love, i.e., the potentiality of perfection in one's own. being.

For Ken Wilber, "Eastern disciplines are not theories, philosophies, psychologies, or religions—rather they are primarily a set of experiments in the strictly scientific sense of that term."[2]

Sadhana as the embodiment of the means and methods of an all-round development for genuine spiritual realisation leads the seeker from finitude to infinitude, i.e., it unfolds the infinity of the finite Spirit within man. Sadhana can be described as a science of spiritual discipline, its means and methods of spiritual realisation aim at the conscious effort of the gradual unfolding of the divine elements which are present in all beings, and the corresponding transformation of one's whole nature. Spiritual progress signifies a process rather than a cognitive state.

The various forms of sadhana—devotion, action and knowledge—are not independent of one another, but mutually supplement each other. Each discipline may be regarded as a different stage which the seeker passes through in the course of sadhana. These different forms of sadhana are only a method, a discipline or way of life, and though closely related to the goal they should not be mistaken for the goal itself. When the means is mistaken for the end, the sadhak may end up in dogmatism and fanaticism.

The perception of the individual concerning an unsatisfactory world marked by suffering, evil and inadequacy is often the starting point of the spiritual urge. However, this imperfect condition of what is manifested to the individual is not the essence of the manifested world, and "the highest wisdom will lie not in escape, but in the urge towards a victory here, in a consenting association with the Will behind the world, in a discovery of the spiritual gate to perfection."[3]

Sri Aurobindo describes sadhana as "the practice by which perfection, Siddhi, is attained."[4] As the discipline of self-perfection, sadhana is a liberation of human bondage. Sri Aurobindo relates sadhana to "a liberation into divine resemblance out of the bondage of the human seeming ... we must form some sufficient working idea of the complex thing that this human nature at present is in the confused interminglings of its various principles, so that we may see the precise nature of the conversion each part of it must undergo and the most effective means for the conversion. How to disengage from this mentalised vital animal man the happy fullness of his submerged hints of Godhead, is the real problem of a human being and living. Life develops many first hints of the divinity without completely disengaging them; Yoga is the unravelling of the knot of Life's difficulty."[5]

By sadhana Sri Aurobindo also means "the purification of the nature, the consecration of the being, the opening of the psychic and the inner mind and vital, the contact and presence of the Divine, the realisation of the Divine in all things, surrender, devotion, the widening of the consciousness into the cosmic Consciousness, the Self one in all, the psychic and the spiritual transformation of the nature."[6]

Perfection in integral Yoga can be attained when each sadhak is able to follow his or her own path of Yoga. This indicates that the practice of sadhana is not a fixed system. Integral sadhana is not constituted by any set of mental teaching or prescribed form of meditation. On the contrary, it proceeds by a broad direction of determined personal effort, experience, aspiration and faith in the power of the divine guide, and by a rejection of all that is foreign to these things.

Sadhana conceives of a divine life upon earth and the liberation of earth-nature itself as part of the complete purpose of the embodiment of the spirit here. It is not an escape from the world to God, but a transformation of the seeker's integral being into the terms of God-existence, i.e., transforming one's entire being into God, "so that in a sense God Himself, the real person in us, becomes the Sadhaka of the Sadhana". It is often the mind and the vital which are dissatisfied, and if they feel the soul's sheer love for the Divine for His own sake, then the sadhana gets its full power.

For Sri Aurobindo, "the Divine can come early or it can come late [during the practice of Sadhana] but come it will if one is faithful to one's call.... The Divine knows best and one has to have trust in his wisdom and attune oneself with his will. Length of time is no proof of an ultimate incapacity to arrive: it is only a sign that there is something in oneself which has to be overcome ... when a demand is there for the Divine, a sincere call, it is bound one day to have its fulfilment. It is only if there is a strong insincerity somewhere, a hankering after something else—power, ambition, etc—which counterbalances the inner call that the logic is no longer applicable."[7]

This optimism is not a mere intellectual or philosophical view, but the soul's aspiration for light and truth. The. spiritual aspiration is innate in man and a sure sign of Nature's will for a higher way to fulfilment. The soul's dissatisfaction with imperfection as a law of life upon earth is a kind of divine dissatisfaction, and spiritual growth aims at the victory over imperfection. The growth of the soul is the growth out of darkness into light, out of falsehood into truth. Imperfection, such as evil, error, falsehood, is relative in its nature and not absolute, like Truth, Good, and Beauty, the inherent aspects of the eternal self-existence. Once the imperfection has been faced and endured it has to be rejected, overcome and transformed.

For Sri Aurobindo knowledge of the truth, "is an aid

and a partial guide. It puts up signposts, gives the names of the main roads and the already explored directions, so that the traveller may know whither and by what paths, he is proceeding."[8]

The process of sadhana, in which the. egoistic state of consciousness in outward appearances is gradually turned into a higher state where the universal and transcendent are able to transform this egoistic state, has three stages: (1) efforts towards an initial self-transcendence and the attempt of the ego to enter into contact with the Divine; (2) a laborious preparation of the whole lower nature to receive the higher Nature in order to transform our whole being; and, lastly, (3) the utilisation of our transformed humanity as a divine centre in the world. These three stages are, to some extent, successive, but each has its own necessity and must be given its place.

For Sri Aurobindo the object in sadhana "is not to remove all 'limitations' on the expansion of the ego or to give a free field and make unlimited room for the fulfilment of the ideas of the human mind or the desires of the ego-centred life-force. None of us are here to 'do as we like', or to create a world in which we shall at last be able to do as we like; we are here to do what the Divine wills and to create a world in which the Divine Will can manifest its truth no longer deformed by human ignorance or perverted and mistranslated by vital desire. ... Our yoga is not for our own sake but for the sake of the Divine."[9]

DIFFICULTIES IN THE PROCESS OF SADHANA

Sadhana, as the indispensable discipline for realising the aim of integral Yoga, is an intensive preparation of every individual wlio aspires for a divine life on earth. It includes the realisation of a rationally definable goal in relation to the world, other men, nature and God, rather than only the exclusive introvert process of self-realisation.

It is of utmost importance to have beforehand a right understanding about the nature of the goal of the path, the full content of the ideal and its immediate implications so that no effort is wasted. "The difficulty of the endeavour is a known thing, but the difficult is not the impossible—it is the difficult that has always been accomplished, and the conquest of difficulties makes up all that is valuable in the earth's history. In the spiritual endeavour also it shall be so."[10]

Sri Aurobindo would relate a spiritual crisis to the difficulty of harmonising the divine life with human living. Joy of the world, ecstasy of the Divine embrace, personal liberation and peace are an imperfect possession if they are dependent on inaction or aloofness, and cannot stand the storm and the battle the sadhak is bound to come across for some time during the practice of sadhana. The sadhak should "not be in too furious a haste to acquire even peace, purity and perfection. Peace must be ours, but not the peace of an empty or devastated nature. ... Perfection is demanded of us, but not the perfection that can exist only by confining its scope within narrow limits."[11]

Passivity of the soul that lives content in transcendent calm has to be fused with the activityof the divine helper and the divine warrior. For Sri Aurobindo renunciation of life and rejection of the world cannot be the goal of life, though an inner renunciation of attachment and the craving of desire are used as an instrument, i.e., a negative means for the removal of obstacles which stand in the way of the positive fulfilment.

Sri Aurobindo maintains that "in their apparent nature the two [the human and the Divine] are opposed; each is the reverse of the other. The divine is infinite and immortal being, the human is life limited in time and scope and form. ... The divine is infinite consciousness transcending and embracing all that it manifests within it; the human is consciousness limited by body and ego. ... The divine is inalienable self-bliss and inviolable all-bliss; the human is sensation of mind and body seeking for delight, but finding only pleasure, indifference and pain. ... The divine founds itself upon unity and is master of the transcendences and totalities of things; the human founds itself on separated multiplicity and is the subject even when the master of their division and fragmentations. ... Between the two there are for the human being a veil and a lid which prevent the human not only from attaining but even from knowing the divine."[12]

Sri Aurobindo's integral sadhana, as a progressive surrender of the ego to the incalculable but always inevitable working of the beyond-ego, is not an easy sadhana. The goal of yoga is always hard to reach, but the goal of integral Yoga is more difficult than any other—it is only for those who have the call, the capacity, the willingness to face everything and every risk, even failure. Failure should be admitted "as a passage as calmly as success until the hour of the divine victory arrives ... to revolt, to condemn, to cry out is the impulse of our unchastened and ignorant instincts."[13]

Everybody can do some kind of Yoga according to his or her nature, but there are few of whom it can be said that they have capacity for this Yoga."[14] A mere restless dissatisfaction with the ups and downs of ordinary life is not a sufficient preparation for integral Yoga. One who has not the courage to face patiently and firmly life and its difficulties will never be able to go through the still greater inner difficulties of the sadhana. Difficulties are to be met in the right spirit, and if the seeker does not come out stronger, then there must be some obstacle within oneself, some impurity or weakness which has to be traced and corrected. Some have to overcome the difficulties of their nature first, others have a splendid beginning but face all the difficulties afterwards.

According to Sri Aurobindo, integral Yoga "is a difficult Yoga to follow and not many can really meet the demands it makes on the nature ... this is a slow and difficult process; the road is long and it is hard to establish even the necessary basis."[15]

The path of integral sadhana is steep and does not avoid regions of darkness: "Fits of depression and darkness and despair are *a* tradition in the path of sadhana—in all Yogas, oriental or occidental, they seem to have been the rule. ... That is why whenever they come in you or others I [Sri Aurobindo]' try to lift up before them the gospel of faith. If still they come, one has to get through them as soon as possible and get back into the sun."[16] These periods of darkness, however acute, are temporary phenomena; those who seek the Divine have to persist in their seeking and after some time the darkness will gradually fade and light will come.

Alternations of states of brightness and darkness are the result of the nature of human condition. Sri Aurobindo knows perfectly well that "pain and suffering and struggle and accesses of despair are natural, though not inevitable on the way, not because they are helps but because they are imposed on us by the darkness of this human nature out of which we have to struggle into the Light."[17]

In some of his letters to sadhaks he describes his own struggle: "My life has been a battle from its early years and is still a battle [1935]. ... I have had [difficulties and doubts] worse than any human mind can think of. It is not because I have ignored difficulties, but because I have seen them more clearly, experienced them on a larger scale than anyone living now or before me that, having faced and measured them, I am sure of the results of my work."[18] "As for the Mother and myself, we have had to try all ways, follow all methods, to surmount mountains of difficulties, a far heavier burden to bear than you or anybody else in the Ashram or outside, far more difficult conditions, battles to fight, wounds to endure, ways to cleave through impenetrable morass and desert and forest, hostile masses to conquer—a work such as, I am certain, none else had to do before us."[19]

The difficult and complex course of integral sadhana is only for those who accept to seek its aim, by the true aid of faith and the guidance of the Guru. The call and aspiration to the necessity of a larger spiritual existence, something higher and beyond, needs the consecration of the sadhak to God. The call of the soul and the heart's aspiration must be genuine. It should not be confused or mixed with the development and satisfaction of the old external order of things or the surface orientation of the sadhak's lower nature. For Sri Aurobindo, "Our whole being—soul, mind, sense, heart, will, life, body— must consecrate all its energies so entirely and in such a way that it shall become a fit vehicle for the Divine. This is no easy task; for everything in the world follows the fixed habit which is to it a law and resists a radical change."[20]

The sadhak's desire for transformation is often coloured by the unwillingness of one's outer nature to surrender to a higher power. This resistance may come from some elements that are not prepared for a change, or from some mental or vital habitual formations, or some temporary inertia of the physical consciousness. The struggle is felt more in integral sadhana, not because these things rise more strongly in such sadhaks than in ordinary men, "but because of the intensity of the struggle between the spiritual mind which demands control and the vital movements which rebel and want to continue in the new as they did in the old life."[21]

The variations of bright and dark periods are almost a universal experience of Yogis, and Sri Aurobindo gives two reasons for this phenomenon: "The first is that the human consciousness either cannot bear a constant descent of the Light or Power or Ananda, or cannot at once receive and absorb it; it needs periods of assimilation. ... The second cause is some resistance, something in the human nature that has not felt the former descent, is not ready, is perhaps unwilling to change."[22]

A full practical self-consecration is a gradual and slow process, and often a long period of preparation may be necessary before there comes the irrevocable consecration. The true essence of sacrifice in the beginning of the practice of sadhana demands an indispensable discipline. However, sadhana includes a discipline far more difficult than mere ethical and physical austerities, and the seeker must enter this path only if he or she is sure of the psychic call. Not all can approach at once the Divine in the pure psychic way and need to be supported in the beginning of the practice by mental and vital approaches. It is for this reason that the seeker ought not to plunge into this path without a fairly long period of preparation and purification. This period of preparation enables the sadhak to arrive at the proper inner psychological condition to face the spiritual battles and sufferings. In one of his Letters on Yoga Sri Aurobindo describes that he" himself does not care to accept many into his path and rejects many more than he accepts."[23] "As for fitness and unfitness, nobody is entirely fit for this Yoga; one has to become fit by aspiration, by abhyasa [practice], by sincerity and surrender."[24]

Difficulties in the spiritual progress are common to all ways and seekers of Yoga. The ordinary Yoga usually concentrates on a single aim and is therefore less exposed .to relapses, but integral Yoga is complex and many-sided, and the seeker cannot expect any immediate smooth progress. As a matter of fact, integral sadhana is not an easy and smooth practice, difficulties seem enormous and radical and even incurable by their continuity. "To have faith enough or enough psychic sight to react at once or almost at once and prevent these attacks is given hardly to two or three in a hundred. But one ought not to settle down into a fixed idea of one's own incapacity or allow it to become an obsession.... Where there is a soul that has once become awake, there is surely a capacity within that can outweigh all surface defects and can in the end conquer."[25] "So long as a man has that faith [in the Divine], he is marked for the spiritual life and I will say that, even if his nature is full of obstacles and crammed with denials and difficulties, and even if he has many years of struggle, he is marked out for success in the spiritual life."[26]

The capacity of the outer nature is not enough, there must be also the call and will to seek the Divine, and persistence in the practice. Not everyone is suited for the practice of integral Yoga as it can be insistently demanding, "it is the way for heroes and strong souls, not for weaklings."27

According to Sri Aurobindo, "There can be for the seeker of the integral Yoga no clinging to resting-places on the road or to half-way houses; he cannot be satisfied till he has laid down all the great enduring bases of his perfection and broken out into its large and free infinities, and even there he has to be constantly filling himself with more experiences of the Infinite."[28]

It is essential for the seeker to go inside oneself with a complete dedication to the spiritual life without clinging to mental preferences or insistence on cravings and attachments. "If the little external personality is to persist in retaining its obscure and limited, its petty and ignoble, its selfish and false and stupid human consciousness, this amounts to a flat negation of the sadhana."[29]

Difficulties in the sadhana such as failures, struggle, lapses or states of darkness are harmful to spiritual progress. The rule in sadhana is not to let any of these difficulties depress the sadhak, but to stand back from them, observe their cause and remove it, for the cause is always the sadhak him or herself. These difficulties are not created by the practice of Yoga; in Yoga the seeker just becomes conscious of their presence. During sadhana, the struggle is transferred to the psychological plane where it will be much easier to sort out the disturbing matter and gradually the sadhak emerges from the struggle; these apparently superficial disturbances may afterwards still touch but not disturb the seeker.

It is not enough to open the inner and higher parts of the being to the Divine Force to change them; this relatively easy accomplishment only occurs in the initial stages of sadhana. The difficulty lies in the transformation of the lower parts, as explained by Sri Aurobindo: "The real difficulty even for those who have progressed is with the external man. Even among those who follow the old ideal, the external man of the Sadhak remains almost the same even after they have attained to something. The inner being gets free, the outer follows still its fixed nature. Our Yoga can succeed only if the external man too changes, but that is the most difficult of all things. ... The internal being of most of the Sadhaks here, however imperfect still, is still different from that of the ordinary man, but the external still clings to its old ways, manners, habits. Many do not seem even to have awakened to the necessity of a change."[30]

In order to get a better understanding of the obstacles in the transformation of the various parts of the being it will be helpful to describe in more detail the difficulties and opposition each part encounters in the process of transformation.

Difficulties of the Physical Being

When sadhana is taking place on the mental or vital plane it is easier to change because these levels are more flexible than the physical plane. In dealing with the physical plane, the working of the Force is slower than when it acts on the mental and vital planes, because the resistance of the physical plane is always greater. "The resistance in the physical nature is very obstinate as it has a constant tendency to despond and despair, to give up, renounce the aims and the endeavour, and to collapse."[31] But the resistance can also come "by attachment to old ideas, to preconceived notions, to mental preferences and partial judgements, to opinions and reasonings which come in the way of higher truth and to which it is attached."[32]

The nature of the physical consciousness is characterised by obscurity, inertia, clinging to habits, forgetfulness, constant repetition of the same thing, and mechanical movements. When the seeker descends into the physical consciousness to complete the preparation of sadhana, one may become too passive, and while neglecting to concentrate one's will to conquer the physical nature, the vital force may take advantage of the inertia of the physical consciousness to assert itself fully. This kind of passivity happens to many sadhaks when there is the descent into the physical nature. The transformation of the physical plane usually lasts for an uncomfortably long time, but need not be at all definitive. According to Sri Aurobindo, "it is the period of darkest night before the dawn which comes to every or almost every spiritual aspirant. ... It is a period when doubt, denial, dryness, greyness and all kindred things come up with a great force and often reign completely for a time. It is after this stage has been successfully crossed that the true light begins to come, the light which is not of the mind but of the spirit.... It is difficult to explain these things because the psychological necessity is difficult for the ordinary human reason to understand or to accept. [33]

To overcome the darkness of the physical consciousness, the sadhak has to understand that it is only a stage and one has to persist in faith. Moreover, "there is no human being whose physical outer consciousness is fit for the Yoga. It is by Grace and a light from above that it can become capable and for that the necessity is to be persevering and open it to the Light."[34]

Difficulties of the Vital Being

Difficulties on this plane are often more numerous and violent than on the mental plane, because the vital is not governed by reason but by the pride of the ego and the desire of pleasure. Like the ego, the vital is a good instrument but a bad master. A strong generative outer vital is full of life-force, a force for action or creation, and this life force is the indispensable instrument for all action of the divine Power on the physical nature and the material world. But the vital is also a force for ambition and the lower passions, and it is often difficult for such a lower vital ego to surrender and be purified.

It is the vital ego which is the main cause of difficulties which afflict the sadhak in many ways. The I or the self regarding ego persistently deflects the sadhak, and many are not able to avoid magnification of the ego when the ordinary limits of nature are broken down and a greater consciousness takes their place. Sri Aurobindo is aware of the dangers latent in the descent of power into an impure nature. This often stirs into activity the lower vital motives such as fear, anger and desire, or the lower mental forces such as doubt, ambition, denial, etc. Violent effort to pull down the. Force "may lead to violent reactions, or it may bring down contrary or wrong or mixed forces which the sadhaka is not experienced enough to distinguish from the true ones. Or else it may substitute the sadhaka's own limited power of experience or his mental and vital constructions for the free gift and true leading of the Divine."[35]

During the practice of sadhana, the sadhak is bound to come across the aggravation of certain lower vital movements, which means that the seeker has come to grips with the basic instinctive aspects of the vital nature, as expressed by Sri Aurobindo: "The exacerbation of certain vital movements is a perfectly well-known phenomenon in Yoga and does not mean that one has degenerated, but only that one has come to close grips instead of a pleasant nodding acquaintance with the basic instincts of the earthly vital nature. ... These things rise up like that because they are fighting for their existence.... I dare say seven sadhaks out of ten have a similar experience. Afterwards when they cannot effect their object, which is to drive the Sadhak out of his Sadhana, the whole thing sinks and there is no longer any vehement trouble."[36]

The purification of the vital takes a long time due to its habit of persistence in the habitual movements of the nature. According to Sri Aurobindo, "The vital ego itself must become conscious of its own defects and willing to get rid of them; it must decide to throw away its vanities, ambitions, lusts and longings, its rancours and revolts and all the rest of the impure stuff and unclean movements within it. This is the time of the greatest difficulties, revolts and dangers. The vital ego hates being opposed in its desires, resents disappointment, is furious against wounds to its pride and vanity; it does not like the process of purification."[37]

It is this magnified image of the seeker's ego which is the Master whom one serves: "This happens only too often in Yoga to strong but crude vital natures or minds too easily exalted when they allow ambition, pride or the desire of greatness to enter into their spiritual seeking and vitiate its purity of motive; a magnified ego stands between them and their true being and grasps for its own personal purpose the strength from a greater unseen Power."[38] To avoid the difficulties in the vital it is better to keep a vigilant connection with the inner and higher levels of consciousness and to prepare oneself for the reception of Light.

It must be clear that the vital part of us is indispensable for our completeness, its life-power is, therefore, not a thing to be rejected for its very nature, but it becomes a true instrument only when its feelings and tendencies have been purified by the psychic touch.

Difficulties of the Mental Being

The mind with its limited knowledge and hesitations and the tendency to cling to established ideas, does not want change. It usually takes a long time and its success at the beginning may be only partial. For Sri Aurobindo: "too great activity of the intellectual mind and its attachment to its own pride of ideas, its prejudices, its fixed notions and its ignorant reason may shut the doors to the inner light and prevent the full tide of bhakti from flooding everything; it may also cling to a surface mental activity and refuse to go inside and allow the psychic vision and the feelings of the inner heart to become its guides."[39] The mind while analysing details and constructing out of them some general results uses this slow and tardy process of concentration. For Sri Aurobindo the higher ranges of the mind have the capacity to rapidly bring about essential change.

It is often the overactivity of the mind that creates an obstacle to spiritual experience; mental ideas or intellectual conclusions are mistaken for realisations. Moreover, the restless activity of the mind blocks the descent of the true illuminating knowledge. This does not mean that a well-trained intellect is not a good preparation of the mind for greater knowledge, but it only creates ideas about greater knowledge and not the experience of knowing the true thing itself. There is also the conflict in the mental man which springs up between the higher and lower elements of nature, when the lower elements revolt consciously against the higher will, when each continually struggles for mastery. The continuous pressure of higher spiritual experiences may over-tax the physical mind and produce a sense of exhaustion or a reaction of dullness.

In sadhana the mind has to be quiet and its energy controlled and turned to a proper purpose. For Sri Aurobindo the intellect functions as a means for the reception of Light or an aid to the experience of spiritual states if it is open, quiet and receptive. When the mind is quiet and pure, inspirations and intuitions can come because the silenced mind is most receptive to the knowledge of the inner and higher consciousness.

Conclusion: Difficulties of the Lower Parts of the Being

During the practice of sadhana, the sadhak discovers that the various parts of the outer being are all mixed up, but when the seeker gets beyond this ordinary surface consciousness one discovers their distinctiveness and their separate forces. Their division or conflict is the cause of most of the more acute difficulties of the sadhana. The forces of the lower mental, vital and physical nature, standing in the way of sadhana, can do what they like by simulating experiences and building up unreal formations. Fluctuations in the power of the sadhana are unavoidable and common to all sadhaks until the whole being has been made ready for the transformation. When the psychic is in front, then the opposing forces of the lower vital or mental with its ordinary movements and ignorant action cannot come in.

It is possible for the mind to accept the Divine, while the vital remains lost in its desires and passions of the ordinary life. The vital or mechanical physical mind can come up and act as the chief disturber of silence when peace descends into the thinking mind, or else the lower vital mind can bring up the ego and passions. If these influences are not eliminated, and the higher powers begin to descend, the lower may come across and cover up the descent, and the stimulation it gives is misused for the purposes of the lower nature. It is mainly due to this reason that many sadhaks fall into a state of magnified ego, upheavals, exaggerated sex or other vital passions after having higher spiritual experiences. As pointed out by Sri Aurobindo, "Although there is no ego in the spiritual planes, yet by the spiritual experience the ego on the lower planes may get aggrandised through the pride and wrong reception of the experience. Also one may by entering into the larger mental and vital planes aggrandise the ego. These things are always possible so long as the higher consciousness and the lower are not harmonised in the being and the lower transformed into the nature of the higher."[40]

Egoism is one of the greatest dangers in sadhana, and in most sadhaks the ego proves to be the stumbling block in the development towards a truly spiritual individuality. "This Yoga can only be done to the end by those who are in total earnest about it and ready to abolish their little human ego and its demands in order to find themselves in the Divine. It cannot be done in a spirit of levity or laxity; the work is too high and difficult, the adverse powers in the lower Nature too ready to take advantage of the least sanction or the smallest opening, the aspiration and tapasya needed too constant and intense. It cannot be done if there is a petulant self-assertion of the ideas of the human mind or wilful indulgence of the demands and instincts and pretensions of the lowest part of the being, commonly justified under the name of human nature.... It cannot be done if you cling to your past self and its old mental, vital and physical formations and habits; one has continually to leave behind his past selves and to see, act and live from an always higher and higher conscious level. It cannot be done if you insist on "freedom" for your human mind and vital ego."[41]

The outer instruments of human nature have no force to carry the seeker through the severe ardour of the spiritual journey; "only his spirit's august and steadfast will and the quenchless fire of his soul's invincible ardour are sufficient for this difficult transformation and this high improbable endeavour."[42]

If our nature is not an instrument which is created for the purpose of condemning it or denying its utility, but if it is considered an instrument for some definite end—say divine purpose, i.e., it is created for the progressive expression or manifestation of the Divine—then its essential unity with the divine counterparts can be brought about and converted into force and light. "The secret reason of man's failure to rise truly beyond himself is a fundamental incapacity in the mind, the life and the body to organise the highest integral truth and power of the spirit. And this incapacity exists because mind and life and matter are in their nature depressed and imperfect powers of the Infinite that need to be transformed into something greater than themselves before they can escape from their depression and imperfection; in their very nature they are a system of partial and separated values and cannot adequately express or embody the integral and the one ... they cannot arrive of themselves at any but a provisional, limited and imperfect harmony and order.... But there is more behind and above, there are greater more unmistakably harmonious values, greater truly perfect powers of the Spirit than mind, life and matter and these wait for their expression and only when they are expressed can we escape from this system of harmony through discords and of a perfection in the whole that subsists by imperfection in the detail."[43]

It is known that the movements of the lower human and higher spiritual nature pull different ways, and that the lower is at first much stronger. Sadhana does not leave the one for the other so that the sadhak can live a double life. The lower realm is gradually remoulded in the light and joy of the higher.

Besides the difficulties in the movements of the outer parts of the being which are attached to the realm of the lower nature, there are also difficulties the sadhak has to face in the transformation of the inner human nature; each of the triple transformations has its own difficulties and dangers.

Difficulties in the Intermediate Zone

In the process of going inwards, two complementary movements take place; the outward-coming of the inner being and the inward-going of. the consciousness to become aware of the inner self and nature. The outer being is not the primary source of the spiritual urge; it is the inner being which seeks union, and when the inner being comes to the fore, all becomes possible which is impossible for the outer nature when left to itself.

The movement of going inward should be natural and carried out without haste. The sadhak has to pass through an intermediate zone before entering the field of pure Truth, Light, Power and Bliss. If this movement is shuffled in an excessive hurry and eagerness, with an exaggerated self-confidence, relying only on the sadhak's mind, all sorts of mental and vital delusions take place.

A very uncertain and mixed beginning is characterised by an excessive pre-occupation with the illusions or rather the incertitude and incompleteness of the supra-physical or subtle worlds. When seekers get in touch with the larger mental or vital world, which pours down with great force, they feel themselves freed from the normal limits, overwhelmed by the first rush of power of a supernormal condition. But this intermediate stage is not definite and final, as it usually lacks the necessary knowledge and experience.

In the intermediate zone the seeker gets out of the personal consciousness and opens to the cosmic consciousness without having yet transcended the human mind levels. One is not in direct contact with the Divine Truth on its own levels, but still can receive some information from them. "It is a borderland where all the worlds meet, mental, vital, subtle physical, pseudo-spiritual—but there is no order or firm foothold—a passage between the physical and the true spiritual realms."[44]

One may cross this zone without being hurt as long as the seeker remains aware of its half-lights and its often mixed and misleading experiences. It is not necessary for every sadhak to struggle through the intermediate zone. Those who follow scrupulously a strict guidance or have the psychic being in front of their nature, or a central sincerity, pass safely. In the words of Sri Aurobindo, "if one has purified oneself, if there is no abnormal vanity, egoism, ambition or other strong misleading element, or if one is vigilant and on one's guard, or if the psychic is in front, one can either pass rapidly and directly or with a minimum of trouble into the higher zones of consciousness where one is in direct contact with the Divine Truth."[45]

However, "one may also go astray in it, follow false voices and mendacious guidance, and that ends in a spiritual disaster; or one may take up one's abode in this intermediate zone, care to go no farther and built there some half-truth which one takes for the whole truth—that is what happens to many sadhaks and yogis."[46]

Many sadhaks wander in this intermediate zone for a long time, and many never get out of it. These sadhaks take all the pseudo-spiritual experiences as true and real without discrimination; they confuse this intermediate consciousness with the supreme realisation, or they mistake a touch of force for the full Divine Force, or mix up an entirely illumined consciousness with a partial illumination of the mental or vital plane. If the purification has not been complete the sadhak may become a prisoner of those inner and wider levels of consciousness. Unfamiliar or supernormal experiences, which may engulf the sadhak before the tranquillising purification of the outer nature has been effected, may create chaos or push the seeker into an obscure battlefield full of secret misleading and violent oppositions.

As mentioned above, the best safeguard against the lures of the intermediate stage in the beginning practice of sadhana is the establishment of an inner purity and sincerity in which the sadhak is only motivated by the higher call until the psychic is in front, and an opening of a higher consciousness from above rather than a larger vital consciousness.

Difficulties of the Subliminal Being

By going inward and living within, the sadhak can find one's true existence: integral Yoga is not possible unless the seeker leaves the outer self and becomes aware of one's inner or subliminal being and inner nature. According to Sri Aurobindo, "What we discover within this secret part of our-selves is an inner being, a soul, an inner mind, an inner life, an inner subtle-physical entity which is much larger in its potentialities, more capable of a manifold knowledge and dynamism than our surface mind, life or body; especially, it is capable of a direct communication with the universal forces, movements, objects of the cosmos, a direct feeling and opening to them, a direct action on them and even a widening of itself beyond the limits of the personal mind, the personal life, the body, so that it feels itself more and more a universal being no longer limited by the existing walls of our too narrow mental, vital, physical existence. This widening can extend itself to a complete entry into the consciousness of cosmic Mind, into unity with the universal Life, even into a oneness with universal Matter."[47]

A certain separation between the outer and inner being is necessary for some time after the seeker has become aware of both the inner and outer parts. Without this separation they may disrupt, invade or confuse either part by the movement of the two separated worlds before they are ready to harmonise.

The subliminal being has also the means of directly distinguishing between what rises from within, and what comes to us from outside. The sadhak has the means to exercise a control over this power of harmonisation, provided the seeker has the right psychic and mental will in the endeavour.

If the vital-ego motive or illusions of the mind seek entry into the subliminal being, then it may result in an exaggeration of ego and desire. When the actions of the inner ranges of the subliminal are subject to the grosser desires of the mind and the vital being, in spite of its wider range of power and capacities, or by distortions of the will and false distorted intuitions and inspirations, the sadhak is lost in a zone of danger. According to Sri Aurobindo, "If there is too much egoism in the nature of the seeker or a strong passion or an excessive ambition, vanity or other dominating weakness, or an obscurity of the mind or a vacillating will or a weakness of the lifeforce or an unsteadiness in it or want of balance, he is likely to be seized on through these deficiencies and to be frustrated or to deviate, misled from the true way of the inner life and seeking into false paths, or to be left wandering about in an intermediate chaos of experiences and fail to find his way out into the true realisation."[48] The change from the surface consciousness to the inner being is difficult, "because the outer nature opposes the movement and clings to its normal accustomed poise and externalised way of existence and, in addition, because there is a long way from the surface to the depths in which the psychic entity is veiled from us, and this intervening space is filled with a subliminal nature and nature-movements which are not by any means all of them favourable to the completion of the inward movement. The outer nature has to undergo a change of poise, a quieting, a purification and fine mutation of its substance and energy by which the many obstacles in it rarefy, drop away or otherwise disappear; it then becomes possible to pass through to the depths of our being and from the depths so reached a new consciousness can be formed."[49]

Difficulties in Psychic Transformation

For a psychic transformation it is essential that the various parts of the lower nature undergo a change through a process of purification and quieting. In the psychic transformation, "All that is ignorant, obscure, perverted or simply imperfect and inferior in the being is raised up, perhaps brought to its acme, dealt with, corrected, exhausted, shown its own disastrous results, compelled to call for its own cessation or transformation or expelled as worthless or incorrigible from the nature. This cannot be a smooth and even process; there afe alternations of day and night, illumination and darkness, calm and construction or battle and upheaval, heights of hope and abysses of despair."[50]

It is difficult to change and purify the various parts of the outer lower nature as it opposes this psychic movement and clings to its old accustomed habits. The sadhak may, before the tranquillising purification, try to break down the wall screening his or her inner being from outer awareness by a strong call and aspiration, or a violent effort and an effective discipline. Such a premature movement is not without its serious dangers. "In entering within one may find oneself amidst a chaos of unfamiliar and supernormal experiences to which one has not the key or a press of subliminal or cosmic forces, subconscient, mental, vital, subtle-physical, which may unduly sway or chaotically drive the being, encircle it in a cave of darkness, or keep it wandering in a wilderness of glamour, allurement, deception, or push it into an obscure battlefield full of secret and treacherous and misleading or open and violent oppositions."[51]

This long and difficult process needs the total surrender of the self and of all the parts of our nature to the Divine, which may be supplemented by the method of detachment from all mental, vital and physical claims and impulses, austerity and the rejection of false needs and false habits. If equality and the psychic light are also there, then this process will be rid of its worst dangers. Guidance and protection will support the sadhak through the difficulties and trials of the psychic transformation, for the inner impulsion will be present throughout. The psychic change may be complete, and can be done by a painless process; still it must be a long and scrupulous programme, "otherwise one has to be satisfied with a partial result or, if one's own scrupulousness of perfection or hunger of the spirit is insatiable, consent to a difficult, often painful and seemingly interminable action."[52]

In a momentary revelation when the psychic being with its Light, Power and Bliss reveals itself, a long comprehensive working will then have begun, sometimes intense, sometimes slow. At times a divine Power comes in front and enlightens, at others it withdraws into the background and seems to leave the seeker to one's own resources.

Difficulties in Spiritual Transformation

The repeated movement of ascent of the lower consciousness enables the mind, the vital and the physical to come into touch with the higher planes up to the supramental and get permeated with their light and power. This upward opening puts the sadhak into direct relation with the whole Divine and is able to create within the seeker a new birth of the Spirit. The repeated movement of descent of the higher spiritual consciousness enables the transformation of the whole being. The descent works at the same time for perfection as well as liberation; it deals with the whole nature, part by part, rejecting and recreating.

However, the upward movement, like the inward movement, has its dangers for the practitioners of sadhana. The higher spiritual zone in the upward movement is related to a confused condition in which the sadhak is stepping into the rarer regions of the cosmic realm without having yet transcended the human mind levels. The sadhak is able to receive indirectly some intimations of divine Truth, but in the process of descent from above the forces of the lower nature are often stimulated and excited and want to mix with it and turn it to their profit.

Sri Aurobindo observes that, "If the human mind or the vital desire seizes hold on the descending force and tries to use it according to its own limited and erring ideas or flawed and egoistic impulses—and this is inevitable in some degree until the lower mortal has learned something of the way of that greater immortal nature—stumblings and deviations hard and seemingly insuperable obstacles and wounds and suffering cannot be escaped and even death or utter downfall are not impossible. Only when the conscious integral surrender to the Divine has been learned by mind and life and body, can the way of the Yoga become easy, straight, swift and safe."[53]

The main difficulty of the errors and stumblings of the higher spiritual zone are its powers to deceive and mislead the sadhak, attributing creations and formations of one's own mind, vital or ego to the power of the Divine. It often happens that some undivine powers present themselves as a supreme authority and demand the seeker's service and surrender. These undivine powers, eager to create a mental and vital formation in the earth life, use the thought and will of the sadhak, making him or her an instrument for some apparently brilliant but ignorant formation. When this is accepted there will be disastrous consequences. If the vaster and more powerful consciousness and its unlimited possibilities are tied to one's ego, then the sadhak becomes much more egoistic than the average man.

A magnified ego becomes one of the most perilous obstacles to liberation and perfection. In the words of Sri Aurobindo,"The Truth is not that God moves, round the ego as the centre of existence and can be judged by the ego, but that the Divine is itself the centre and that the experience of the individual only finds its own true truth when it is known in the terms of the universal and transcendent. Nevertheless, to substitute this conception for the egoistic without an adequate base of knowledge may lead to the substitution of new but still false and arbitrary ideas for the old and bring about a violent instead of a settled disorder of right values."[54]

But even if there is an entire dissolution of the old egocentric order, when the outer nature continues by a mechanical movement of past energies it may become a field of an apparent incoherence, although the inner nature is luminous with the Self. Only the descent of the Supermind can establish in the outer as well as the inner existence the harmony of the Spirit. According to Sri Aurobindo, "Obstacle, inner struggle, disparity, difficulty, discord of parts and movements continues in the transformation of mind to supermind only so long as the action, influence or pressure of the mind insisting on its own methods of construction continues or its process of building knowledge or thought and will of action on the foundation of a primal ignorance resists the opposite process of supermind organising all as a luminous manifestation out of the self and its inherent and eternal self-knowledge."[55]

It is, therefore, indispensable for the universal man to undergo a thorough process of self-purification and eliminate the ego from every segment of life in order to avoid the aggrandisement of the ego. When the ego is still not eliminated it may impose itself on the environment or it may glorify the vital and the mind into convincing the sadhak that its interests are the interests of others.

Difficulties in Supramental Transformation

As has already been indicated, a restless mind which endeavours to make the Supermind an immediate aim is full of dangers, for the vital desire may very well bring in an action of dark or vehement vital powers which hold out before it a promise of immediate fulfilment of its impossible longing; the consequence is likely to be a plunge into many kinds of self-deception, a yielding to the falsehoods and temptations of the forces of darkness, a hunt for supernormal powers, ...a fatal self-inflation into an unnatural inhuman and undivine bigness of magnified ego... or a deviation into some kind of morbid abnormality of the nature may be the untoward consequence. This is not a Yoga in which abnormality of any kind, even if it be an exalted abnormality, can be admitted as a way to self-fulfilment or spiritual relisation."[56]

Like the obstinate difficulties in the psychic and spiritual transformation, the lower parts of our nature are still subject to the lower automatism of habit, and these parts refuse to give up their response to the lower laws of nature. They remain attached to the old mechanical reactions and seek to reaffirm them as the eternal rule of Nature. The mind, accustomed to act within limits, may try to supramentalise itself or may develop a considerable power of intuitive half- supramentalised. knowledge, but the will may remain untransformed; the other emotional and nervous parts of the being may continue to be equally unregenerate. There may be the development of an inspired will but no corresponding uplifting of the mental or the emotional being. Or the vital and the physical mind may try to supramentalise themselves, but the thinking mind may remain as it was. For Sri Aurobindo, "this pilgrimage of ascension and this descent for the labour of transformation must be inevitably a battle, a long war with ourselves and with opposing forces around us which, while it lasts, may well seem interminable. For all our old obscure and ignorant nature will contend repeatedly and obstinately with the transforming Influence, supported in its stark resistance by most of the established forces of environing universal Nature."[57]

Conclusion Difficulties in Sadhana

"The road of Yoga is long, every inch of ground has to be won against much resistance and no quality is more needed by the sadhak than patience and single-minded perseverance with a faith that remains firm through all difficulties, delays and apparent failures."[58]

An integral transformation is obviously often strewn with obstacles of every kind; dark periods are relieved by bright ones. In a straightforward passage in *The Hour of God* Sri Aurobindo explains the difficult process of sadhana as follows: "The outer instruments of mortal man have no force to carry him through the severe ardours of this spiritual journey and Titanic inner battle or to meet its terrible or obstinate ordeals or nerve him to face and overcome its subtle and formidable dangers. Only his spirit's august and steadfast will and the quenchless fire of his soul's invincible ardour are sufficient for this difficult transformation and this high improbable endeavour. Imagine not the way is easy; the way is long, arduous, dangerous, difficult. At every step is an ambush, at every turn a pitfail. A thousand seen or unseen enemies will start up against thee, terrible in subtlety against thy ignorance, formidable in power against thy weakness. And when with pain thou hast destroyed them, other thousands will surge up to take their place ... each step forward is a battle. ... But thou sayst God's hand will be with me and the Divine Mother near with her gracious smile of succour? And thou knowest not then that God's Grace is more difficult to have or to keep than the nectar of the Immortals? ... And if his presence is felt behind the veil, yet is it like the winter sun behind clouds and saves not from the rain and snow and the calamitous storm and the harsh wind and the bitter cold and the atmosphere of a sorrowful grey and the dun weary dullness. Doubtless the help is there even when it seems to be withdrawn, but still is there the appearance of total night with no sun to come and no star of hope to please in the darkness. Beautiful is the face of the Divine Mother, but she too can be hard and terrible. Nay then, is the divine life a prize without effort, or the crown for a weakling?"[59]

Sadhana cannot be successfully undertaken unless there is a strong awakening to the necessity of the larger spiritual existence. "If the change [in the seeker of the Divine consecrating oneself to God] comes suddenly and decisively by an overpowering influence, there is no further essential or lasting difficulty…But this is not always the manner of the commencement. The Sadhaka is often led gradually and there is a long space between the first turning of the mind and the full assent of the nature to the thing towards which it turns. .... In such cases, a long period of preparation may be necessary before there comes the irrevocable consecration; and in some instances it may not come. There may be some advance, there may be a strong effort, even much purification; but the life will either be spent in preparation or, a certain stage having been reached, the mind pushed by an insufficient driving-force may rest content at the limit of the effort possible to it. Or there may even be a recoil to the lower life,—what is called in the ordinary parlance of Yoga a fall from the path. This lapse happens because there is a defect at the very centre. The intellect has been interested, the heart attracted, the will has strung itself to the effort, but the whole nature has not been taken captive by the Divine ... here has been an experiment, perhaps even an eager experiment, but not a total self-giving to an imperative need of the soul to an unforsakable ideal. Even such imperfect Yoga has not been wasted; for no upward effort is made in vain. Even if it fails in the present or arrives only at some preparatory stage or preliminary realisation, it has yet determined the soul's future."[60]

In the complicated process of purification and growth latent imperfections need to be raised up into the light where they can be combated and eradicated. All sadhaks who practice sadhana and who commit themselves to the

Light need not feel discouraged when confronted with periods of darkness. The sadhak has to face them and pass through, and it is a misapprehension to imagine that a high stage of advancement in sadhana automatically protects the sadhak from running into disaster. This does not mean that everyone is exposed on a major scale to these dangers, yet nearly everyone experiences them in a certain way.

THE SUNLIT PATH

The path of integral Yoga is not a short cut to the Divine, spiritual victory often needs the struggle and labour to reach the heights; "There is a long stage of preparation necessary in order to arrive at the inner psychological condition in which the doors of experience can open and one can walk from vista to vista ... this Yoga is bitter like poison in the beginning because of the difficulty and struggle, but in the end sweet as nectar because of the joy of realisation, the peace of liberation."[61]

It is necessary from the beginning of the practice to understand and accept the arduous difficulties the sadhak has to face. If the sadhana fails in its immediate aim it has to be understood that it is because the Divine has 'intended' the failure. If difficulties return, the sadhak has to go through them. "To all sadhaks, even to the best and strongest there come interruptions in the flow of the sadhana; that is not a cause for thinking oneself unfit and wanting to go away with the idea that there is no hope. A little quietude would bring back the flow.... These difficulties always come and have to be overcome. Once overcome by the working of the Force, the sadhana goes on as before. ... No sadhak ought ever to indulge thoughts of unfitness and hopelessness—they are quite irrelevant because it is not one's personal fitness and worthiness that makes one succeed, but the Mother's grace and power and the consent of the soul to her grace and the workings of her Force."[62]

A present inability should not create a sense of incapacity for the practitioner. "If imperfection were a bar, then no man could succeed in Yoga; for all are imperfect, and I am not sure from what I have seen, that it is not those who have the greatest power for yoga who have too, very often, or have had the greatest imperfections. ... Imperfections can be stumbling-blocks and give one a bad fall for the moment, but not a permanent bar."[63]

In spite of all these difficulties Sri Aurobindo is clear that all those who are sincere and faithful in heart and rely on the Divine Will arrive at the kingdom. If the call of the soul is there, although not yet full, there can be no irretrievable failure. This long battle with ourselves and with opposing forces around us may seem interminable, but they are only temporary difficulties which can be overcome by faith in the Divine. The Divine does not throw aside all difficulties and sufferings, but carries the seeker through them and out of them. It is the illimitable power of the divine universal Shakti that is behind our aspiration, and which does not fail to pour itself into us "for the times and durations of our struggle while they depend at first, instrumentally and in part, on the strength of our faith and our endeavour, are yet eventually in the hands of the wisely determining secret Spirit, alone the Master of the Yoga, the Ishwara."[64]

The spiritual optimist, trusting the inner guidance, does not escape difficulties, but is able to meet them, without pain and despondency. When this faith is not there the seeker has to undergo a hard and difficult discipline to overcome constant fluctuations, disappointments and failures. "The circumstances that provoke our first entry into the path are not the real index of the thing that is at work in us ... outward circumstances are only a cover for the real workings of the spirit, and if it is the spirit that has been touched, the inward soul that has received the call, the sraddha [a wide spiritual and intelligent faith] will remain firm and resist all attempts to defeat or slay it. It is not that the doubts of the intellect may not assail, the heart waver, the disappointed desire of the life mind sink down exhausted on the wayside. That is almost inevitable at times, perhaps often... a battle between the powers of ignorance and the lower nature and the higher powers that have to replace them. ... But the Divine holds our hand through all and if he seems to let us fall, it is only to raise us higher."[65]

The initial stages of sadhana may be accompanied by periodic violent storms which almost all sadhaks have to face, but as long as the practitioner sticks to the path then after a certain period these storms diminish in frequency and force. "In Yoga, as in every great or serious human effort, there is always bound to be an abundance of adverse interventions and unfavourable circumstances which have to be overcome. To give them too great an importance increases their importance and their power to multiply themselves, gives them, as it were, confidence in themselves and the habit of coming. To face them with equanimity—if one cannot manage a cheerful persistence against them of confident and resolute will—diminishes, on the contrary, their importance and effect and in the end, though not at once, gets rid of their persistence and recurrence. It is therefore a principle in Yoga to recognise the determining power of what is within us, to set that right and establish the inward strength as against the power of outward circumstances ... for the difficulty is truly inside, not outside. Outside circumstances only give it the occasion to manifest itself and so long as the inner difficulty is not conquered, the circumstances will always crop up one way or another."[66]

For those who are perfectly confident .in the Divine Presence supporting them, the path is less turbulent. Sri Aurobindo is aware that the vital being has a tendency to cling to suffering, which has to be firmly expelled by the practitioner, of integral sadhana. Once the causes of suffering (signs of disharmony and imperfection) are removed the sadhak is able to attune to the nature of the working of the Divine Power.

Much of the struggle of sadhana is due to the lack of direct guidance of the psychic being. When the mind takes the lead in the sadhana and strains to force the whole nature into its preconceived moulds, then it often ends in disconsolation. For Sri Aurobindo the soul in us has nothing but a one-pointed orientation towards the Divine, and the sunlit path is the path of the psychic leading the seeker to God.

Sri Aurobindo describes the sunlit path thus: "do not be always thinking of your defects and wrong movements. Concentrate more upon what you are to be, on the ideal, with the faith that, since it is the goal before you, it must and will come.... Turn your eyes more to the coming light and less to any immediate darkness."[67]

The sunlit path can be followed by those who are able to practice surrender, trusting the inner guidance or, in the absence of these two, the habitual practice of turning one's face to the sun. This does not mean that the practitioner has no difficulties, but with confidence in the ultimate victory the sadhak regards them cheerfully as "all in the day's work."

In all, it can be said that there will always be difficulties in the beginning of the sadhana and they will last as long as is necessary for the change. However, they are bound to disappear if they are met with a persistent aspiration and faith in the Divine Shakti, which will guide the sadhak through the difficulties. Obstacles should be encountered as something wrong in the machinery of human nature, which has to be changed, and not as wrongdoings which make the sadhak despair of completing the sadhana. Defects must be looked at as wrong movements of the lower nature, which must be rejected calmly, firmly and persistently with full confidence in the Divine Power. It is of no use allowing failure to depress the sadhak unduly; the one thing that matters is keeping oneself open to the Force rather than constantly observing failures.

PREPARATORY PROCESS OF PURIFICATION —THE METHODS OF THE SUNLIT PATH

A more or less prolonged period of purification and preparation of the instrument is recommended so that the nature is ready to make a good use of the descending spiritual forces. Actually "suddhi [purification] is the most difficult part of the whole yoga; it is the condition of all the rest... To prevent suddhi the lower nature in you and around you will exhaust all its efforts, and even when it cannot prevent it will try to retard...When you have once found calm, peace of mind, firm faith, equality, and be able to live in it for some time, then and only then, you may be sure that suddhi is founded; but you must not think it will not be disturbed. It will be, so long as your heart and Prana are still capable of responding to the old movements. The one thing necessary when the renewed trouble comes, is to stand back in your mind and will from it, refuse it the sanction of your higher being even when it is raging in the lower nature."[68]

By purity Sri Aurobindo means freedom from all desire, egoism and attachment but later, as the process of purification proceeds, its negative aspect of renunciation is replaced by a positive method of purifying and harmonising the instruments of Nature.

The triple effort of aspiration (the call), equality (opening) rejection and surrender are the main supports of integral sadhana. These intrapsychic processes form the core of spiritual practice and a combination of these primary factors, together with the descent of the divine Grace and the sadhak's faith, ensures a more or less unimpeded progress on the long and difficult path of the integral sadhana.

Aspiration and Faith

Integral Yoga can be successfully undertaken and followed, only if there is a strong aspiration to the necessity of a larger than life existence. Aspiration has in it the conviction that spiritual progress is not so much a personal affair but a work for the Divine and of the Divine. Aspiration, which is more effective than capacities, is not a form of desire but the feeling of the inner soul's need to turn towards the Divine.

The call for the Divine is not a mere challenge or a self- indulgent alternation between spirituality and 'consumerism'. Nor is it the mistaking of the dissatisfactions of ordinary life and relationships, and the wish to be cared for and guided by a kind of superhuman power, for 'the call'. It is also not just an idea or intellectual seeking of something higher and beyond, but needs the motive of the soul for a deep and vast change of consciousness through self-consecration to God.

The call for a higher life must be genuine and proceed from the depth of the being. Impulses from the surfaces of the mental and vital nature—as a result of some dissatisfactions in life or ambition—is not a sufficient reason to enter the difficult path of integral sadhana. The seeker should have a thirst for the Divine and feel a real need to change the ordinary way of living. This call will act as a solid foundation and help the individual to stand firm in moments of personal crises.

Sri Aurobindo describes faith as "the soul's witness to something not yet manifested, achieved or realised, but which yet the Knower within us, even in the absence of all indications, feels to be true or supremely worth following or achieving. This thing within us can last even when there is no fixed belief in the mind, even when the vital struggles and revolts and refuses." [69] This dynamic intuitive conviction is not born of ignorance but reflects luminous faith.

Without a strong faith in a divine Guidance the seeker has at first to go by small steps and face the difficulties of his or her nature, and the immediate appearance of failure that the Divine Will is leading us by perseverance, until one makes a sufficient opening. Such faith is there even when the mind doubts, the vital despairs and the physical collapses; it accepts what happens not definitively but as something that has to be gone through on the journey.

"So long as a man has that faith.... I will say that even if his nature is full of obstacles and crammed with denials and difficulties, and even if he has many years of struggle, he is marked out for success in the spiritual life."[70]

Equality and Self-opening

Calmness is indispensable during the initial movement of introspection. Inner quietude and equality are two of the first conditions of a secure and successful sadhana. By equality Sri Aurobindo means an unmoved mind and vital which are free from the distortions created by personal feeling, i.e., to have an equal view of men and their nature, and the acts and forces that move them. Without equality and increasing purity the seeker cannot receive perfectly all that comes down, even if the sadhak opens to the Divine.

The whole principle in integral Yoga is to open oneself to the Divine influence and this self-opening to the Divine Power above and the Divine Presence in the heart can only come by faith, aspiration and surrender. The object of the self-opening is to allow the force of the Divine to flow in and do the work of transformation. If there is sincerity in the aspiration, and a patient will to arrive at a higher consciousness—in spite of all obstacles, the opening in one form or another is sure to come.

The self-opening is of two kinds; the inward self-opening and upward self-opening. The former consists of opening oneself to the subliminal and the psychic within, in which a personal relation is established with the individual Divine, the latter lies in opening oneself to the ranges of the superconscient above, where the seeker is put in active touch with the Universal and Transcendent Divine. The self-opening specifies the direction in which the surrendered consciousness is moving for an encounter with the Divine. Without a sufficient opening and receptivity to the action of the Divine Force within, all the sadhak's external efforts during the practice of sadhana may produce only meagre results.

Surrender

In order to overcome all the difficulties during the practice of sadhana, Sri Aurobindo advises the beginner practitioner to be patient and develop the indispensable condition of sincerity, a quiet mind and the will to surrender.

A complete surrender with no demand in return and no personal preference is not possible in one day, but the sadhak can begin with an attitude, a will to surrender imposed on the entire being. This will to surrender involves an inner or passive submission of increasing self-giving, trust and confidence in the Divine and ceasing to rely on one's own efforts alone. In this passive surrender, the individual will is no longer exercised and the entire being is ready to be acted upon by the divine Will. However, this passivity proves often to be a kind of self-deception, which is likely to cause an inflow of ignorant forces; in passive surrender, everything is left entirely to the Divine and it often turns out that the seeker surrenders to the lower nature under the pretext of surrendering to the Divine. Sri Aurobindo insists therefore that surrender should be active, in which everything is given up that is found to be in conflict with the needs of the sadhana. In this active surrender the individual will is sought to be harmonised and identified with the divine Will and there is a conscious effort to accept everything that is divine and reject all that is undivine. Such an active surrender involves, on the one hand, a vigilant watch over the forces of darkness, and, on the other hand, a ready cooperation with the guidance of the Divine, either directly through the psychic being or through the guidance of the Guru.

In difficult phases and periods of discouragement, when the personal efforts of the sadhak seem to fail, the Guru can intervene and give the seeker support, as the Guru is a channel or representative of the manifestation of the Divine. A complete surrender demands no egoistic clinging to preconceived ideas or acting in the half-truth of our own theories. In the words of Sri Aurobindo, "A complete surrender means to cut the knot of the ego in each part of the being and offer it, free and whole, to the Divine. The mind, the vital, the physical consciousness (and even each part of these in all its movements) have one after the other to surrender separately, to give up their own way and to accept the way of the Divine."[71]

But such surrender is not easy. In the initial stages surrender is often a doubtful kind of self-giving with a demand in it; formations of the mind, impulses of the vital and instigations of the ego may easily betray the sadhak into a false experience. Sri Aurobindo describes this situation as: "the impulse of the egoistic sense in us is to lay hold on it and use this increased might for our egoistic purpose. This is a most dangerous thing, for it brings with it a sense and some increased reality of a great, sometimes a titanic power, and the rajasic [vital] ego, delighting in this sense of new enormous strength, may instead of waiting for it to be purified and transformed throw itself out in a violent and impure action ... using the strength given him for his own and not for the divine purpose ... for, when a strong ego meddles in the matter, it falsifies the spiritual relation and under cover of making itself an instrument of the Divine is really bent on making instead God its instrument. The only remedy is to still the egoistic claim of whatever kind, to lessen persistently the personal effort and individual straining and instead of laying hold on the Shakti and using it for its purpose, rather to let the Shakti lay hold on us and use us for the Divine purpose."[72]

But later on, in the more advanced and more developed stages of sadhana, when the seeker puts oneself in the hands of the Divine rather than relying on one's own human efforts a progressive self-giving takes place.

There are other dangers that beset the path before the surrender is complete. Each individual finds different resistances in one's own nature; some sadhaks are faced with stubborn obstacles in surrendering the mind (doubts), and others in surrendering the vital being (impatience, restlessness, fear, desire or ambition). Then there is the danger when the mind is split in two directions: one part may turn itself towards God, whereas the other part still secretly obeys the demands of the vital nature; one part of the life is given to the Divine, whereas the rest of it is reserved for the old ways. It is only when the surrender takes place in all parts of the being that the divine Shakti begins gradually replacing personal effort.

It seems that surrender does not come easily to all at an early stage of sadhana; many have to go through a long journey of purification and discipline. Egoistic forces are always with the seeker tempting one to follow any alluring call; only if the heart centre is fully opened and the psychic in control, then everything is safe. However, "the psychic can at any moment be veiled by a lower upsurge. It is only a few who are exempt from these dangers and it is precisely those to whom surrender is easily possible."[73]

Sri Aurobindo nevertheless admits that, "it depends on certain conditions, which have nothing to do with superior or inferior yoga-capacity, but rather with a predisposition in the heart to open to the Sun of the Divine Influence."[74]

Grace

The movement of the three intrapsychic processes as described above needs to be supplemented by faith in the descent of the divine Grace. For Sri Aurobindo all evolutionary progress is mediated by the cooperation of an upward tending force from below (aspiration, self-opening and surrender), and an upward-drawn and downward-pressing force from above (Grace). "There are two powers that alone can effect in their conjunction the great and difficult thing which is the aim of our endeavour, a fixed and unfailing aspiration that calls from below and a supreme Grace from above that answers."[75]

Transformation is not an easy thing to achieve; it needs a tremendous amount of individual effort and the help of the divine Grace. As long as the soul does not come to the front of our consciousness, it is always the ego that is the organiser and ruler of our nature. It is the ego that is the initiator for the unfailing aspiration, an exclusive self-opening, a sincere surrender to the divine Power, personal detachment and self-discipline. All these processes require the full cooperation and strength of the ego. However, this same ego is also an organ of craving, attachment, passions and desires, and as such an obstacle or limitation for spiritual development. But where does the individual effort end, and when is this human effort replaced by the descent of the divine Grace? For Sri Aurobindo they occur simultaneously; there is no precise line of demarcation where individual effort ends and when the divine Grace takes over.

Though the seeker is not able to merit Grace, yet one is able to develop capacities in order to receive it; though it cannot be commanded, it can be invited and reveal its immense gift to those who are prepared to receive it. A relinquishment of personal desires, ambitions, will, likes and dislikes are some of the preconditions for the Grace to descend in its completeness. The sadhak should be ready so that the Grace is able to fully manifest itself, i.e., one's being needs to be prepared, purified and made sufficiently strong to receive, contain and collaborate with its workings, otherwise the Force of Grace will pass by. Though Grace comes first, if aspiration does not answer to it then no progress is possible. For Sri Aurobindo personal effort, the stringent self-discipline which is required to practice sadhana, is less effective than one's opening to the divine Grace or surrender to God's spiritualising energy.

However, as long as sadhaks remain subject to their lower nature their personal effort remains indispensable; in proportion as one rises over it and places oneself in the charge of the higher Powers, one's effort is gradually replaced by the working of the divine Grace. A strong personal effort is therefore essential in the early stages of sadhana before the Divine Presence takes up the sadhana itself. But not too much reliance must be placed on this effort, as with unaided human effort alone, however Herculean, man can never reach the supreme goal of yoga; the Divine must sprinkle Her Grace on the seeker as without this Grace the sadhana can never fully succeed. For Sri Aurobindo, in the process of integral Yoga there will be first "the personal endeavour of the human being, as soon as he becomes aware by his soul, mind, heart of this divine possibility and turns towards it as the true object of life, to prepare himself for it and to get rid of all in him that belongs to a lower working, of all that stands in the way of his opening to the spiritual truth and its power, so as to possess by this liberation his spiritual being and turn all his natural movements into free means of its self-expression. It is by this turn that the self-conscious Yoga aware of its aim begins. ... The second stage of this Yoga will therefore be a persistent giving up of all the action of the nature into the hands of this greater Power, a substitution of its influence, possession and working for the personal effort, until the Divine to whom we aspire becomes the direct master of the Yoga and effects the entire spiritual and ideal conversion of the being."[76]

Howsoever hard the sadhak tries to bring down the higher Forces into the lower parts of one's being, they will not flood the lower being unless the divine Grace descends into the lower levels and transforms them. To overcome the forces of the lower nature by one's own efforts may end in disaster. Too great a reliance on personal effort may lead to pride and other forms of self-assertive egoism. Similarly, too early an abandonment of individual effort may lead to inertia or inactivity—the belief that the Divine will take up the work.

It is the divine Grace that will take the seeker's struggling soul safely across the surging waves of disturbing mental processes during the development of spiritual discipline. For ultimately it is the divine Grace that carries the seeker over every obstacle and steadily changes the lower nature into the higher, rather than the personal exertions of the human will. Grace as a responsive gesture of the Unseen often descends in the form of miraculous intervention at times of acute danger or during a grave crisis in the seeker's life. It is often the main factor responsible for success in the spiritual enterprise.

By an inner condition of aspiration, openness and surrender the seeker calls the Divine for help, as it is the Divine Force which is doing the sadhana, though often secretly and invisibly. In each circumstance, within and without, the seeker works out the imperfections, and with the help of the Divine wisdom and love that are at work in the sadhana the sadhak is uplifted. Those who have not been able to establish direct contact with the Divine influence are advised to have faith and aspire for the opening. If the sadhak lacks surrender, then aspiration for the higher Truth and quietness can make up for it to a certain point. Most important however is the opening of the psychic being, because when the psychic being is in control, then all is safe. In moments of despondency the sadhak is reminded of two things: the call of the Divine Power to one's nature and the truth of one's divine potentialities.

THE TRIPLE PATH AS AMEANS TO THE OBJECT SADHANA

Corresponding to the three principal faculties of the human being—will, knowledge and love—there are three corresponding Yogas; *Karma* Yoga or the Yoga of works, *Jnana* Yoga or the Yoga of knowledge, and *Bhakti* Yoga or the Yoga of love and devotion.

The Yoga of knowledge seeks fulfilment in the intellectual being of man, the Yoga of works envisages union with the Will, and the Yoga of devotion in the eternal Delight. In traditional Yogas one main power of the being or one group of its powers is made the means on the path, but in Sri Aurobindo's synthetic Yoga all powers are included and combined in the transforming instrumentation. An integration of the whole human being through action, knowledge and love will have the unique result of an integral self-fulfilment. Sri Aurobindo's integral Yoga absorbs this cardinal principle of the Gita, but adds the ideal of higher planes and the supramental Truth-Consciousness, as a means of the complete transformation of earthly life.

In integral sadhana, it is not only the heart that has to turn to the Divine, but also the mind and the will of action. But since men differ in nature each sadhak will approach the sadhana in one's own way—one through work, one through devotion, one through meditation, and those who are capable of it through all together. Each method is a preparative help towards the proper direction of the realisation of the sadhana in the three parts of the being.

The three paths succeed only if they are done with the right spiritual aspiration, gathering up the whole life and nature and turning it towards the Divine, rather than work done for the service of humanity, a life-fleeing exclusive meditation or an emotional devotion shut up in its own ecstasy.

Sadhana Through Work

Karma Yoga selects for its instrumentation the will as the doer of action; by purification, concentration, and some form of discipline it becomes a means for contact of the sadhak's soul with the divine Soul of the universe.

Sri Aurobindo refers to work not as an action of philanthropy, which the mind of man substitutes for the deeper truth of works, but as action done for and in union with the Divine. Any work done as a sacrifice to the Divine, as a means of selfdedication through karma, is a field of inner training. Such self-dedication depends on the spirit in which all work is done and not on the nature of the work itself. As expressed by Sri Aurobindo, "All depends on the spirit in which a thing is done ... a man by doing in the right way and in the right spirit the work dictated to him by his fundamental nature, temperament and capacity can move towards the Divine.... It is quite possible for a man to do business and make money and earn profits and yet be a spiritual man, practice yoga, have an inner life."[77] Work done as a training in the spirit of Karma Yoga aims, as the Gita insists, not at the work done for its own sake but at the dedication of every human activity to the supreme Will. When the human will becomes the servant of the Divine Will, the sadhak is no longer limited in its dynamics by the imperfection of one's nature.

In the path of works, action is the knot to be loosened first, and the sadhak must endeavour to loosen it where it is centrally tied, in desire and in ego. The first law of action—egoistic indulgence of desire—in order to be exhausted, must be put away from the sadhak. Through purification or the renunciation of egoistic self-motivation and total indifference to the fruits of action and through complete absorption in the action itself, the practitioner of the Yoga of works becomes conscious of the universal Energy as the true doer of all one's actions. The choice and direction of the act is more and more consciously left to this universal Energy. There is no need to flee from action or take refuge in a blissful inertia. For Sri Aurobindo, the elimination of desire does not mean the extinction of the energy that impels it, but the egoistic form it takes and which has to be dissolved; the force and energy that feeds them must not be abandoned but offered to the Divine.

Desireless work carries along with it three results that are of central importance for the sadhak's spiritual ideal: (1) It leads inevitably towards the essence of an integral devotion, (2) it turns by communion with the Divine Will and Force into a way of knowledge more integral than any human intelligence can construct or discover, (3) in renouncing the egoism of the sadhak's mind, will and action, all these actions become now directed towards the Divine. In this way all works become a dynamic worship and source of the Divine. According to Sri Aurobindo, "All action must be done in a more and more Godward and finally a God-possessed consciousness; our works must be a sacrifice to the Divine and in the end a surrender of all our being, mind, will, heart, sense, life and body to the One must make God-love and God-service our only motive. This transformation of the motive-force and very character of works is indeed its master idea; it is the foundation of its unique synthesis of works, love and knowledge."[78]

Ordinary men work from the usual motives of the vital being—their needs, desires and the pleasure of manifesting their capacities—but in the practice of sadhana these ordinary motives have to be replaced by higher motives in which the sadhak no longer works for oneself but for the Divine. The outer form of work can vary according to the different nature of the sadhak, but for Sri Aurobindo "it is not, certainly, the superficial temperament or the character or habitual impulses that are meant, but in the literal sense of the Sanskrit word our 'own being', our essential nature, the divine stuff of our souls. Whatever springs from this root or flows from these sources is profound, essential, right; the rest opinions, impulses, habits, desires—may be merely surface formations or casual vagaries of the being or impositions from outside ... In proportion as we are purified, the true being within declares itself more clearly. Egoism renounced, the nature purified, action will come from the soul's dictates, from the depths or the heights of the spirit."[79] By constantly attributing all one's works to the Divine, the psychic being comes forward and spiritually purifies all works. Works done in this spirit are quite as effective as devotion or meditation.

For Sri Aurobindo, Karma Yoga is, therefore, not only practised as a means for liberation, but also a very effective and indispensable means for transformation. If the sadhak follows the lead of the Divine, opening to its guidance and inspiration, one is able to heighten the powers and faculties of one's nature and transform the whole instrumentation of one's personality. "The end of the path may be a perception of the divine in all energies, in all happenings, in all activities, and a free and unegoistic participation of the soul in the cosmic action. So followed it will lead to the elevation of all human will and activity to the divine level, its spiritualisation and the justification of the cosmic labour towards freedom, power and perfection in the human being."[80]

Sadhana Through Knowledge and Meditation

In Sri Aurobindo's Yoga psychology knowledge does not mean mental knowledge; mental knowledge refers to the sum total of objects that the mind grasps, but it never penetrates into the essential unity of things. The mind can know only the surface of things and not their essential substance and reality. Sri Aurobindo assumes that it is evident that "the knowledge for which Yoga strives must be different from what men ordinarily understand by the word. For we mean ordinarily by knowledge an intellectual appreciation of the facts of life, mind and matter and the laws that govern them ... But 'all life' includes not only, not even mainly life as humanity now leads it. It envisages rather a higher truly conscious existence. ... It is this greater consciousness and higher existence which is the peculiar and appropriate object of Yogic discipline ... Yogic knowledge seeks to enter into a secret consciousness beyond mind which is only occultly here, concealed at the bases of all existence."[81] In the spiritual life the ultimate aim of knowledge is not understanding or enlightenment, but being and becoming. The central aim of knowledge is the recovery of the Self, the Self as a reality, and the universe as a reality of the Self and not of mere material force. This aim presupposes the admission that one's present mode of being is not one's true self-existence. The Self is not only the reality behind the movement of one's psychological being, but also behind the transcendent and universal Existence.

For Sri Aurobindo the path of knowledge first leads to "God-possession, it is to possess God and be possessed by him through consciousness, through identification, through reflection of the divine Reality.... it is to possess oneness with God and through that to possess also oneness with the universal, with the cosmos and all existences.... Secondly, it is to raise our being into the divine being, our consciousness into the divine consciousness, our energy into the divine energy, our delight of existence into the divine delight of being. And it is not only to lift ourselves into this higher consciousness, but to widen it in all our being."[82] Integral Yoga does not proceed by the elimination of the lower parts of the being in order to merge into the quiescent Self, but the only thing that has to be eliminated is ignorance. The method of sadhana through knowledge must be regarded as a process of turning inward—a penetration into surface appearances of outer things, arriving at the one eternal reality within. Psychological analysis is a great and effective introduction to this turning inwards and therefore an important part of the Yoga of knowledge, but its object is only to remove a difficulty rather than to arrive at the final and positive result of this path. Besides, psychological self-knowledge is merely an intellectual conception or an enlightened psychological experience of the modes of the Self, but integral knowledge is based on 'realisation', the realisation of the Self in its pure being. As a first approach, psychological self-knowledge has to be followed till the wide infinite level is attained.

Besides turning inwards into the core of one's being, purification and concentration are two other important means for the attainment of knowledge. Purity and concentration are two aspects of the same status of being in the path of knowledge and a necessary preparation for the Divine Truth. Purity helps to bring about concentration, as without purification concentration would only lead to a state of eternal repose.

Traditionally, concentration, as the removal of the thought from all distracting activities, implies a release from the world and an ascent into the absolute and transcendent state of Samadhi [trance]. Thus Sri Aurobindo observes, "The traditional Way of Knowledge proceeds by elimination and rejects successively the body, the life, the senses, the heart, the very thought in order to merge into the quiescent Self or indefinite Absolute. The way of integral knowledge supposes that we are intended to arrive at an integral self-fulfilment and the only thing that is to be eliminated is our own unconsciousness, the Ignorance and the results of the Ignorance."[83] What has to be eliminated is the falsity of the being which figures as the ego, the falsity of life which figures as a mere vital craving, the falsity of the heart with its passions and desires. In an integral self-fulfilment, the heart, life and thought transcend themselves and find their own absolutes and harmonies beyond measure.

For Sri Aurobindo, Samadhi has a more profound meaning; it is not merely a state withdrawn from all consciousness of the outward into the absorbed bliss or peace of the supracosmic Undifferentiated, but a unified state of consciousness in which the connections with the outside world are not eliminated. These experiences of trance have their utility for opening the being, but it is only when the realisation is constant in the waking state that it becomes the condition for the spiritual transformation of the inner and outer being. To use Sri Aurobindo's own words, "The end of the path may be a perception of the divine in all energies, in all happenings, in all activities, and a free and unegoistic participation of the soul in the cosmic action. So followed it will lead to the elevation of all human will and activity to the divine level, its spiritualisation and the justification of the cosmic labour towards freedom, power and perfection in the human being."[84]

Meditation

Concentration, when the mind is fixed in a particular state or movement, must be distinguished from meditation, where the inner quiet mind remains concentrated on a single series of ideas which work out a single subject. To use concentration as the means for unification with the Divine is the first condition for the attainment of divine knowledge. In integral Yoga concentration means the fixation of consciousness in a particular state (e.g. peace) or movement (e.g. aspiration), whereas in meditation the inner mind is looking at things to get the right knowledge.

Meditation, as a method for calling down the true consciousness in a process leading to knowledge, is one of the means of approach to the Divine. According to Sri Aurobindo, "the way to knowledge is the meditation in the head by which there comes the opening above, the quietude or silence of the mind and the descent of peace, etc. of the higher consciousness generally till it envelops the being and fills the body and begins to take up all the movements. But this involves a passage through silence and a certain emptiness of the ordinary activities."[85]

Sri Aurobindo distinguishes four forms of meditation.

In the first form of concentrated meditation the discursive mind is accustomed to a settled pursuit of a single course of connected thought on a single subject, i.e., a dwelling of the mind on one line of thought or series of ideas constituting a single subject. This process of concentrated meditation is common in the sadhak's ordinary life, but it becomes more difficult when it has to be practiced by inward concentration.

The second process is related to the fixation of the whole mind on the essence of one idea only, so as to reach the very essence of the thing behind the idea rather than the psychological experience of the subject, i.e., the strenuous concentration of the mental faculties on a single object. However, as already discussed in the trance state, this state into which the sadhak rises must be called down to take possession of the lower being.

The third process is related to the tranquillisation of the mind altogether, which can be done in two ways: a) to stand back from the mental action altogether, watching it until it falls into an absolute quiet, and b) to reject all thought-suggestions and firmly hold to the peace of the being which always exists behind the trouble of the mind. On the basis of this calm the sadhak penetrates into the deeper truth of the divine manifestation and is no longer dependent on the external phenomena of things. This third form of meditation is described by Sri Aurobindo as the process where "you stand back from your thoughts, let them occur in your mind as they will and simply observe them and see what they are. This may be called concentration in self-observation. This form leads to another, the emptying of all thought out of the. mind so as to leave it a sort of pure vigilant blank on which the divine knowledge may come and imprint itself, undisturbed by the inferior thoughts of the ordinary human mind."[86] The first two forms are the condition of any Yoga, but for Sri Aurobindo they are only a subsidiary helpful process. The third form of meditation is a more direct and powerful process for the integral sadhana, as by now the strenuous concentration is replaced by a free concentration on the divine Will which gives light to the lower members, remoulding these in the forms of the Divine.

In the fourth form of meditation there is an attempt to fix the mind on the object of adoration, which is often done with the aid of a mantra or a physical image. In the intense devotion the sadhak does not seek "to pass into the being of. the Divine, but to bring the Divine into ourselves and to lose ourselves in the deep ecstasy of his presence or of his possession ... one comes to see the Divine everywhere and in all and to pour out the realisation of the Divine in all one's inner activities and outward actions."[87]

The above-mentioned four main forms of meditation can also be distinguished as two modes of meditation, passive and active meditation. In passive meditation the seeker withdraws him or herself from the surface and concentrates on the upcoming thoughts without getting attached to these thoughts. In this meditation, the active mind learns to look at itself without any sanction from within until its habitual or mechanical activities begin to fall quiet for want of support from within. While detaching oneself, the sadhak receives the power to listen to something other than the thoughts of the external mind. This passive meditation is quite necessary to silence the mind in the beginning of sadhana, but in the more advanced stages of sadhana this meditation does not create a solution to incoming external influences, and the inner silence which the sadhak has experienced will be disturbed in the outer life of the active world.

In active meditation the seeker experiences under any circumstance and situation the silence and reality of this world, i.e., the silence of mind in all situations. In this active meditation the seeker need not run in search of solitude for silencing the mind, and as the practice continues the old world of mental narrowness is gradually replaced by inner visions in which the sadhak discovers that one's thoughts come from outside and can be evaluated or rejected. When the sadhak attains an inner silence all one's actions become meditation.

A harmonised concentration of the whole being is the essence of sadhana. Meditation is a purely mental activity. In integral Yoga the inclusion of the outer consciousness in the transformation is of supreme importance; meditation cannot do this as it is a purely mental activity and deals only with the inner being. In mastering the mind nothing is directly done for the other parts of the being, and meditation, therefore, needs to be supplemented by the path of work and devotion. Integral Yoga excludes a life-fleeing exclusive meditation; it is one means of approaching the Divine, i.e., it is only a device but not a shortcut. The true movement is to continue the practice of sadhana whatever one is doing. For Sri Aurobindo, "a complete cessation of work and entire withdrawal into oneself is seldom advisable; it may encourage a too one-sided and visionary condition in which one lives in a sort of mid-world of purely subjective experiences without a firm hold on either external reality or on the highest Reality and without the right use of the subjective experience to create a firm link and then a unification between the highest Reality and the external realisation in life."[88]

Nevertheless, each of the four forms of meditation has its value in spiritual life, as its central object is to summon the various faculties of the being and gather them round the object of one's quest. Meditation trains the being in this direction and puts the sadhak in a condition of increased receptivity to the working of the Divine Grace.

Sadhana Through Love and Devotion

Aiming at the unity of the human soul with the supreme Spirit, devotion taps the emotional powers of the soul and turns them all Godwards. Bhakti Yoga, as a culture of spiritual emotions, exclusively turns the human heart towards love of the Divine.

Traditional Bhakti Yoga rejects a complete union with God, as it does not want to abolish all one's individuality in the absorbed rapture of the union; this would only mean a dissolution of the individual.

Sri Aurobindo's approach to love is more comprehensive as compared to the orthodox principles and practice of Bhakti Yoga. In integral Yoga it is the integral Divine who is the object of the sadhak's love and devotion. Love, as the greatest power of the Divine, delivers the seeker from all egoistic limitations, but this love must be expanded through knowledge. Though love and bhakti are two aspects of the psychic feeling, Sri Aurobindo distinguishes them as follows; "The nature of Bhakti is adoration, worship, self-offering to what is greater than oneself; the nature of love is a feeling or a seeking for closeness and union. Self-giving is the character of both; both are necessary in the yoga and each gets its full force when supported by the other."[89]

Bhakti proceeds by worship, and in this particular stage of experience there is a difference, an insufficient unity between the human soul and the Divine. Worship is only a first step on the path of devotion. Real Bhakti begins where external worship changes into adoration, which deepens in intensity with time. In the transformation of worship into pure Bhakti a development takes place from the motivated worship of popular religion into a principle of motiveless and self-existent love.

In the path of Bhakti, the seeker approaches the Divine by means of one s humanity, i.e., with human emotions, and the Yoga of devotion aims at a divine satisfaction of the emotional being of man.

In the beginning of sadhana the love offered by the sadhak to the Divine is not always of the purest kind. When turned towards the Divine, the emotions are often mixed with the egoistic desires and needs of the seeker's unpurified nature. The purest and most spontaneous love comes from the psychic, which seeks an integral divine union in the context of terrestrial existence. Its love for God is capable of bringing down the transforming light of divine Love upon earth. When the psychic love unites with the divine Love it can draw freely upon the latter's omnipotence.

Psychic love, as a form taken by divine Love in the human being, has its own personal bhakti, whereas the love that belongs to the spiritual plane is more universal and impersonal; the two are united in the highest divine Love. The psychic element is the love of the inmost being for self-giving and union. In itself psychic love is pure, but it is usually not left pure in the attraction of human beings to one another. Human love can nevertheless take a pure and unselfish form if it is touched by the psychic.

For Sri Aurobindo, "psychic love can have a warmth and a flame as intense and more intense than the vital, only it is a pure fire, not dependent on the satisfaction of ego-desire.... It is true that the psychic love does not usually get its full play in human relations and human nature; it finds the fullness of its fire and ecstasy more easily when it is lifted towards the Divine. In the human relation the psychic love gets mixed up with other elements which seek at once to use it and overshadow it."[90]

In sadhana emotion itself is not a bad element, it is a necessary part of human nature, but the sadhak has to be on guard against yielding to a vital attraction or attachment.

If love and bhakti are too vital, then there is likely to be a whirling around the sadhak's own ego instead of a straight flight towards the Divine. This vital love is a passion good enough to serve a temporary purpose, but it doesn't last as it never gets satisfied and brings only suffering and disappointment. Real Bhakti comes when the psychic is awake and when the purified emotions are all turned towards the Divine. Unlike unpurified emotionalism, Sri Aurobindo insists on the aspiration for the purification of emotions which, once purified, become one of the most powerful aids in integral Yoga.

Human love is mostly founded on a vital and physical basis with a mental support. It is often blended by the confusion of the individual's complex consciousness stumbling on one's frailties. When the consciousness deepens and heightens then the greater eternal love is able to transform human love into divine Love. All the parts of the being are used as a means of expression and share in the full play of divine Love, provided they have the right movements of pure expression without the vital mixture of ego and desire. The ecstatic experience of Love is not like the silent contemplation of the way of knowledge; the crown in the way of Love is bliss of union and not peace of unity. Usually the divine Love first enters the seeker through the psychic, but in integral sadhana the seeker has to realise the union of love not only in one's psychic depth, but in all parts of the being.

This transformation of the nature of love from the character of a limited human emotion to an all-embracing Divine Love is not only applicable to the individual but also to universal Love. All expressions of sympathy, universal empathy, love of mankind, are at first used as instruments of expression of human nature. As consciousness changes it is able to grow into a greater eternal love. The unity of this divine Love takes hold of all living relations and turns them Godwards. As expressed by Sri Aurobindo, "The principle of Bhakti Yoga is to utilise all the normal relations of human life into which emotion enters and apply them no longer to transient worldly relations, but to the joy of the All-Loving, All-Beautiful and the All-Blissful."[91]

In the Bhagavad Gita's triple path of Yoga, neither Karma Yoga (work), nor Bhakti Yoga (love), nor Jnana Yoga (knowledge) can be separated, each needing the incorporation and fusion of the others for its fullness. In the integral view, these three paths are one; works fulfil themselves in knowledge, knowledge is not complete without work, and the crown of the union of knowledge and works is love; for love is the delight of union. As the power of divine self-delight it brings richness and fullness. Fulfilled love includes knowledge and is not inconsistent with divine works.

According to Sri Aurobindo, "We can see also that in the integral view of things these three paths are one. Divine Love should normally lead to the perfect knowledge of the Beloved by perfect intimacy, thus becoming a path of Knowledge, and to divine service, thus becoming a path of Works. So also should perfect Knowledge lead to perfect Love and Joy and a full acceptance of the works of That which is known.... It is in this triple path that we come most readily to the absolute knowledge, love and service of the One in all beings and in its entire manifestation."[92]

In the practice of integral Yoga the sadhak may begin with knowledge or with devotion or with works, or may combine them all in one movement; there is no single rule for it, all depends on the sadhak's personality and nature. In the words of Sri Aurobindo, "integral Yoga is a turning of all the being in all its parts to the Divine. It follows that there must be knowledge and works as well as bhakti, and in addition, it includes a total change of the nature, a seeking for perfection, so that the nature also may become one with the nature of the Divine. It is not only the heart that has to turn to the Divine and change, but the mind also—so knowledge is necessary, and the will and power of action and creation also—so works too are necessary."[93]

It is possible to start with Godward emotion or with knowl- edge, but these subjective experiences create a tendency to live too exclusively within, and it becomes difficult later on to apply to life the sadhak's gains in the higher Nature, and transforming the outer life and body. The outer actions follow their old confused imperfect paths, which do not correspond with the inner light.

Sri Aurobindo, therefore, advises the sadhak to start from works and proceed by works, although at each step works are supposed to be moved more and more by a divine Love and divine Knowledge. According to Sri Aurobindo; "Action is the first power of life ... therefore it is that by turning his action Godwards the life of man best and most surely begins to become divine. It is the door of first access, the starting- point of the initiation. When the will in him is made one with the divine will and the whole action of the being proceeds from the Divine and is directed towards the Divine, the union in works is perfectly accomplished."[94]

The difficulty any sadhak feels about sadhana is not really a question of meditation versus bhakti versus works. It is a difficulty of the attitude or approach to be taken. In the words of Sri Aurobindo, "work done as sadhana—done as an outflow of energy from the Divine and offered to the Divine or work done for the sake of the Divine or work done in a spirit of devotion is a powerful means of sadhana and that such work is especially necessary in this yoga. Work, bhakti and meditation are the three supports of yoga. One can do with all three or two or one. There are people who can't meditate in the set way that one calls meditation, but they progress through work or through bhakti or through the two together. By work and bhakti one can develop a consciousness in which eventually a natural meditation and realisation becomes possible."[95]

Each individual has to follow the unique inner law of one's own inner being. Though the general lines are common to all, each nature is unique and has its own way of treading the path, and each sadhak must choose the method which suits him or her best. In love the sadhak aims at purification of the heart and intellect, in action at self-surrender in all things to God; in knowledge at realisation of the One within and beyond all manifested existence.

The sadhak can start the sadhana in any part of one's being that he or she knows is more awakened than the others; in some it is the mind, in some the will, in others it is the heart. Whichever way one takes it is essential that the foundations of sadhana are laid firm to avert the dangers of a breakdown on the way due to the incessant pressure of the divine Force at work for the growth and reconstruction of the various parts of the being. The various steps in laying th proper foundation are quietude, purity and equanimity. It is not easy to attain these states within a short time; it demands patience and a steady will. The development of these essential parts of the foundation of integral Yoga requires a spiritual atmosphere in which the sadhana can thrive.

The mental perfection rendered by the Gita, through a synthesis of knowledge, love and works can resolve many discords of the human, nature. The practice of sadhana in integral Yoga raises this synthesis from a spiritual-mental to an integral perfection, and aims at an ascent beyond the mind.

This integrality is described by Sri Aurobindo as follows: "this integral Yoga of knowledge, love and works has to be extended into a Yoga of spiritual and gnostic self-perfection. As gnostic knowledge, will and Ananda are a direct instrumentation of spirit and can only be won by growing into the spirit, into divine being, this growth has to be the first aim of our Yoga. The mental being has to enlarge itself into the oneness of the Divine before the Divine will perfect in the soul of the individual its gnostic outflowering. That is the reason why the triple way of knowledge, works and love becomes the keynote of the whole Yoga, for that is the direct means for the soul in mind to rise to its highest intensities where it passes upward into the divine oneness. That too is the reason why the Yoga must be integral."[96]

Conclusion: Sadhana and its Difficulties

Sri Aurobindo's sadhana can be understood as the repeated effort to become aware of the Divine within, a quest which is ultimately undertaken for its own sake. The practice of integral Yoga brings the seeker in contact with the extraordinary complexity of one's own being and the artificiality of one's surface personality. The average human being who lives in the waking surface psychological existence appears fairly simple, but as soon as seekers go deep within themselves they discover that their being is "a roughly constituted chaos, surrounded by a whole complex world into which we have to introduce the principle of a divine order." During sadhana the sadhak becomes aware of the different parts of being— the physical, vital and mental—each of which has a separate individuality. Through sadhana they can be separated from one another and gradually experienced as independent entities.

Sri Aurobindo leaves scope for many different paths of spiritual development; each of the different paths may be useful and appropriate for some people. Although he has laid down a general path for integral self-development, every sadhak has to find out one's own line of development in accordance with one's nature. Men differ in their capacities for spiritual development and each seeker differs in his or her achievements in self-development. The pragmatic differences among men and the various demands of the sadhak's nature require a different path for each seeker.

Sadhana aims at the replacement of the automatism of natural habits by the power of self-control. Rejection of the natural habits does not mean suppression, in which the desire is eliminated but remains latent at the level of the subconscious. It implies the attitude of detachment towards the desire, i.e., each desire is observed with detachment and is allowed to pass and is rejected from the consciousness. In this process of dis-sociation the sadhak seeks to withdraw the will from wrong motivation by bringing down the light and purity from above. During the practice the seeker is therefore advised not to suppress, hide or fight repressed impulses but allow them to come up to the surface consciousness, to step back and allow some interval, observe them detached and impartially, and finally establish a control over them. The seeker does not have to renounce the movements of the lower unregenerate nature but has to master them gradually and connect them to the Divine. After this mastery, the seeker is able to go further and transform the very substance of the primary impulses. Sri Aurobindo wants the sadhak to reject all egoism, yet all one's energy should not be used solely for rejection but should also be directed to the positive replacement of them by the higher consciousness. Just as there are forces that may depress the seeker, there are also forces that restore and strengthen, and the sadhak is advised to develop the power to draw upon these restorative resources.

Integral sadhana is not an easy escape from the inordinate misery of everyday life. According to Sri Aurobindo, "This is an exceedingly difficult aim and difficult Yoga; to many or most it will seem impossible. All the established forces of the ordinary ignorant world-consciousness are opposed to it and deny it and try to prevent it, and the Sadhak will find his own mind, life and body full of the most obstinate impediments to its realisation. If you can accept the ideal whole-heartedly, face all difficulties, leave the past and its ties behind you and are ready to give up everything and risk everything for this divine possibility, then only can you hope to discover by experience the Truth behind it."[97]

Integral sadhana, as a radical transformation of one's nature, does not pretend to be an easy process. The magnitude of the change it aims at makes it more difficult than any of the older Yogic systems. The endeavour of the attainment of a Divine Life creates immense difficulties, dangers and problems for the sadhak; its attainment requires for most sadhaks an exercise of utmost complexity. It is a mistake to over-simplify the various problems that confront seekers in their attempt to take the Divine Life by storm.

Each individual is a unique spiritual being, but to discover this uniqueness Sri Aurobindo urges the sadhak to follow certain strict guidelines of behaviour, and to conform to the spiritual attitudes that he specifies to be important. It seems that the seeker needs to change one's life radically in order to overcome the difficulties on the way.

According to P.T. Raju, "Almost all systems of Indian Philosophy recognize this change [the change from an ordinary man into a spiritual man] and emphasize its importance. But only one man out of a thousand can make up his mind to follow the path of inwardness; and out of a thousand who make up their minds, only one can accomplish it."98

The search for the deepest truths is often accompanied by tormenting uncertainty and restless groping. The methods of integral Yoga are not always useful for those seekers who are more in need of the guidance of a psychotherapist. It could be dangerous to suggest that someone with deep-rooted unconscious conflicts or severe emotional distortions practice integral Yoga.

Sadhana forces the concealed dark elements to come out into the open and be exposed to the inner Light, and in this process there are those who feel an intense need to find the guidance of one's psychic being. But a constant faith, aspiration, rejection and surrender do not guarantee in return the descent of the inner Light. The sadhak's failure in his or her attempt may even add to one's difficulties, as the divine Consciousness within is often hidden behind the veil of unresolved psychological issues, which need the same intense personal will to be conquered as the intense need to find the inner and psychic being. Sri Aurobindo is aware of these unresolved psychological issues, but he wants to replace the psychological methods used in Western psychotherapeutic models by spiritual methods of his supramental Yoga. He knows quite well that spiritual methods are not easy, but he insists that "if people become disciples, they are supposed to follow spiritual aims and endeavours, however hard and above ordinary nature and not the things that are easy and natural."[99]

What the sadhak aims at in the practice of Yoga can only come by the opening of the being to the divine Force and a persistent rejection of all egoism, demand, desire and all other vital motives except the aspiration for and the opening and surrender to the Divine Truth.

The spiritual dimension certainly has to be included as a separate factor with regard to health, but could it be that Sri Aurobindo overemphasises the spiritual dimension in psychological health, as if spiritual heights alone are able to solve all kinds of psychological disorders and conflicts that afflict humanity?

In difficult stages the influence of the Guru is invaluable, and one can imagine that if the implementation of integral sadhana was difficult with the benefit of Sri Aurobindo's and The Mother's constant guidance, it will be significantly more difficult in their physical absence.

Could B. Cortright's view on the integrative way of working with the transpersonal approach be usefully applied in such difficult situations? For him and many other transpersonal psychologists, transpersonal psychotherapy reaches its full stature when "it has synthesized into itself the most powerful insights and techniques that the behavioral, psychoanalytic and humanistic schools have discovered."[100]

NOTES

1. Troy Wilson, The Hindu Quest for the Perfection of Man, p.22-23.
2. Ken. Wilber, The Spectrum of Consciousness, p.23.
3. Sri Aurobindo, Letters on Yoga p.24.
4. Sri Aurobindo, The Synthesis of Yoga, p.40.
5. Ibid., p.597.
6. Sri Aurobindo, Letters on Yoga, p.1271.
7. Ibid., p.792-793.
8. Sri Aurobindo, The Synthesis of Yoga, p.51.
9. Sri Aurobindo, Letters on Yoga, p.1313.
10. Ibid., p.578.
11. Sri Aurobindo, The Synthesis of Yoga, p.234.
12. Ibid., p.377.
13. Ibid., p.213.
14. Sri Aurobindo, Letters on Yoga, p.551.
15. Ibid., p.848-849.
16. Sri Aurobindo, On Himself, p.156.
17. Ibid., p.465.
18. Ibid., p.153-154.
19. Ibid., p.464.
20. Sri Aurobindo, The Synthesis of Yoga, p.66.

21. Sri Aurobindo, Letters on Yoga, p.1297.

22. Ibid., p.1666.

23. Ibid., p.1052

24. Ibid.,p.1318.

25. Ibid., p.559.

26. Ibid., p.573.

27. Sri Aurobindo, The Hour of God, P-154.

28. Sri Aurobindo, The Synthesis of Yoga, p.748.

29. Sri Aurobindo, Letters on Yoga, p.1306.

30. Sri Aurobindo, On Himself, p.140.

31. Sri Aurobindo, Letters on Yoga, p. 88

32. Ibid., p. 288.

33. Ibid., p.1426.

34. Ibid., p.1449.

35. Sri Aurobindo, Bases of Yoga, p.42.

36. Sri Aurobindo, On Himself, p.157.

37. Sri Aurobindo, Letters on Yoga, p.1626.

38. Sri Aurobindo, The Synthesis of Yoga, p.236-237.

39. Sri Aurobindo, Letters on Yoga, p.1623.

40. Ibid., p.1368.

41. Ibid., p.1310.

42. Sri Aurobindo, Essays Divine and Human, p.163.

43. Sri Aurobindo, The Problem of Rebirth, p. 171-172.

44. Sri Aurobindo, Letters on Yoga, p.1053.

45. Ibid.,p.1053.

46. Ibid.,p.1041.
47. Sri Aurobindo, The Life Divine, p.276.
48. Ibid., p.905.
49. Ibid., p.904.
50. Sri Aurobindo, The Synthesis of Yoga, p.169.
51. Sri Aurobindo, The Life Divine, p.905.
52. Ibid., p.914.
53. Sri Aurobindo, The Hour of God, p.72.
54. Sri Aurobindo, The Life Divine, p.54.
55. Sri Aurobindo, The Synthesis of Yoga, p.817.
56. Ibid., p.268.
57. Ibid.,p.123.
58. Sri Aurobindo, Bases of Yoga, p.39.
59. Sri Aurobindo, The Hour of God, p.39-40.
60. Sri Aurobindo, The Synthesis of Yoga, p.64-65.
61. Sri Aurobindo, Letters on Yoga, p.1630.
62. Ibid.,p,1704.
63. Ibid., p.1665.
64. Sri Aurobindo, The Synthesis of Yoga, p.752.
65. Ibid., p.746-747.
66. Sri Aurobindo, Letters on Yoga, p.1696-1697.
67. Ibid., p.1687.
68. Sri Aurobindo, The Hour of God, p.155-156.
69. Sri Aurobindo, Letters on Yoga, p.573.
70. Ibid., p.573.

71. Sri Aurobindo, Bases of Yoga, p.27.

72. Sri Aurobindo, The Synthesis of Yoga, p.738-739.

73. Sri Aurobindo, Letters on Yoga, p.1169.

74. Ibid., p.785.

75. Sri Aurobindo, The Mother, p. 1.

76. Sri Aurobindo, The Synthesis of Yoga, p.592-593.

77. Sri Aurobindo, Letters on Yoga, p.675.

78. Sri Aurobindo, The Synthesis of Yoga, p.97.

79. Ibid., p.261-262.

80. Ibid., p.35.

81. Ibid., p.286-287.

82. Ibid.,p.490.

83. Ibid., p.277.

84. Ibid., p.35.

85. Sri Aurobindo, Letters on Yoga, p.534.

86. Ibid., p.721.

87. Sri Aurobindo, The Synthesis of Yoga, p.549.

88. Sri Aurobindo, Letters on Yoga, p.531.

89. Ibid., p.776.

90. Ibid.,p.817.

91. Sri Aurobindo, The Synthesis of Yoga, p.33.

92. Ibid., p.35.

93. Sri Aurobindo, Letters on Yoga, p.525.

94. Sri Aurobindo, The Synthesis of Yoga, p.521.

95. Sri Aurobindo, Letters on Yoga, p.536.

96. Sri Aurobindo, The Synthesis of Yoga, p.588.

97. Sri Aurobindo, Lights on Yoga, p.l.

98. P.T. Raju, Spirit, Being and Self, p.39.

99. Sri Aurobindo, Letters on Yoga, p.864.

100. B. Cortright, Psychotherapy and Spirit, p.22.

Part III :

A Dialogue between Ken Wilber's Integral Views and Sri Aurobido's Metaphysical Vision

Chapter Nine

The Transpersonal Psychology Movement and Integral Sadhana

CONVENTIONAL SYSTEMS OF PSYCHOTHERAPY AND INTEGRAL SADHANA

Psychotherapy aims at understanding the individual as a whole, and helps the person to improve one's life through increasing self-knowledge and insight. As a voyage of discovery into various unknown aspects of the personality, it enables the individual to gain psychological insight into one's inadequate manner of dealing with life's problems, sense of insecurity, and the underlying deep-rooted origins of psychological disturbances. The process is accompanied by the exploration of and venturing into unknown areas of the self. As such, psychotherapy examines self-concepts, removes distortions of this self-concept, and restores psychological health through creating a realistic assessment of the selflimitations and potentialities of the individual. The goal of psychotherapy is not only to free the individual from the sense of isolation and estrangement from oneself, but also to help the person in adjusting to a rapidly changing society. For the therapist, consciousness is a function dependent on the mind, and as a consequence the client can never study one's psychological processes directly.

In integral Yoga the mind is a vehicle for consciousness

and it is not subject to the forces of the external material world. This transpersonal consciousness—in the form of Pure Awareness—could be used for therapeutic aims. In the experience of this transpersonal self, the seeker transcends conditioning and becomes unaffected by the flow of mental and emotional events. By becoming less emotionally involved, clients or seekers become more of an observer and while these events are still happening, they no longer disturb them.

Psychotherapy as an art or science of the psyche tries to establish the fundamental knowledge of the nature of man and one's relation to the environment. In its methods of investigation, it leads mainly toward the natural sciences and leaves out a universal Spirit which realises itself in the multiple concrete phenomena. It does not conceive the relationship of divinity to man.

The common element in each system of psychotherapy is based on a greater awareness and integrity of the various aspects of the being. Many systems of psychotherapy agree that individuals are able to change themselves by increasing their self-consciousness, though such changes are only related to the client's psychological disturbances. Systems of psychotherapy and Sri Aurobindo's sadhana include development of insight and deepening of awareness pertaining to the aspects of behaviour of which the seeker is more or less unaware. A genuine insight into the unconscious dynamics of the individual's psychological disturbance has in itself a strong therapeutic effect. But awareness gained through psychotherapy does not, in itself, bring about the psychological state of total well-being. For Sri Aurobindo consciousness is also power or will-force and to attain psychological health is, therefore, not only to be aware of one s being but also to recognise and possess the full force of consciousness.

Integral sadhana and conventional systems of

psychotherapy try to delve into the hidden nature of the suffering being through illuminating insight, but in their capacity and degree of illuminating power they differ widely.

Psychotherapy is concerned with the ideal of human life, to establish a control of a rational and strong mind, a right will, a mastery of one's emotional life and the development of man s capacities to be fulfilled in life. The goal in most Western systems of psychotherapy is to strengthen the ego and utilise the positive aspects of the ego for overcoming psychological disturbances. For Sri Aurobindo, psychological disturbances and illnesses are different forms of an exacerbated egoistic state, in which the seeker is too much occupied with oneself. In integral Yoga, healing takes place by the process of focusing on the Divine within, rather than the continuous placing of one's attention on the importance of the ego; true well-being can come only from the true Self. To enter integral Yoga demands an infinite trust in the Divine, patience and self-discipline.

A mental control can certainly effect a change, but it usually takes a long time and the success at the beginning may be only partial and is often accompanied by many failures. The psychotherapist is successful if the client becomes aware of certain aggressive, impulsive drives so that one is able to get control over them. However, the client is still not liberated from these forces. The client has not yet freed oneself from selfish actions or repressed impulses.

In sadhana mental control has to be gradually replaced by spiritual mastery, as true mastery not only controls but also liberates and transforms. The sadhak in sadhana does not solely rely on one's personal effort alone, but also places reliance on the Grace and the power of the Divine.

For Sri Aurobindo psychological difficulties do not dis-, appear by the mind's brooding on them. These difficulties, no doubt, have to be observed but if the mind stresses psychological difficulties then they tend to stick without a solution and may even increase. Sri Aurobindo wants the seeker to put one's whole stress on faith and aspiration, to bring about a change in the poise and attitude of the mind, as it is from something above and outside the difficulties that the solution must come. This does not mean that the mind has no role to play in solving psychological difficulties, but the mind's task of concentrating on details and putting them right should be a subsidiary process.

Catharsis as a method of expressing repressed affects, at times, allows for a release of suppressed anger and fear, and this release may be necessary. But expression of or indulgence in emotions need not always lead to a release of destructive energies. They often lead to negative habit patterns. The temporary feeling of well-being through emotional catharsis may not be lasting enough to bring about an inner change towards a new direction. The release of repressed affects may be purifying, but without rational insight there may be other motives which subsequently cause the same accumulation of feelings. In integral Yoga catharsis aims at the understanding of the causal elements which underlie the disturbing emotions i.e., the observation of the multiplicity of possible causes of the emotional and cognitive faculties. This process of self-awareness through non-attached observation leads to a certain degree of self-control, and with the help of renunciation of various kinds of attachments, the seeker is gradually able to rise above one's physical, vital and mental restrictions.

Western psychotherapeutic techniques do bring underlying causes of mental problems to consciousness, but the psychological incompatibilities of the underlying forces often remove only secondary causes, e.g., anxiety. Psychotherapy analyses and explores the nature of inner conflicts and tries to give solutions for the removal of these conflicts. The psychotherapist explains certain mental processes and the cure of various related abnormalities that are related to these mental processes, but this does not necessarily create an adequate philosophy of life. Sri Aurobindo's integral Yoga, on the other hand, tries to fathom the essence of creation and the meaning of life, i.e., it tries to find truths on which the seeker can focus one's *Weltanschauung* and way of life.

Actually, the object of sadhana is not to make unlimited room for the fulfilment of the ideas of the human mind or the desires of the ego-centred life force, but to enable the sadhak to discover the divine within. Sadhana as a living thing is not a set method of mental principles, and each sadhak has to be dealt with according to one's nature, capacities, real needs and according to what is best for one's spiritual welfare. It should be clear that integral sadhana is essentially the art or discipline of living a spiritual life and it is not so much concerned with healing psychopathological symptoms. As such it cannot be seen as a form of therapy, but as a methodical process of surrendering the ego-self to the larger spiritual Self. Integral Yoga is not a system developed for psychologically disabled clients; Sri Aurobindo is primarily interested in the area and development beyond the ego. Those seekers who are able to become aware of and work out their attachments and who are able to face intense psychological crises may benefit from integral Yoga.

Integral yogic methods and concepts aim at the ultimate union with the Divine and are not meant to be palliatives for psychological problems. However, the integral yogic methods can, on the one hand, have beneficial effects in reducing various types of stress-related disorders and in promoting individual growth. On the other hand, the yogic methods may involve certain risks, when the balance between the different parts of one's being is disrupted, sometimes leading to some serious psychopathological disorders.

THE EGO IN TRANSPERSONAL PSYCHOTHERAPY AND INTEGRAL SADHANA

In Western psychotherapy the development of the ego as an essential stage of human development and stability receives all the attention. The ego functions as an adaptive organ, it adapts itself to a complex biological and psychological environment. The ego takes care that the individual's perceptions are related to thoughts, feelings, emotions and prejudices, so one sees what one expects to see. The positive aspects of the ego are utilised for overcoming psychological disturbances, and a well-developed ego is often equated with psychological health. However, this psychological health simultaneously requires a contrary reaction of the ego; the release of the I, a trans-ego state within the realm of the individual's actual experience. The ego functions as an instrument for this world but is not able to go beyond this world into the Kingdom of God. Only by the victory over the limitations of the egocentric self, when the ego breaks several barriers and can experience a union with the cosmic Self, can it become a fit instrument for the real Self.

Although the transpersonal psychotherapist uses transpersonal experiences as an integral part of the therapeutic process and although he or she aims beyond the traditional ego-goals, some of the therapists emphasise the importance of establishing the ego-identity before it can be relinquished. Ego development is viewed as a stage along the way, and confusion in one's normal ego-centred life may be the starting point for the process of awakening. Surrendering to something greater than oneself requires a degree of self-autonomy and self-determination. This surrender of egocentricity in transpersonal psychotherapy is related to altruism or selfless service in the world by which the individual ego becomes progressively less all-important. After all, the principal focus of transpersonal effort remains more or less centred on growth into a fuller human functioning.

Sri Aurobindo, however, very clearly distinguishes the cosmic Self from this collective existence; the former is spiritual in essence and in experience, whereas the latter is unable to break connections with the life of human society or human mankind, i.e., the collective ego.

The ego as a false centre of unity tries to find completeness of one's being in an identification with a changing surface personality, but is unable to come to terms with the eternal self or one's total existence. The ego in its self-enlargement may perceive its unity with others, but this perception is ephemeral and not based on experience in totality. It is only in the spiritual self that the sadhak is able to find and possess true unity. The dissolution of this limited ego is, therefore, the necessary means for the cosmic Life to arrive at its divine fruition. By abolishing successively this practical ego-sense the sadhak comes to the realisation of the true self and is able to make this self one with the cosmic Spirit, and with the inexpressible but not unknowable Transcendence. The disappearance of the ego does not bring with it the destruction of one's true individuality, one's spiritual existence, but the estranged ego is replaced by the true spiritual Person, and the sadhak can become a pure instrument of the Divine.

Transpersonal psychotherapists and Sri Aurobindo presume that the seeker has already achieved a certain degree of adult maturity and individuality; Without prior resolution of developmental tasks, such as social adjustment, personal identity and interpersonal relationships, these matters may overlap the deeper aims of psycho-spiritual disciplines. Nevertheless, the ego as a tool of great importance within its own frame of reference, becomes a hindrance when misapplied and, for this reason, it has to be kept in perspective. However, for some of the transpersonal psychotherapists, the transcendence of the ego should not be confused with mere loss of ego-strength. In exceeding the ego, the individual stops over-valuing the needs of the inflated ego; the latter is not dissolved but remains intact with all its essential strength and weaknesses, i.e., not the loss or destruction of the ego, but rather seeing through the ego or the ego's surpassing itself. In giving up the desire for egocentric gratification the individual is not being deprived of desires, but learns to acknowledge them without being driven to gratify them. That's why some of the transpersonal psychotherapists do not aim at dissolving the ego but at relativating it; the seeker stops identifying with one's ideas about this ego as there is no need any longer to defend one's identification with ideas of oneself as a separate identity. Once the process of disidentification with the ego has started, the individual is aware that the ego-functions are still available if one needs to deal with earthly matters, but by now one has better things to do, i.e., re-establishing an intimate relationship with one's true self. In this way, ego-transcendence does not mean loss of one s ego- oriented rules of social behaviour, but the individual can see through them and accept responsibility for one's willed action.

Some of the transpersonal psychotherapists would advise the forthcoming spiritual practitioners to work through personal psychodynamic issues first, (childhood traumas and other unresolved emotional matters) in order to clarify and purify underlying psychological problems before spiritual awakening takes place. This view is thus described by Ken Wilber: "Most neurotics suffer not because of a lack of ego transcendence, but from the prior lack of ego-esteem, and therapy must be, first and foremost, the facilitator of strong ego-esteem, and then—but only then—the facilitator of egotranscendence."[1] Only a strong psychological grounding, a mature level of ego-organisation, allows the practitioner to enter into those spiritual practices which aim at the manifestation of mature psycho-spiritual development, i.e., transcending various personality structures as well as the development of awareness to deal with the powerful energies in the transegoic realm.

When the ego has not yet come to terms with its less respectable instincts, it may get possessed by the strongly repressed unconscious. There is always the danger of disorder when the position of the ego is called into question. But when the ego is first balanced, before it is transcended, the 'invasion' of the conscious by the unconscious contents will be smoothly integrated. By now, when the tamed ego surpasses itself there is an integration and no invasion of the conscious by primordial, repressed contents. This does not mean that people with unstable egos are not fit for spiritual growth; for people still working on their disturbed unconscious realms spiritual growth means fortifying the ego.

From the point of view of sadhana, the ego is the main obstacle and one of the greatest pitfalls in the process of spiritual development. However, it is essential to place the characteristic role of the ego in the process of evolution, understand its origin, and analyse its limitations and transcendence.

The fundamental law of the ego is making a distinction between the me' and the 'not me'. Objects and persons are experienced as if they have a separate, distinct and independent reality. The ego, as a practical constitution of the individual's consciousness, is devised to centralise the activities of Nature in the individual, and its function is meaningfully described by Sri Aurobindo: "Man the individual has to affirm, to distinguish his personality against Nature, to be powerfully himself, to evolve all his human capacities of force and knowledge and enjoyment so that he may turn them upon her and upon the world with more and more mastery and force; his self-discriminating egoism is given him as a means for this primary purpose."[2]

The I or ego, however, as a formation of the physical, vital and mental nature, is only constituted for the purpose of centralising and individualising the outer consciousness and action. This egocentric individualisation is only a superficial formation. It is simultaneously the source of imperfection, as it builds up a wall of division. It is separated by ignorance from other-selves and from the inner Divinity. For Sri Aurobindo, the ego is more related to the enslavement to the need for satisfaction of desires, wants, needs and ambitions. The ego-sense has its value at the lower levels of existence, and it is indispensable for the evolution of the lower life but a hindrance for the development of the higher levels.

In order to be a possessor of one's being, the sadhak must find out one's highest Self, the real man within rather than one's mental, vital and physical ego. The individual soul, as the true spiritual being, appears in its complete truth when the sadhak gets rid of the ego and of one's false separative sense of individuality. When the true being, a comprehensive and unifying centre from within, is discovered, the utility of the ego is outgrown. But how could the ego be abolished? Could a society survive if the majority of its people become entirely selfless? Does the annihilation of the ego necessarily imply the giving up of hope or the giving up of ambition or the striving for a better future? It will take thousands of years, but it will be necessary in the process of evolution that the person without an ego identifies oneself with the greatest common good, first with humanity as a whole, later with the Divine Will beyond humanity.

The subordination of the ego to the progress and happiness of the human race belongs to the mental and moral world of ethics and not to a spiritual ideal. Humanitarian interests may have a purifying effect but can only remove the grosser forms of the ego. According to Sri Aurobindo, "The greatest service to humanity ... is to prepare or find the way by which the individual and the collective man can transcend the ego and live in its true self, no longer bound to ignorance, incapacity, disharmony and sorrow."[3]

In all sadhaks, the ego is proven to be a stumbling block and it is not possible to get rid of the ego movements all at once. The ego and its desires are one of the main causes of the spiritual casualties that take place in sadhana. Even the possibility of detachment from and sublimation of the ego are not entirely free from serious dangers. It is not very difficult to starve the ego by rejecting all its impulses of action or to exalt it to a trance of peace and ecstacy, but sadhana aims to arrive at a divine manhood which shall be the perfect instrument of a divine action; each difficulty has to be entirely experienced and entirely mastered.

The first stages of sadhana, with almost all sadhaks, are egocentric. One's own endeavour is inevitable for most, as without it there would be no sufficient push or will to bring about the first necessary changes. However, the expulsion and rejection of the ego cannot be done only by the will and its efforts. At a certain stage of preparation, the negative attempt by a denial of the reality of the ego and its rejection must be replaced by the positive side of the sadhana, i.e., fixing one's thoughts constantly upon the One and the Infinite everywhere. During the progress in sadhana the sadhak becomes gradually able to get rid of the ego altogether through an uncompromising rejection of all egoistic habits, along with a constant and exclusive aspiration to feel the presence of the Divine Force in one's life and an unreserved surrender to that Divine Force. Another means of release from the ego is the control of the psychic being within, exerting its influence directly upon the rebellious parts. For a complete elimination of the ego-sense, the sadhak has to rise into the Supermind and bring down its supramental consciousness into the lower active nature.

GOD IN TRANSPERSONAL PSYCHOTHERAPY AND INTEGRAL SADHANA

Is God used as a projected salvation against despair borne of the absurd, and does man create a God in his or her emotional need for immortality? Is God being used as a replacement for unsatisfied human life on earth, and as a psychotherapeutic means against the vagueness regarding the meaning of life as presented to humans?

Man has an innate urge to transcend the apparently real and the element of godhead lies dormant in many people. God as infinite Truth is experienced by each person in the light of one's own tendencies and temperament. These individual tendencies propel different individual to see only that aspect of the infinite that is in tune with their temperaments. However, that God is only one's projection of God.

God is in danger when He/She is at the mercy of the hurdle of human motives, of which one's own well-being is perhaps the most noble one. God is still alive as a psychological status, but this same God is not a reality within the seeker's *Weltanschauung.* With one's psycho-social problems, meaninglessness, and metaphysical fears, one turns towards wordly salvation, as if man is the measurement of everything. The individual accepts one's wordly involvement as the highest welfare and life itself becomes the ultimate aim rather than experiencing and loving God from within. By prioritising the intellectual and emotional faculties over the spiritual ones, there remains nothing more important and bigger than man himself. The absolute reason of everything remains exclusively human and God is merely a psychological necessity, a deep-rooted human wish fulfilment, and such a projected pseudo-god may create confidence and security. By allowing oneself to reject such beliefs new insights into the unknown are able to rush in. Psychologizing God and using this within a therapeutic perspective is to take away God's metaphysical meaning. Encompassing God through preconceived categories of thought reduces God's experiential significance; making God something which the seeder can comprehend by one's thoughts and feelings is to take away God's spiritual essence. The belief in God as a support for one's own salvation, as a healer of one's loneliness on earth is not the same as loving or knowing God as an end in itself, as a reality present in one's life. Such a God as the subject of an existential realm need not become a mere conceptual abstraction.

When God is used as a speculative, theoretical psychological concept—all that which can be seen—then this God is related conceptually with worldly ideas, which can be experientially verified. But such theoretical concepts omit the individual involvement in a higher transcendental dimension and the intuitive communion with God or faith in His existence. The psychological God-image of concepts and theories is not the same God who is hidden behind this image, the Being of all Being and the Ground of all life. The naturalistic vision of a personal God can become an indulgent emotionalism confirming our prejudices rather than compelling us to transcend them. A God who does not transcend the personal category may in some profound sense be a product of the imagination of the human mind, and by creating an idol it pushes God outside the human condition. To look at the reality of things behind man's projected idea about God reveals God as the Source of everything. When God is no longer viewed from the limited psychological realm, but as this Source of the One and the All, then God is able to manifest itself in the individual's life. Again, God when used as a practical utility may remove obstacles but such a psychological God gives birth to passive and blind faith. The effort to gain faith is not a mere matter of belief in the Divine, but also an effort to realise the presence of the Divine within us. Men have the attribute of divinity within themselves and men and God do not remain distinct orders of being.

The practical interest of transpersonal psychotherapy in God does not really aim at the spiritual realisation of the union with God. Transpersonal psychology acknowledges mystical and spiritual experiences as symbols which indeed point to what we know as God, though many of the transpersonal psychologists often remain searching for the absolute ground of everything almost exclusively in man rather than the Divine. The transpersonal exploration of the mystical dimensions of life and its preoccupation with man's spiritual aspirations for a 'human spirituality' could be a highly valuable self-preparation for Sri Aurobindo's aim and destiny of human life.

Sri Aurobindo is aware of the pragmatic God-image which is at the mercy of the bundle of human needs and he writes, "It may be asked how is that devotion high and noble, which seeks God only for the worldly boons he can give or as a refuge in sorrow and suffering, and not the Divine for its own sake? ... where there is not knowledge, the devotee does not approach the Divine in his integral all-embracing truth, but constructs imperfect names and images of the Godhead which are only reflections of his own need, temperament and nature, and he worships them to help or appease his natural longings. He constructs for the Godhead the name and form of a divinised Christ or Buddha, or else some composite of natural qualities ... and to that he raises his altars without and in his heart and mind and falls down before it to demand from it worldly good and joy or healing of his wounds. ... Still the supreme Godhead does not at all reject these devotees because of their imperfect vision. For the Divine in his supreme transcendent being, unborn, imminuable and superior to all these partial manifestations, cannot be easily known to any living creature. ... Therefore, according to their nature, as they approach him, he accepts their bhakti [devotion] and answers to it with the reply of divine love and compassion. These forms are after all a certain kind of manifestation through which the imperfect human intelligence can touch him, these desires are first means by which our souls turn towards him nor is any devotion worthless or ineffective, whatever its limitations. It has the one grand necessity, faith. ... By the force of that faith in his worship he gets his desire and the spiritual realisation for which he is at the moment fitted ... By knowing the Divine in his forms and qualities, he shall come to know him as the All and the Transcendent who is the source of all things."[4]

Integral sadhana aims at giving ourselves wholeheartedly to the attempt at possessing the fullness of God, to be as perfect and pure as God is pure and perfect, and afterwards when we are ourselves perfect souls, to bring all mankind to the same divine perfection. For Sri Aurobindo God is in His ultimate existence beyond all manifestation; in relation to the world He is that which transcends all universal existence, but also that which contains and upholds the universe. As the supreme Personality, "the Personal God is not limited by His qualities, He is capable of infinite qualities and beyond them and lord of them to use them as He will, and He manifests Him in various names and forms of His infinite godhead to satisfy the desire and need of the individual soul according to its own nature and personality. It is for this reason that the normal European mind finds it so difficult to understand Indian religion as distinct from Vedantic or Sankhya philosophy, because it cannot easily conceive of a personal God with infinite qualities, a personal God who is not a Person, but the sole real Person and the source of all personality. Yet that is the only valid and complete truth of the divine Personality. ... Through the realisation of higher and higher principles of being and states of conscious existence we arrive ... at the transcendent Existence itself which is also the Existent who transcends all definition by personality and yet is always that which is the essence of personality."[5] God is both the

Personal Brahman and the Impersonal Brahman. There is no difference between these two stages, for every impersonal State depends upon a manifest Personality.

As soon as man is assured of a natural existence, he or she is able to move upwards to God. Humanity's spiritual fulfilment or God-attainment implies exceeding man's present apparent manhood and becoming what one really is, divine in the nature of the world. For Sri Aurobindo, man and the universe are veiled aspects of God; in the spiritual experience the experiencer is one with God and this oneness is the characteristic of Spirit. In integral Yoga, God is not a mere extra-cosmic being or only a static transcendent absolute entity, dominating man and the world as something foreign to His nature. God is related to the supra-cosmic, He/She embraces and includes the universe, the Cosmic Self that upholds all beings but He/She is also the Self of each individual. Thus Sri Aurobindo observes that, "in order to fulfil God in the individual we must exceed the individual. The removal of limited ego and the possession of cosmic consciousness is the first aim of our sadhana. In order to fulfil God in the cosmos, individually, we must transcend the universe. The ascension into transcendent consciousness is the second aim of our sadhana."[6] If God represents some Being totally different from man or life, completely outside the universe, then it might be averred that man can never be transformed into the Divine being. Sri Aurobindo maintains that God, out of pure self-delight, replicates Himself in the universe, and by the Grace of God man can rise from one's present condition. Integral sadhana prepares the seeker for the reception of this Divine Grace. According to Sri Aurobindo, "In order to exceed our Nature and become Divine we must first get God; for we are the lower imperfect term of our being. He is the higher perfect term.... The attainment of God is the true object of all human effort for which all the other efforts, political, social, literary, intellectual are only a necessary condition and preparation of the race."[7]

The bedrock of Sri Aurobindo's Yoga is the potential divinity of every soul. Spiritual endeavour consists in striving to manifest this divinity. For Sri Aurobindo man stands in an integral relation to God and has the attribute of divinity within oneself. He has given the human aspiration for the Divine a new vigour as man's unquenchable thirst for God, immortality and bliss. Man is the living and thinking laboratory in whom and with whose conscious cooperation nature will work out the hidden Godhead within the individual. This realisation of God within and without, the manifestation of the Divine in oneself becomes the ultimate aim and destiny of man. As pointed out by Sri Aurobindo, "God exists in Himself and not by virtue of the cosmos or of man, while man and the cosmos exists by virtue of God and not in themselves except in so far as their being is one with the being of God. But still they are a manifestation of the power of God.... What appears here as man is an individual being of the Divine; the Divine extended in multiplicity is the Self of all individual existences. Moreover, it is through the knowledge of self and the world that man arrives at the knowledge of God and he cannot attain to it otherwise. It is not by rejecting God's manifestation, but by rejecting his own ignorance of it and the results of his ignorance, that he can best lift up and offer the whole of his being and consciousness and energy and joy of being into the Divine Existence. He may do this through himself, one manifestation, or he may do it through the universe, another manifestation."[8] Though the quest itself has specific dangers and inevitable paradoxes, for several reasons the progress of being in our youngest solar system is not without contraries.

TRANSPERSONAL PSYCHOTHERAPY AND INTEGRAL SADHANA

Transpersonal psychotherapy and integral sadhana take consciousness as the true subject matter of psychology. Both approaches are concerned with the development of the latent possibilities of human nature, man's potential for spiritual growth and higher states of consciousness. The purpose of transpersonal psychotherapy is to widen the concept of what constitutes human nature and bring about a synthesis into human psychology of the modern scientific approach and traditional Eastern and Western contemplative insights and wisdom. It provides a basis for cross-cultural psychology, emphasising the study of transcendental and religious experiences and man's higher functions in order to be able to grasp the unifying and universal elements characteristic of all cultures.

Transpersonal psychotherapists in general attempt to find adequate answers to the fundamental questions of life. Some of the therapists examine the various psychological processes in the context of spiritual development and guide the seeker towards an opening beyond the psychological structures of the self, effecting healing and/or growth. Those transpersonal psychotherapists maintain that there is a higher state of being than the mere psychological state; our true identity is not only a psychological self but also a spiritual Self, and psycho-spiritual development aims at realising our true identity with the Self's spiritual Ground.

Transpersonal psychotherapists who are dealing with spiritual issues during psychotherapy are often confronted with the seeker's psychological difficulties. The search within is not without psychological risks. Almost every seeker in one's search for the Divine will be confronted with one's unresolved psychological problems. On the way to inner freedom the seeker is irrevocably bound to encounter one's aggression, fears, limitations, insecurities, pains, loneliness, etc., but simultaneously he or she also discovers new unknown areas within, which often creates a sense of inner fulfilment. As a technique for self-exploration and self-analysis; transpersonal psychotherapy can be seen as a form of self-healing, when it supplies the seeker with the necessary tools for inner freedom and release from human suffering due to one's bondage to one's own acquired nature. As such, it actualises the inner reality of man and one's craving for the Divine.

Sadhana often generates an intense effect and also has its potential risks of phases of chaos. However, in the course of practice the psychic transformation enables the sadhak to tackle one's problems in a more orderly manner, and the disintegrated mental structure gets united into a synthetic entity. For Sri Aurobindo the divine Guide of the sadhana is the psychic being; a mental rule or mental consciousness cannot be its leader. It is always the psychic being that is the real cause of man's turning to spiritual life and one's greatest help in it. It is the psychic being which opens the entire lower nature to the Divine.

In Sri Aurobindo's Yoga of self-perfection, intellectual, volitional ethical, emotional, aesthetic and physical training and improvement are all so much to the good, but they are only in the end a constant movement in a circle without any last delivering and illumining aim, unless they arrive at a point when they can open themselves to the power and presence of the Spirit and admit its direct workings. This direct working effects a conversion of the whole being which is the indispensable condition of our real perfection ... So long as there is only an intellectual, ethical and other selftraining for the now normal purposes of life which does not travel beyond the ordinary circle of working of mind, life and body, we are still only in the obscure and yet unillumined preparatory Yoga of Nature; we are still in pursuit of only an ordinary human perfection ... By personal effort a precursory change, a preliminary conversion can be effected ... That is as far as man can go by his unaided or indirectly aided effort, because that is an effort of mind and mind cannot climb beyond itself permanently."[9]

Integral Yoga aims at a divine perfection where the Divine becomes the direct guidance of the sadhana. Unlike transpersonal psychology, the yoga of integral perfection aims not only at the realisation but also at the perfection of the seeker's divine nature.

"In order that this spiritual being may not be something vague and indefinable or else but imperfectly realised and dependent on the mental support and the mental limitations, it seeks to go beyond mind to the supramental knowledge, will, sense, feeling, intuition, dynamic initiation of vital and physical action, all that makes the native working of the spiritual being. ... It rejects nothing that is essential in the mundane aim, but enlarges it, finds and lives in its greater and its truer meaning now hidden from it, transfigures it from a limited, earthly and mortal thing to a figure of intimate, divine and immortal values."[10]

Could it be that the transpersonal techniques need a more deep-rooted metaphysical approach to man in order to transform human life into a divine life?

For Sri Aurobindo, and Indian psychology in general, man is in his or her very essence a divine or spiritual being: each and every seeker is a portion and manifestation of the divine with latent possibilities. His integral sadhana emphasises the genuineness of the sadhak s own divine nature. The transpersonal psychotherapist assumes that man possesses sparks of the soul, which are spiritual 'substances', and with this substance man is able to commune with God. But in doing so the therapist is mixing up the word soul with the psyche, seeing the former as an epiphenomenon of the latter. As such there remains a qualitative difference between the human being and the Divine, whereas for Sri Aurobindo man is by his/her entire nature a divine being, i.e., the seeker *is* a searching soul rather than only *having* a soul.

In transpersonal psychology the soul is often only a hypothesis, but in integral sadhana the realisation of the soul is pursued as a matter of experience. The soul-entity in the transcendental realm is not identical with the chemical components of the body, although without them it would have no means of material expression. The individual can realise and conceptualise the psychic being for him or herself but can never localise it on the laboratory table i.e., one cannot dissect the soul under a microscope.

Sri Aurobindo would agree with the transpersonal psychotherapist that the lower nature and its obstacles have to be seen and purified; the more the lower nature is purified the easier is the descent of the higher Nature, although excessive preoccupation with the lower realm may not be very helpful. The seeker must become conscious of one's defects, "lay oneself before the light, see, reject, and change." Sri Aurobindo advices the sadhak not to react whenever he or she is confronted with stressful situations or problematic circumstnces, but to "step back", allow some time interval to go deep within, observe the situation in an impersonal calm and detached way and seek for the Divine intervention. He emphasises the importance of the descent of the spiritual Nature, "it is more true that the more the higher Nature descends, the more the lower is purified. Neither the complete purification nor the permanent and perfect manifestation can come all at once, it is a matter of time and patient progress. The two (purification and manifestation) go on progressing side by side and become more and more strong to play into each other s hands that is the usual course of the sadhana."[11]

Some transpersonal psychotherapists agree with Sri Aurobindo's views, but they also maintain that, in certain cases, purification needs an initial preoccupation on the lower nature, in order to avoid the various problems and dangers related to obstinate and hidden resistances and ego-enlargement, i.e., a deep-rooted investigation and working out of wrong movements rather than laying oneself before the light and waiting for the descent of the spiritual Nature. Sri Aurobindo is aware of such cases where stubborn resistances of the lower nature "have to be fought out or worked out— fought out if the nature is unsteady or insists violently, worked out if the will is steady and the nature moderate in its reactions."[12]

Could transpersonal psychotherapy be of any assistance during this "fighting it out" process? After such preparation where the resistances of the lower nature have been adequately dealt with, the psychic or enlightened mental will can guide the seeker quietly through all remaining difficulties.

As Sri Aurobindo's integral sadhana is not an easy practice and is often very difficult, especially in the initial stages, some seekers may need a few preliminary steps before they are ready to face all these difficulties. However, transpersonal psychotherapists must be aware of the aim of integral Yoga, and their psycho-spiritual methods should fit in and not contradict the path of integral sadhana.

Sri Aurobindo and the transpersonal psychotherapist look at the spiritual or mystical experience as something different from the normal waking consciousness. Both wish to give the spiritual experience a place in the natural area of experience within the human personality. The individual in the transcendent experience transcends the psychodynamic level and enters into the transpersonal realm, unifying spiritual and psychological perspectives. Though the transpersonal psychotherapist deals with the experience of an extension of identity beyond the usual limits of the ego and personality, beyond space and time, and enquires into the essential nature of Being, these explorations remain mostly confined to the highest reaches of human nature, and it seems that many transpersonal psychotherapists are often more concerned with the concept of 'human' instead of the 'divine'.

For most of the transpersonal psychotherapists, the primary focus remains centred on the growth towards a fuller human functioning, but in doing so they ignore the comprehending essence of man, i.e., to move to the divine to meet the needs of the soul. For Sri Aurobindo, the various ways to inner freedom are accompanied by a surrender to a higher Power and not a surrender of the psyche to the potential of the individual.

For Sri Aurobindo the transpersonal experience, as a specific mode of human comprehension, cannot be the complete and highest possible experience; these experiences may have a transcendental dimension but are not necessarily integral and spiritual (they pertain to or concern the Spirit). In transcending the ego, the transpersonal experience creates the universalisation of being, an expansion of consciousness towards the dimensions of the entire universe. But this universalisation of being is for Sri Aurobindo not an objective extension of the empirical consciousness. It is the collective ideal of the Divine that carries with it the solution and remedy to the disharmonies of existence as encountered by humans. Sri Aurobindo's sadhana aims at the transformation or divinisation of the values of humanity with the realisation of spiritual self-perfection; the values of humanity will be subordinated to those of the Spirit, as it is the soul, which is the source of all values.

Transpersonal psychology envisages the possibility of developing higher areas of awareness through transpersonally oriented therapeutic activities. These therapeutic activities play an important role in stimulating the individual's effort in the process of psycho-spiritual growth, but are not meant to stimulate behaviour modification.

However, transpersonal psycho-spiritual methods such as meditation, imagination, bodywork, etc., have a much deeper meaning for Sri Aurobindo. In integral sadhana, these methods are founded on a system of psycho-spiritual thought and are seen in a wider context including the paths of *Karma* and *Bhakti*. Moreover, the results of the transpersonal investigations can be questioned on the ground that spiritual issues cannot be investigated in isolation but need to be contextualised, viewing them in the light of classical ancestry. Such a task can be undertaken only by those skilled investigators who are directly involved in, or at least familiar with the specific spiritual discipline and its actual practices. The transpersonal intellectual quest for truth should be distinguished from Sri Aurobindo's practical realisation of truth, including the means that lead to this realisation. Transpersonal psychotherapists, attempting to explore the spiritual realm using therapeutic and scientific methods should therefore not omit the context in which spiritual disciplines are developed, and they should also describe its intent or purpose as well as the conditions for its rightful application.

In the application of transpersonal-therapeutic models, the transpersonal psychotherapist might abolish all the individual's ego limitations, but this does not automatically lead to the experience of unity with the Divine. As long as the individual lacks a proper spiritual attitude—aspiration for, as well as an opening and surrender to the Divine—then all psychological methods may be very valuable for the integration of the personality, but need not bring the individual into direct contact with one's spiritual development.

At present, the approach of transpersonal psychology leans more towards a mutual influence and relationship between the spiritual and psychological realms, than to the merely sequential link of the linear model in which spiritual development emerges only after psychological development is completed. Psychological integration need not always be completed before spiritual realisation, and the latter need not always include psychological integration. Spiritual realisation cannot always be measured or evaluated in terms of psychology; at times, psychological wholeness may be disintegrated but this may not affect the realisation of the Divine soul within.

Psychological development and spiritual development are not the same thing, and even though there might be a correlation and mutual interaction between the two, yet spiritual development may have different complex pathways and is, therefore, not identical to psychological development. Sometimes, these paths intermingle but at other times they remain separate. Depending upon the psycho-spiritual make-up of the seeker, the transpersonal psychotherapist assumes that psychological and spiritual healing can be pursued simultaneously and need not take place sequentially.

For Sri Aurobindo, however, the sadhak will find a complete resolution to the psychological obstacles of his egoic existence only by entering into the spiritual realm. It is in the connection with the spiritual realm that the sadhak will find a transforming significance, and a full transformation of psychological difficulties occurs only when the sadhak opens oneself to the spiritual realm. A purely psychological approach to the spiritual inner and higher parts of the being, cut off from Sri Aurobindo's metaphysical vision reduces the latter to the former, but the sources of the spiritual realm go well beyond psychological processes.

Integral Yoga is not primarily concerned with the attainment of a particular psychological state, and though psychological health is a necessary preliminary step towards perfection and integration, it is in the elaboration of the goals of the spiritual, liberated individual that Sri Aurobindo sharply diverges from any form of Western psychotherapy.

In psychological development, the seeker is allowed to focus more clearly on the various psychological aspects of human experience which may have certain consequences for spiritual development. Sri Aurobindo is aware that, in the transformation of the being, psychological self-analysis has an immense value and is practically indispensable and certainly will affect the process of purification. However, such psychological self-knowledge is only an intellectual conception or enlightened psychological experience of the modes of our being, but not a realisation of the Self as a pure Being. Psychological self-knowledge is only a key or first approach to the ascent which the seeker has to make till higher or deeper levels are attained. With the help of spiritual practices and Divine Grace, the seeker aims at the manifestation of the soul or the Divine Power within.

Integral sadhana and transpersonal psychotherapy are, therefore, not contradictory to each other, rather they are complementary, representing different levels of health and growth, and are simply dealing with different ranges of human development. Many of the analysis and insights of transpersonal psychology could be useful in helping the individual become stable and strong, and in providing the spiritual seeker with a first illuminating insight, before one enters the difficult path of Sri Aurobindo's integral sadhana.

When transpersonal psychotherapy and integral sadhana are well combined in their true balance, then their views, each with its own reality, are correlative. The combined insight of integral sadhana and transpersonal psychotherapy will contribute further to the progress of psychology, and their combined wisdom might accomplish what neither can do alone.

NOTES

1. R. Walsh and Fi Vaughan, *Paths Beyond Ego* p. 129.
2. Sri Aurobindo, *The Life Divine*, p. 692 - 694.
3. Sri Aurobindo, *The Synthesis of Yoga*, p. 344.
4. Sri Aurobindo, *Essays on the Gita*, p.285-287.
5. Sri Aurobindo, *The Synthesis of Yoga*, p.365-366.
6. Sri Aurobindo, *The Hour of God*, p.49.
7. Ibid., p.54-55.
8. Sri Aurobindo, *The Life Divine*, p.690-691.
9. Sri Aurobindo, *The Synthesis of Yoga*, p.592-593
10. Ibid., p.594.
11. Sri Aurobindo, *Letters on Yoga*, p. 906.
12. Ibid., p.1641.

Chapter Ten

A Critical Evaluation of Ken Wilber's Commentary on the Limitions of Sri Aurobindo's 'Individual' Integral Yoga

Ken Wilber admits that Sri Aurobindo has had and still continues to have a profound influence on his work, and that Sri Aurobindo was instrumental in his moving from Wilber I to Wilber II model. However, he refines these models later, into Wilber III and IV, and by now he comments on the limitations of Sri Aurobindo's integral view. Actually, Ken Wilber's criticism of Sri Aurobindo is not a repudiation of Sri Aurobindo's vision but a refinement. Ken Wilber states that Sri Aurobindo's 'individual' integral Yoga and practice is "especially focused on integrating the Ascending and Descending currents in the human being, thus embracing the entire spectrum of consciousness in both a transcendental/ascending and immanent/descending fashion. ... But that approach is really just the beginning of a much more integral view. ... A truly integral Yoga needs to take a much fuller account of the Western contributions of psychology, psychotherapy, and personal transformation (Ken Wilber III), and it needs most especially to be set in the context of the four quadrants and their historical unfolding (Ken Wilber IV)."[1]

For Ken Wilber these refinements are crucial, "especially as we begin the actual and specific details of integrating Eastern and Western models." He claims that without this refinement Sri Aurobindo's integral Yoga is limited and partial. In Ken Wilber's opinion, Sri Aurobindo's model lacks the developmental details of the transitional structures and self-sense which are associated with the basic structures and levels of the Upper-left quadrant (consciousness) and upperright quadrant (body). But it also lacks an understanding of the cultural and social influence on individual consciousness and behaviour.

Ken Wilber maintains that none of the Romantics (from Schelling, Fichte and Hegel to the Romantic poets) would have understood the four quadrants very well, and their comprehension of the transpersonal stages would have been rather limited. He assumes that these shortcomings were mainly due to the failure to develop transpersonal practices. Their systems were mistaken for metaphysics, as they lacked an experiential methodology to reproduce in consciousness the spiritual insights of their founders. Another failure of the idealist movement was related to the misidentification of the transpersonal domain with vision-logic.

For Ken Wilber a truly integral practice puts an equal importance on the upper-left quadrant (consciousness in its broadest sense) and on the upper-right quadrant (body in its broadest sense). This integration then acts as a quickening process of evolution from the gross bodymind to the causal bodymind. But the lower-left and lower-right quadrants, the cultural and social dimensions in their broadest sense, are also part of the overall integral practice. In this context, a balanced 'all-level, all-quadrant' programme can be developed for integral practice

In his *Integral Psychology,* Ken Wilber writes again, in a similar way, on the shortcomings of Sri Aurobindo's integral system. He admits the magnitude of Sri Aurobindo's achievements, but Sri Aurobindo's greatest shortcoming is a shortcoming faced by all theorists, namely, the unavailability of the important discoveries made since his time. "Aurobindo was most concerned with the transformations of consciousness (Upper Left) and the correlative changes in the material body (Upper Right). Although he had many important insights on the social and political system, he did not seem to grasp the actual interrelations of cultural, social, intentional, and behavioral aspects, nor did his analysis at any point proceed on the level of intersubjectivity (Lower Left) and interobjectivity (Lower Right)."[2]

But how could Sri Aurobindo have been aware in his time of the discoveries of modern cognitive science made many years after his time? It seems, therefore, that Ken Wilber's criticism regarding Sri Aurobindo's shortcomings is more applicable to the followers of Sri Aurobindo, who are not paying sufficient attention and making sufficient effort .to integrate contemporary scientific discoveries within the context of Sri Aurobindo's integral Yoga. They are often not convinced of the necessity of looking critically at Sri Aurobindo's spiritual views and attuning themselves to the most recent revolutionary developments in fields such as physics, biochemistry, genetics, cognitive science, neurobiology and brain science.

Could it be that Ken Wilber, in his integral vision, often analyses and synthesises various concepts, ideas and insights which were already extensively elaborated upon by Sri Aurobindo? Is Ken Wilber only using a different language to explain concepts and ideas similar to those developed in Sri Aurobindo's model? No doubt, Ken Wilber's achievement lies in his ability to analyse and integrate these concepts with the discoveries of contemporary science.

Did Sri Aurobindo's integral approach recognise that the various levels of inner consciousness have correlates with other quadrants? Was he aware that transcendental modes have correlates in the material domain, and that individual consciousness does not arise on its own, but that it has cultural contours and arises due to intersubjective events? Did he take into account that social determinants, like the social system in its objective sense, or techno-economic development, also penetrate into the contents of individual consciousness? In other words, did Sri Aurobindo make a sufficiently strong link between his spiritual objectives and social, economic, cultural and scientific goals which can be tested by any social or scientific criteria? Did he overlook the fact that the different levels of body, mind, soul and spirit each have four aspects: intentional, behavioural, social and cultural, i.e., an 'all-level, all-quadrant' approach, integrating consciousness, culture and nature?

An answer to these questions needs a detailed description of Sri Aurobindo's views on science, metaphysics, the relation between the individual and the collectivity, sociology, culture, religion, ethics, and his future vision.

SRI AUROBINDO'S VIEWS ON SCIENCE

Science has brought to man an increased mastery over one's physical surroundings, but it does not provide adequate self- knowledge or true life-unity and spiritual oneness. The present state of scientific knowledge is characterised by Sri Aurobindo in this way: "Science pursuing its cold and even way has made discoveries which have served on one side a practical humanitarianism, on the other hand supplied monstrous weapons to egoism and mutual destruction; it has made possible a gigantic efficiency of organisation which has been used on one side for the economic and social amelioration of the nations and on the other for turning each into a colossal battering-ram of aggression, ruin and slaughter. It has given rise on the one side to a large rationalistic and altruistic humanitarianism, on the other it has justified a godless egoism, vitalism, vulgar will to power and success. It has drawn mankind together and given it a new hope and at the same time crushed it with the burden of a monstrous commercialism."[3]

Science has always been considered primarily as a means of gaining knowledge of reality, and practical utility comes afterwards as a secondary by-product. However, science itself cannot explain the ultimate reality, it can only at best describe phenomena. In order to comprehend the total reality, it requires an integral vision. Physical science cannot claim anything on these higher and inner regions as it does not have the means of enquiry or any possibility of arriving at any valid decision. Sri Aurobindo does not deny the worth of the achievements and the positive knowledge of science, but he wants to complete it by gaining knowledge of the essential truth of things as distinguished from their phenomenal appearances. To do so, he suggests that scientists probe upward and inward' rather than remaining content with only surface scrutiny. As expressed by Sri Aurobindo, "the physical scientist probing into phenomena erects formulas and standards based on the objective and phenomenal reality and its processes; he has to act as if matter and energy alone existed and mind were only an observer of an independent physical reality.... The psychologist, probing independently into mind consciousness and mind unconsciousness, discovers another domain of realities, subjective in its character, which has its own law and process; to him Mind may even come to appear as the key of the real, Matter as only a field for mind, and spirit apart from mind as something unreal. But there is a farther probing which brings up the truth of self and spirit and establishes a greater order of the real in which there is a reversal of our view both of the subjective mind realities and objective physical realities so that they are seen as things phenomenal, secondary, dependent upon the truth of self and the realities of the spirit. In this deeper search into things mind and matter begin to wear the appearance of a lesser order of the real and may easily come to appear unreal ... an original and ultimate consciousness embracing all the terms of existence in a single integral view would see the whole in its spiritual essential reality and the phenomenon as a phenomenon or manifestation of that reality."[4]

For Sri Aurobindo science is nothing more than a support for the mind, extremely practical and useful in dealing with physical energies in the material world. But while these practical aspects of science are valid in their own field they do not represent the whole truth of things. The scientist, finding out more and more about the processes of the physical field, may now be able to gain repossession of mental and psychic knowledge. Before arriving at supraphysical certitudes, the seeker still has to adhere to the rigorous methods of science, though not to its purely physical instrumentation. The preoccupation with physical existence is in the beginning necessary, but it is only a preliminary step.

"The gospel of materialism, in spite of the dazzling triumphs of physical Science, proves itself always in the end a vain and helpless creed, and that too is why physical Science itself with all its achievements, though it may accomplish comfort, can never achieve happiness and fullness of being for the human race. Our true happiness lies in the true growth of our whole being, in mastery of the inner as well as and more than the outer, the hidden as well as the overt nature; our true completeness comes not by describing wider circles on the plane where we began, but by transcendence."[5]

However much we may analyse the physical realm with the help of mechanical methods, we will not arrive at the knowledge or the workings of the Self or God, as this Self is a Reality not obvious to the senses. Spiritual life does not cut at the roots of science, but lifts it out of its limitations, and in the end science is compelled to perceive the Infinite, the divine Intelligence and Will in the material universe. Sri Aurobindo insists that the marvels of science and technology need to be pressed into the service of the Divine Will to self-manifestation in material conditions. "The Yogin's aim in the practical sciences, whether mental and physical or occult and psychic, should be to enter into the ways of the Divine and his processes, to know the materials and means for the work given to us so that we may use that knowledge for a conscious and faultless expression of the spirit's mastery, joy and self-fulfilment."[6]

For Sri Aurobindo, "Yoga is scientific to this extent that it proceeds by subjective experiment and bases all its findings on experience; mental intuitions are admitted only as a first step and are not considered as realisation—they must be confirmed by being translated into and justified by experience."[7]

The experiences of Yoga belong to an inner domain and go according to their own laws, have their own method of perception and criteria which are not of the domain of rational or scientific inquiry. It is impossible to test the data of spiritual experience and prove their existence, their law and nature by the aid of ordinary reason. In the words of Sri Aurobindo, "The physical scientists have their own field with its own instruments and standards. To apply the same tests to phenomena of a different kind is as foolish as to apply physical tests to spiritual truth. One can't dissect God or see the soul under a microscope."[8] The only way to test spiritual experience is through accumulation of experience and use of an intuitive discrimination which compares the experiences with the methods laid down by the Guru or by the spiritual systems of the past.

For science the Ultimate Truth is physical and objective and the objective Ultimate explains all the subjective phenomena, but in integral Yoga, the Ultimate Truth is spiritual and subjective, and subjective phenomena are viewed in the light of spiritual Truth. The broad lines of Yogic experiences have something identical and universal and run everywhere the same, i.e. the intuitions and experiences are the same in the various systems all over the world.

It is clear for Sri Aurobindo that "subjective discovery must be pursued by a subjective method of enquiry, observation and verification; research into the supraphysical must evolve, accept and test an appropriate means and methods other than those by which one examines the constituents of physical objects and the processes of Energy in material Nature ... most spiritual experiences of any value, cannot be brought before the tribunal of the common mentality which has no experience of these things and takes its own absence or incapacity of experience as a proof of their invalidity or their non-existence. Physical truth of formulas, generalisations, discoveries founded upon physical observation can be so referred, but even there a training of capacity is needed before one can truly understand and judge ... all men can have a spiritual experience and can follow it out and verify it in themselves, but only when they have acquired the capacity or can follow the inner methods by which that experience and verification are made possible."[9]

Ken Wilber expresses a similar view when he explains the concept of 'category error,' where facts of physical truth try to replace principles of mental truth and the latter tiy to replace contemplative truths. A category error occurs when the knowledge of empiricism attempts to usurp the domain of the knowledge of rationalism and transcendentalism. Such category errors can occur in any direction; the eye of reason cannot adequately disclose the realm of contemplation, and the eye of contemplation is not able to disclose the facts of the realm of space, time and matter.

For Ken Wilber, "a higher eye cannot be reduced to nor explained in terms of a lower eye; each eye is valid and useful in its own field, but commits a fallacy when it attempts, by itself, to fully grasp higher or lower realms."[10] Ken Wilber's transcendental paradigm integrates all the three realms—matter, reason and transcendental insight. In a similar way, Sri Aurobindo's valid solution of the truth of cosmic and individual existence involves not only the knowledge of matter and its processes, but also the knowledge of mind, life, spirit and soul and their processes, as well as all that is behind the material universe.

Ken Wilber's three modes of knowing, which disclose a different type of world—sensibilia, intelligibilia and transcendelia—are all valid types of knowledge. To justify the validity of each type of knowledge he suggests the three strands of instrumental injunction (experimental evidence), intuitive apprehension (experiential illumination) and communal confirmation/rejection. A similar approach to the validity of knowledge is described by Sri Aurobindo: "All truth supraphysical or physical. must be founded, not on mental belief alone, but on experience—but in each case experience must be of the kind, physical, subliminal or spiritual, which is appropriate to the order of the truths into which we are empowered to enter; their validity must be scrutinised, but according to their own law and by a consciousness which can enter into them and not according to the law of another domain or by a consciousness which is capable only of truths of another order."[11]

For Ken Wilber and Sri Aurobindo, the supraphysical is as real as the physical, but the reality of the supraphysical planes adapts a different system and ordering of its principles than the reality of the physical and mental planes. According to Sri Aurobindo, "demand for physical valid proof of a supraphysical fact is irrational and illogical ... A supraphysical fact may impinge on the physical world and produce physical results; it may even produce an effect on our physical senses and become manifest to them, but that cannot be its invariable action and most normal character or process. Ordinarily, it must produce a direct effect on our mind and our life being, and can only indirectly and through them, if at all, influence the physical world and physical life. If it objectivises itself, it must be to a subtler sense in us and only derivatively to the outward physical sense."[12]

Sri Aurobindo foresees that "the outposts of scientific Knowledge come more and more to be set on the borders that divide the material from the immaterial, so also the highest achievements of practical Science are those which tend to simplify and reduce to the vanishing-point the machinery by which the greatest effects are produced. ... The sensible physical means for the intermediate transmission of the physical force is removed; it is only preserved at the points of impulsion and reception. Eventually even these must disappear; for when the laws and forces of the supraphysical are studied with the right starting point, the means will infallibly be found for Mind directly to seize on the physical energy ... there lie the gates that open upon the enormous vistas of the future."[13]

Sri Aurobindo's science of the new Man transcends its present limitations and gets transformed into a meta-science, "a new science not yet developed, which deals directly with the forces of the life-world and of Mind and so arrives at what is beyond Mind: but present-day science cannot do that."[14]

Ken Wilber wants 'real science' to expand from its narrow empiricism to a broad empiricism which does not only rely on sensory experience but also includes direct experience. He aims at a broad science of all quadrants which includes the exteriors of 'its', but also the interiors of 'I' and 'we'. The four quadrants can be integrated with the help of a deep science that is operative in spiritual experience as well as in physics. Nevertheless, the strict orthodox empirical science can also be helpful for the investigation of higher states of consciousness, i.e., these higher states can be investigated with the help of physical instruments as the physical world is not merely the lowest world in a series of spheres, but runs parallel to these spheres. In this way, science becomes the exterior or 'it' of Spirit, like Spirit seen subjectively becomes the 'I' of Spirit, and Spirit seen intersubjectively becomes the 'we' of Spirit. Science (broad or narrow) is therefore only one of the four quadrants and helps the individual to investigate the immediate data or experiences that are the raw material of the body realm, subtle realm or causal realm. However, there is also the 'I' and 'we' in the body, the subtle and causal realm, and science is therefore only one-third of the full story. Ken Wilber claims that his integral view is applicable to research with the help of the 'all-level, all-quadrant' model. Such research investigates the various phenomena in each of the four quadrants and correlates each with the others, without reducing one to the others. A future science will be enormously widened if it does not only make use of the world of the senses, but also pays attention to the mental and spiritual worlds which necessitate their own methodologies and validity claims.

Present scientific development in biology and medicine, in neurochemistry, genetics, clinical psychology and information technology are advancing rapidly. These developments are one of the ways in which science is attempting to answer the fundamental questions that could benefit the searching souls. It may not always be clear how Sri Aurobindo's spiritual evolutionary model is at present applicable to this revolution of scientific development.

For Sri Aurobindo, however, "Neither the laws nor the possibilities of physical Nature can be entirely known unless we know also the laws and possibilities of supraphysical Nature; therefore, the development of new and the recovery of old mental and psychic sciences have to follow upon the perfection of our physical knowledge, and that new era is already beginning to open upon us. But the perfection of the physical sciences was a prior necessity and had to be the first field for the training of the mind of man in his new endeavour to know Nature and possess his world."[15]

SRI AUROBINDO'S METAPHYSICAL VISION

As long as science remains concerned with the truth of processes and the conditions under which they happen in nature, it will not give the rationale of the whole, as it misses the Divine Reality which cannot be put into a single formula. For Sri Aurobindo, true understanding of Yoga does not come by the exercise of the logical mind and sadhana can reach its goal when the intellectual and logical mind is stilled and opens itself to the deeper consciousness, vision and knowledge. The experiences of the Divine are not mental constructions or vital movements but essential experiential processes felt in our underlying substance and essence. "One has to arrive at spiritual knowledge through experience and consciousness of things which arises directly out of that experience or else underlies or is involved in it. This kind of knowledge, then, is fundamentally a consciousness and not a thought or formulated idea."[16]

Reason is not in possession of Truth, it leaves Truth rendered into mental representations and an ideative scheme. Its field is the finite and its concepts start from sense data, but it cannot move into the realm of the Infinite. Sri Aurobindo does not deny reason or discourage the intellect, but he does want reason to be *receptive* to a higher kind of perception. Reason can enhance its capacities by opening itself to higher categories of truth. By doing so it can function' as a bridge between the superconscious truth and the ordinary perception of the human mind. Spirituality does not discourage human mental activity, but lifts the faculty of reason up, out of its imperfection, and transforms it by its touch so that it becomes an instrument of the light and power of the divine being and the divine nature.

For Sri Aurobindo, like Ken Wilber, metaphysical

reasoning should establish its generalisations from spiritual experiences and, on the basis of that experience together with the seeker's own evidence, it arrives at a supreme proof in which the reasoning intellect comes in only on the second line as a judge of the generalised statements drawn from the experience. In the words of Sri Aurobindo, "As there is a category of facts to which our senses are our best available but very imperfect guides, as there is a category of truths which we seek by the keen but still imperfect light of our reason, so according to the mystic, there is a category of more subtle truths which surpass the reach both of the senses and the reason but can be ascertained by an inner direct knowledge and direct experience. These truths are supersensuous, but not the less real for that: they have immense results upon the consciousness changing its substance and movement, bringing especially deep peace and abiding joy, a great light of vision and knowledge, a possibility of the overcoming of the lower animal nature, vistas of a spiritual self-development which without them do not exist."[17]

Ken Wilber says exactly the same thing when he writes, "Physics has told us all sorts of significant things about that last level [the physical plane]. Of its predecessors, it can say nothing (without turning itself into biology, psychology, or religion). To put it crudely, the study of physics is on the first floor, describing the interactions of its elements; the mystics are on the sixth floor describing the interaction of all six floors ... Further, physics and mysticism are not two different approaches to the same reality. They are different approaches to two quite different levels of reality, the latter of which transcends but includes the former."[18] He maintains that it is of no use to confuse temporal scientific facts with timeless contemplative realms and for Ken Wilber, "Let them [physics and mysticism] appreciate each other, and let their dialogue and mutual exchange of ideas never cease. But unwarranted and premature marriages usually end in divorce, and all too often a divorce that terribly damages both parties."[19]

Like Ken Wilber, Sri Aurobindo sees that the generalisations of science cannot be made the basis for a sound metaphysical thinking; the mystic has one's own domain and instruments. A scientific generalisation is valid in the limits of the domain of scientific observation and the measurement of physical processes and motions, whereas a metaphysical generalisation transforms the limited physical result into an unlimited allembracing formula. For Ken Wilber and Sri Aurobindo, the problem of the absolute/relative cannot be solved by using empiricism and rationalism; its truth can only be disclosed by contemplative unfolding. The conflict between science and metaphysics arises from a misunderstanding of each other's role, position and fields of study; the conflict arises due to the overstepping of the respective spheres.

Sri Aurobindo would agree with Ken Wilber's suggestion about the continuation of their dialogue regarding the possibility of a future co-operation between science and metaphysics in the pursuit of truth; the truth of the physical universe is able to throw some light on the phenomena of the inner world and vice versa. As described by Sri Aurobindo, "Nothing can be more remarkable and suggestive than the extent to which modern Science confirms in the. domain of Matter the conceptions and even the very formulae of language which were arrived at, by a very different method, in the Vedanta. And these, on the other hand, often reveal their full significance, their richer contents only when they are viewed in the new light shed by the discoveries of modem Science."[20]

Ken Wilber relates metaphysics to thought with evidence. The contemplative endeavours of great saints, yogis, mystics and gurus all aim at going within and beyond reason. However, they all start with reason in establishing truth by evidence through experimental contemplative methods tested by individual experience. Thus metaphysical claims are conclusions based on the long practice of experimental introspection and communal verification, which are directly disclosed to immediate awareness under proper conditions.

Metaphysics, according to Ken Wilber, needs contemplative practices or experimental methods which reproduce the spiritual insights of its founder. As such, metaphysics implies a contemplative development grounded in genuine spiritual experience rather than the utilisation of symbolic mental experiences to stand for spiritual experiences.

In appreciating Sri Aurobindo's metaphysical system, Ken Wilber writes, "Scholars usually take Plotinus's system (and Aurobindo's and all such similar transpersonal holarchies) to be primarily a form of philosophy or 'metaphysics': the various levels, particularly the higher ones, are imagined to be some sort of theoretical construct that is deduced, logically, or postulated, speculatively, to account for existence and manifestation. It dawns on few interpreters that these systems are, through and through, from top to bottom, the results of actual contemplative apprehensions and direct developmental phenomenology. The higher levels of these systems cannot be experienced or deduced *rationally,* and nobody from Plotinus to Aurobindo thinks they can. However, *after the fact* of direct and repeated experiential disclosures, they can be rationally reconstructed and presented as a 'system'. ... Not a single component of these systems is hidden to experience or nestled safely away in a 'metaphysical' domain that cannot be checked cognitively with the appropriate tools. There is absolutely nothing 'metaphysical' about these systems: they are empirical phenomenological developmental psychology at its most rigorous and most comprehensive, carried straightforwardly and openly into the transpersonal domains via the experimental instrument of contemplation."[21]

For Ken Wilber, any real future metaphysics should be based on actual contemplative development in which direct spiritual experiences replace abstract metaphysical thought. This involvement in the higher dimensions of existence, potentially inherent in each and every being, can be directly actualised and realised by anyone. These higher and deeper grades of development exist within, they are experimental, experiential and need not be explained by otherworldliness or metaphysical postulates.

Ken Wilber agrees with Sri Aurobindo regarding the actualisation of transpersonal potentials, "if they aren't actualized they are merely *projected horizontally* into utterly futile schemes to turn this finite world into a utopian world of infinite wonderment; an infinite above collapses into an infinite ahead, and whether that infinite ahead be endless scientific progress or boundless material possessions or political utopianisms as ultimate salvation, they are all fundamentally ways of fussing about in the finite looking for the infinite."[22]

However, it seems to this author that the psychological interpretations of Sri Aurobindo's metaphysical vision have to be primarily understood from the depth of the unifying heart, rather than merely being investigated by the synthesising mind on the vision-logic level. Sri Aurobindo's metaphysical claims are grounded in his spiritual practice and in the realisation of his reproducible spiritual experiences. In this context, D. Rothberg notices that "Part of carrying out transpersonal inquiry may thus be not only to examine the validity of reasons and evidence in relation to particular claims and theories. It may also be to explore more 'internally' (perhaps even as a kind of contemplative practice) the experiential background of ideas."[23]

Ken Wilber admits that "transpersonal studies in

themselves are not necessarily a spiritual practice although, of course, the two are intimately connected. ... It is from the community of those who have displayed a *competence* in any of these fields that the reconstructive science of transpersonal psychology draws its subjects. The theory of transpersonal psychology depends upon those who have practiced and achieved competence in a transpersonal spiritual discipline."[24]

SRI AUROBINDO'S VIEWS ON THE INDIVIDUAL AND COLLECTIVITY

When individuals intuit the Higher Self, Inner soul or Transcendental consciousness, and interpret such manifestations merely in the personal I terms, they often leave out the social, cultural and objective manifestations of these intuitions, as if they were aspects of the Self's manifestation that could be avoided. However, as mentioned before, according to Ken Wilber, "Spirit manifests always and simultaneously *as* the four quadrants of the Kosmos."[25] For Ken Wilber, "the more you contact the Higher Self, the *more* you worry about the world, as a component of your very Self, the Self of each and all. Brahman is the World. To finally contact Brahman is to *ultimately* engage the World."[26]

Spirit manifests as a self in a wider intersubjective community with objective correlates, i.e., "intuitions touching the I and We and the It domains ... to see it embraced in culture, embodied in nature, and embedded in social institutions."[27]

Ken Wilber, as well as Sri Aurobindo, does not want the individual to withdraw from social engagements and intersubjective actions, but for Sri Aurobindo all these actions, howsoever based on lofty ideals, are taken in the service of humanity and not in the service of the Divine. Sri Aurobindo's Higher Self includes the Universal and Transcendental dimensions of the Divine, and this Higher Self does not focus on the worries of the mundane world.

This does not mean that Sri Aurobindo ignores the mundane world, but instead of worrying about it, he emphasises its transformation. By bringing down the divine consciousness to the world the necessity of service to man in distress will be eliminated.

For Sri Aurobindo the individual cannot be human without society and vice versa, and the same individual cannot be what he or she is without the integral character of one's relation to society. There is an isomorphic relation [a similarity in structure in unrelated forms] between the development of the individual and society, where one influences and in turn is influenced by the other. Sri Aurobindo writes, "Since our divine perfection embraces the realisation of ourselves in being, in life and in love through others as well as through ourselves, the extension of our liberty and of its results in others would be the inevitable outcome as well as the broadest utility of our liberation and perfection."[28]

Man is both individual and social at the same time, and his or her individuality and social nature are the two indivisible aspects of one's being. Individual characteristics such as uniqueness, purposiveness or self-consciousness are also found in society, but only in a non-manifested form. The individual provides the dynamics of the collective progress, but it seems for Sri Aurobindo that the need for the organisation of the parts of a whole is more difficult to achieve, when done by the collectivity than by the individual.

For Sri Aurobindo, the collective consciousness can develop only through the illuminating consciousness of its individuals. He observes that, "The individual is indeed the key of the evolutionary movement; for it is the individual who finds himself, who becomes conscious of the Reality. The movement of the collectivity is a largely subconscious mass-movement; it has to formulate and express itself through the individuals to become conscious: its general mass-consciousness is always less evolved than the consciousness of its most developed individuals, and it progresses in so far as it accepts their impress or develops what they develop."[29]

In his primary emphasis on the individual as the key to the evolutionary movement he focuses his attention *initially* to a greater extent on the individual than on the collective being, though *the chief aim of integral Yoga includes society in a unique way—that of increasing levels of knowledge among all.* The principal individual laws which can be applied to individual existence can also be applied to social existence; both have a common nature and explore an identical goal.

The nature of human society is closely related to the nature of the individual human being; both follow a similar parallel curve of evolution on earth, but for Sri Aurobindo the collectivity is more dependent on the individual than the individual on the collectivity, i.e., the individual is not confined within the community and a mere cell of the collective existence; the individual would not cease to exist if separated from the collective mass.

It is through the individual that the cosmic spirit organises its collective units and through the individual that it raises Nature from its inconscience to the Superconscience and exalts it to meet the Transcendent.

The emergence of a new principle occurs first in a few exceptional individuals from whom it afterwards widens into larger parts of the collectivity. This is described by Sri Aurobindo as: "it is through the progressive and formative individual that it [the Spirit] offers the discovery and the chance of a new self-creation to the mind of the race. For the communal mind holds things subconsciently at first or, if consciously, then in a confused chaotic manner: it is only through the individual mind that the mass can arrive at a clear knowledge and creation of the thing it held in its subconscient self. ... All great changes therefore find their first clear and effective power and their direct shaping force in the mind and spirit of an individual or of a limited number of individuals. The mass follows, but unfortunately in a very imperfect and confused fashion which often or even usually ends in the failure or distortion of the thing created. If it were not so, mankind could have advanced on its way with a victorious rapidity instead of with the lumbering hesitations and soon exhausted rushes that seem to be all of which it has yet been capable."[30]

For Sri Aurobindo, "The perfect society will be that which most entirely favours the perfection of the individual; the perfection of the individual will be incomplete if it does not help towards the perfect state of the social aggregate to which he belongs and eventually to that of the largest possible human aggregate, the whole of a united humanity."[31]

In the integral spiritual society, the free individual can realise the deeper unity and potentiality of one's being, beyond the mental being. When individuals realise the unity of mankind in their own spiritual depth then these individuals can be assured of a deeper unity of existence. Nevertheless, Sri Aurobindo does not ignore the importance of a collective social life. Man does not live as an isolated being and does not grow in an isolated freedom. Man develops by one's relation with others and one's freedom expresses itself in a progressive self-harmonisation with the freedom of one's fellow-beings. "Collectivism may itself in the end realise this aim [freedom on the basis of unity] if it can modify its own dominant principle far enough to allow for a free individual development on the basis of unity and a closely harmonised common existence. But to do that it must first spiritualise itself and transform the very soul of its inspiring principle: it cannot do it on the basis of the logical reason and a mechanically scientific ordering of life."[32]-

For Sri Aurobindo, "the solution lies not in the reason

but in the soul of man, in its spiritual tendencies. It is a spiritual, an inner freedom that can alone create a perfect human order. ... It is in the soul that it must find its roots; the love which is founded upon a deeper truth of our being ... the spiritual comradeship which is the expression of an inner realisation of oneness."[33]

A perfected life upon earth includes the perfection of the collective being, but this collective perfection remains short of attainment so long as the individuals constituting it remain imperfect themselves. The race of Supermanhood implies not only the bringing into play of the Supermind in man, transforming him or her into an image of the Divine, but also the dynamic manifestation of God in the material circumstances of our human life. The object of integral Yoga is not to create an individual superman, but to bring down the supramental consciousness on earth, to create a new race with the principle of the supramental consciousness governing the inner and outer individual and collective life.

When rightly conceived supermanhood is not only an ideal of individual growth or the isolated realisation by a few individuals of the true inner life, but also an ideal of collective transformation or racial evolution. For Sri Aurobindo, the spiritual life bases its action in the collective life upon an inner experience and inclusion of others in our own being, an inner sense and reality of oneness. ... A realisation of spiritual unity, a dynamisation of the intimate consciousness of one-being, of one self in all beings, can alone found and govern by its truth the action of the divine life. In the gnostic or divine being, in the gnostic life, there will be a close and complete consciousness of the self of others. ... The gnostic being finds himself not only in his own fulfilment which is the fulfilment of the Divine Being and Will in him, but in the fulfilment of others; his universal individuality effectuates itself in the movement of the All in all beings towards its greater becoming."[34]

Sri Aurobindo does not regard Supermanhood as one single rigidly fixed pattern of living, there is sufficient wealth of differences and variations which characterise the race of Superman, although the basic consciousness will be the same in all of them. Every member of the Superman collectivity will realise the Divine not only in him or herself, but also in all the other members, in the All of existence. The inner harmony in every individual will be reflected in the common life of the society and the harmony of the collective existence will enrich the harmonised life of the individual. But the sole true supermanhood and the one real possibility of a step forward in evolutionary Nature is "not an egoistic supermanhood seizing on a mental and vital domination over humanity, but the sovereignty of the Spirit over its own instruments, its possession of itself and its possession of life in the power of the spirit, a new consciousness in which humanity itself shall find its own self-exceeding and selffulfilment by the revelation of the divinity that is striving for birth within it."[35]

The relationship between the individual and the collective being is meaningfully described by Sri Aurobindo: "The collectivity is a mass, a field of formation; the individual is the diviner of truth, the form-maker, the creator. In the crowd the individual loses his inner direction and becomes a cell of the mass-body moved by the collective will or idea or the mass-impulse. He has to stand apart, affirm his separate reality in the whole, his own mind emerging from the common mentality, his own life distinguishing itself in the common life-uniformity, even as his body has developed something unique and recognisable in the common physicality. He has, even, in the end to retire into himself in order to find himself, and it is only when he has found himself that he can become spiritually one with all; if he tries to achieve that oneness in the mind, in the vital, in the physical and has not yet a sufficiently strong individuality, he may be overpowered by the mass-consciousness and lose his soulfulfilment, his mind-fulfilment, become only a cell of the mass-body. The collective being may then become strong and dominant, but it is likely to lose its plasticity, its evolutionary movement: the great evolutionary periods of humanity have taken place in communities where the individual became active, mentally, vitally or spiritually alive."[36]

The ideal of human life unites the preservation of the individuality of man and the fulfilment of one's spiritual possibilities in this world, and simultaneously actively participating in the affairs of the society. It is the achievement of this two-fold ideal of man which is able to establish the Divine Life here upon earth.

Nevertheless, any attempt at a large scale collective spiritual life is always liable to be vitiated by the imperfections of the individuals themselves. Sri Aurobindo points out that, "Our nature, our consciousness is that of beings ignorant of each other, separated from each other, rooted in a divided ego, who must strive to establish some kind of relation between their embodied ignorances; for the urge to union and forces making for union are there in Nature."[37] Sri Aurobindo is aware that usually this union in our present human existence is only "a physical collectivity held together by the common physical life-fact and all that arises from it, community of interests, a common civilisation and culture, a common social law, an aggregate mentality, an economic association, the ideals, emotions, endeavours of the collective ego with the strand of individual ties and connections running through the whole and helping to keep it together. Or, where there is a difference in these things, opposition, conflict, a practical accommodation or an organised compromise is enforced by the necessity of living together; there is erected a natural or a constructed order."[38] But this is not Sri Aurobindo's view of the divine way of collective living, where all will be united by the evolution of the Truth- Consciousness in them.

At present, the relations formed in the collectivity are deformed by imperfections, misunderstandings, strife, discord and unhappiness. As long as the collectivity builds a constructive unity on the basis of interests and egos which impose an artificial constructed order by enforced law and custom, there cannot be a "true union of consciousness founded upon a nature of self-knowledge, inner realisation of unity, concord of our inner forces of being and inner forces of life."[39]

At the same time, for Sri Aurobindo it is a certainty that for the effectuation of a real spiritual change of human life and nature the combination of the individual and the collectivity must happen some day, "but none can tell how many attempts will have to be made and how many sediments of spiritual experience will have to be accumulated in the subconscient mentality of the communal human being before the soil is ready. For the chances of success are always less powerful in a difficult upward effort affecting the very roots of our nature than the numerous possibilities of failure."[40]

Sri Aurobindo does not conceive of the individual's relation to the society as merely that of the part to the whole; their relation is quite complex and many-sided and cannot always be expressed in a single formula of a well-ordered character. The integral man concerns oneself with the political, social, economical and spiritual aspects of life, as the spiritual life comprises all possible aspects of life and concerns itself with all other beings and their lives, i.e., the spiritual life integrates the individual, collective and the whole of mankind.

For Sri Aurobindo the question is not either individuality or collectivity but is more related to what comes first, and his dictum that "from the individual therefore we have to start; he is our index and our foundation"[41] can be disputed.

According to D.P. Chattopadhyaya, "One may

argue that a man is not human at all unless and until he is the member of a group. ... If human personality is shaped and we think it is, by some definite and necessary social institutions like language, traditional behavioural responses, conventions and customs, there is no reason for man to be surprised at the discovery of similarity between personality structure and social structure. But this account of individual-social isomorphism clashes with the view that man comes first and the group next."[42]

Though Sri Aurobindo does not neglect the social, economic, cultural and political liberty in the spiritual synthesis of the individual and the collective being, he nevertheless emphasises only spiritual freedom. Spiritual life does not necessarily mean only something metaphysical or transcendental; man, society and humanity are all graded aspects of the same dynamic spiritual event. But does the creative freedom of the Spirit expresses itself only in terms of some metaphysical or transcendental process, or can it also be realised in the planning of a free, prosperous and just society? Spiritual life does not necessarily mean only something metaphysical or transcendental; man, society and humanity are all graded aspects of the same dynamic spiritual event

Sri Aurobindo tackles these problems in the light of spiritual intuition, the logic of the infinite, i.e., the spiritual intuition which is able to grasp the complex relation of the seemingly opposite characteristics of the future divine life and the facts of the present human life

SRI AUROBINDO'S VIEWS ON SOCIOLOGY

Sri Aurobindo's view of society is not a biological one, but essentially spiritual, even though he admits a close identity between the biological organism and society. The organic unity of society is only a characteristic of its external self; it is the external self of society which has an organic structure.

But for Sri Aurobindo, the human collectivity is not a mere mechanical combination; the truth of the individual and of the collectivity and their true synthesis can be discovered only in a deeper unitary principle of Being within the individual.

Sociology as a science pays almost all its attention to external data, institutions, rites, customs, economic factors and development, but it often neglects man's deeper psychospiritual elements. The surface laws of life and their practical utilities are not difficult to understand and are sufficient for a superficial life. But the knowledge of the secret all-determining laws of the depth of life are more difficult to comprehend, yet it is these depths and their unseen forces that we ought to know in order to understand existence. It is most difficult for man to understand these hidden laws, when they are working obscured in the collective life, and "Sociology does not help us, for it only gives us the general story of the past and the external conditions under which communities have survived ... our whole thought and action with regard to our collective life is shallow and empirical; it does not seek for, it does not base itself on a firm, profound and complete knowledge."[43]

Man is unaware of the secret forces and influences which are at work at the subtler levels and which are shaping the effects and results of human striving in the peripheral world. All the advancements of scientific and technological development notwithstanding, man has failed to create a humane society. It is not only in social and political devices that the unity of the human race can be fruitfully accomplished. Intellectual and material circumstances, especially scientific discoveries, may fail to bring about the unity of mankind, unless man accepts an inner change along with the external judgement. Sri Aurobindo is aware that the perfection of this ideal human unity still waits to be discovered: "at present the human intellect has been so much mechanised by physical Science that it is likely to attempt the revolution it is beginning to envisage principally or solely through mechanical means, through social and political adjustments."[44]

The normal society treats man essentially as a physical, vital and mental being. Its system of mental growth and efficiency, its intellectual, ethical and scientific culture is mainly based on the development of the vital side of human life, creating an ever-growing system of economic efficiency and vital enjoyment. More and more science and more mechanical devices attempt to save man by machinery and substitute complex nature for 'arbitrary logical reason'. The radical defect of such a developmental society is its neglect of the spiritual element.

For Sri Aurobindo the spiritual society will regard man not as a mind a life and a body but as a soul incarnated for a divine fulfilment upon earth. The imperfect instruments are not ends in themselves, they need not be destroyed but their destiny lies in their spiritualisation. All one's physical, vital, mental, ethical, intellectual and psychic parts are seen as instruments for growth. But before such a spiritual society can take shape, the common mind of man must be prepared and become more favourable to this change, for the unpreparedness of society has always been the chief stumbling-block of spiritual change. "If mankind is to be spiritualised, it must first in the mass cease to be the material or the vital man and become the psychic and the true mental being."[45]

Sri Aurobindo describes the task of sociology in a spiritualised society as follows: "A spiritualised 'society would treat in its sociology the individual, from the saint to the criminal, not as units of a social problem to be passed through some skilfully devised machinery and either flattened into the social mould or crushed out of it, but as souls suffering and entangled in a net and to be rescued, souls growing and to be encouraged to grow, souls grown and from whom help and power can be drawn by the lesser spirits who are not yet adult."[46]

Such ideals about a spiritualised society, the idea of the kingdom of God on earth, is only a necessary beginning. Man has to go beyond the mere holding of the ideal and its influence in human life; it needs to be worked out and lived out by each man inwardly. It may take millennia before the spiritual change becomes part of the communal life of humanity, and it may even be questioned whether such a mass progress or conversion is possible, but for Sri Aurobindo, "if it is not, then the spiritualisation of mankind as a whole is a chimera."[47] He sees the predominant lead and influence of developed spiritual individuals as the only hope for a divine guidance of the race. And only a spiritualised society can bring about a reign of individual harmony and communal happiness.

For Ken Wilber, modern Western sociology is still not much concerned with the insights of the Perennial Philosophy, because sociology is a recently developed science, which came into existence when reductionism and materialism were dominant. Besides the technical interests of the natural sciences in the domination of the external world and the practical interest in the sciences of humanity, which aim at understanding human life, there is also in modem Western society an interest in the knowledge about spirituality and actual spiritual development. In Ken Wilber's non-reductionistic transcendental sociology, the progress of modern development is characterised by an increase of rationalisation and, as evolution continues, it moves from the rational to the psychic to the subtle, causal and finally the ultimate, i.e., rationality is a step in the direction of spirituality and the process of rationalisation is therefore not anti-spiritual.

SRI AUROBINDO'S VIEWS ON CULTURE

A true culture needs to be valued to the extent of the

discovery of the right maintenance and harmony of spirit, mind and body, and its living aim is the realisation on earth of the kingdom of heaven. Sri Aurobindo describes culture as, "the expression of a consciousness of life which formulates itself in three aspects. There is a side of thought, of ideal, of upward will and the soul's aspiration; there is a side of creative self-expression and appreciative aesthesis, intelligence and imagination; and there is a side of practical and outward formulation. A people's philosophy and higher thinking give us its mind's purest, largest and most general formulation of its consciousness of life and its dynamic view of existence. Its religion formulates the most intense form of its upward will and the soul's aspirations towards the fulfilment of its highest ideal and impulse. Its art, poetry, literature provide for us the creative expression and impression of its intuition, imagination, vital turn and creative intelligence. Its society and politics provide in their forms an outward frame in which the more external life works out what it can of its inspiring ideal and of its special character and nature under the difficulties of the environment... None of them express the whole secret spirit behind, but they derive from it their main ideas and their cultural character. Together they make up its soul, mind and body."[48]

Ordinary culture is related to the pursuit of the mental life and its intrinsic values and ideas, but for Sri Aurobindo culture in its full sense ought to include the pursuit of "a Truth greater and truer than the knowledge given by Reason and Science, a Right larger and more divine than the moralist's scheme of virtues, a Beauty more profound, universal and entrancing than the sensuous or imaginative beauty worshipped by the artist, a joy and divine sensibility which leaves the ordinary emotions poor and pallid, a Sense beyond the senses and sensations, the possibility of a diviner Life and action which man's ordinary conduct of life hides away from his impulses and from his vision."[49]

For Sri Aurobindo it is not a mere intelligently mechanised civilisation supporting a rational, materialistic and utilitarian culture which serves man's existence, but the future hope of the race lies more in the preservation of a spiritual culture where everything else in it is derived from or dependent upon an inward looking spiritual conception of life.

The value of a culture cannot be judged by material and economic capacity and prosperity, intellectual reason or the practical environment; they are necessary though not the highest part. For Sri Aurobindo science, practical reason and efficiency, an economic production or a huge mechanism of a political and social organisation is not really the whole truth and complete ideal of any culture. A culture must be judged first by its essential spirit in which the spiritual aspiration is the highest aim of life. This does not mean that culture only gives man some kind of insight into a greater spiritual consciousness which exceeds all earthly life. Knowledge, science, education, politics, religion, philosophic enquiry, art, poetry, technology, architecture etc., are all instruments and powers of the Spirit and valuable not for their own sake but because of the Spirit within them. Though "the first value of a culture is its power to raise and enlarge the internal man, the mind, the soul, the spirit, its soundness is not complete unless it has shaped also his external existence and made of it a rhythm of advance towards high and great ideals. This is the true sense of progress and there must be as part of it a sound political, economic and social life, to grow and to move securely towards a collective perfection, and a vital elasticity and responsiveness that will give room for a constant advance in the outward expression of the mind and the spirit. If a culture does not serve these ends, then there is evidently a defect somewhere either in its essential conceptions or its wholeness of in its application that will seriously detract from its claims to a complete and integral value."[50]

The full development of the intellectual, volitional, ethical, aesthetic, social and economic being of man are indispensable preliminaries for a spiritual culture. However, a culture which is mere intellectual, secular and materialistic aims at a strong culture of the vital and the physical man. According to Sri Aurobindo, "the pursuit of the mental life for its own sake is what we ordinarily mean by culture; but the word is still a little equivocal and capable of a wider or a narrower sense according to our ideas and predilections."[51] Man's intelligence is not entirely composed of the rational intellect and rational will. There exists a deeper more intuitive light and force of the developed spiritual consciousness, a knowledge of intimate inner contact with the truth of things and beings. This knowledge reveals a truth greater then the knowledge given by reason and science. The ultimate goal and aim of our being is to reach this spiritual consciousness; culture, as it is understood ordinarily, cannot be the directing light and harmonising principle of all our life and action. "Culture in order to attain the Transcendent and Infinite must become spiritual culture, something much more than an intellectual, aesthetic, ethical and practical training."[52] That is why the future of humanity does not lie in a culture founded merely upon reason and science; it should include contemplative insight and wisdom. Cultural phenomena then become a framework within which man can seek and grow.

When culture is turned to a higher end, and when it is transmuted and becomes spiritual it can be admitted as a part of a Yogic life. It is for this reason that cultural phenomena have to find a new spiritual base, a deeper inspiration.

As pointed out by Sri Aurobindo, "To have made the discovery of our deepest being and hidden spiritual nature is the first necessity and to have erected the living of an inmost spiritual life into the aim of existence is the characteristic sign of a spiritual culture. ... A wider spiritual culture must recognise that the Spirit is not only the highest and inmost thing, but all is manifestation and creation of the Spirit. It must have a wider outlook, a more embracing range of applicability and, even, a more aspiring and ambitious aim of its endeavour. Its aim must be not only to raise to inaccessible heights the few elect, but to draw all men and all life and the whole human being upward, to spiritualise life and in the end to divinise human nature. Not only must it be able to lay hold on his deepest individual being but to inspire too his communal existence. It must turn, by a spiritual change, all the members of his ignorance into members of the knowledge; it must transmute all the instruments of the human into instruments of a divine living."[53]

In all, it can be said that the various cultural pursuits such as science, philosophy, art, literature, sculpture, painting, music, etc., do not fall outside the scope of integral Yoga, they are all modes of divine self-manifestation. But in integral Yoga these cultural activities are not pursued for their own sake of intellectual or emotional gratification, but as different modes of self-offering to the Divine. Scientific investigation, social reconstruction, literary creation and religious purification are not pursued for their cultural ideals, but these lines of activities will function as an open channel for the self-expression of the Spirit. Sri Aurobindo's concept of culture is, therefore, essentially spiritual in character; his view of an integral spiritual culture harmonises vitality and intellectuality. He proposes to integrate the inner spiritual depth of a culture with its material forms and behavioural manifestation; he does not glorify the spiritual inner depth at the expense of the outer material forms.

However, as long as man remains obsessed with the practical use of reason, one is bound to produce a set of egoistic practical values, which consequently create a vitalistic culture. The developing culture of objective modern technology as a new way of life seems to be the present measure of human achievement, which could pose a threat to traditional art, literature, philosophy, religious values and spiritual ideology. What is the impact of the intrusion of the new system of technology upon the above-mentioned old subjective ideals? How does Sri Aurobindo solve the problem of the apparent dichotomy between holding strong commitments to the values of his tradition and, at the same time, embracing the culture of technology? Did he bring them closer together? Sri Aurobindo is not in favour of technological determinism, where human life is dominated by the dictates of technology. He maintains that there is a higher Conscious Power *(Brahman)* that determines the fate of the earth and humanity. This Conscious Power exposes itself in the world as *Sachchidananda:* everything in this world is an extension and expression of *Brahman,* and this One Power manifesting itself in the world resides even in matter, though matter is the furthest expression of *Brahman.* For Sri Aurobindo, the various traditional systems of Hindu philosophy and modem science are not in conflict with each other. They are a part of the divine purpose in life as long as technology promotes the development towards divine perfection.

In Ken Wilber's theory of sociocultural evolution, he uses his four quadrant model in order to explain that evolution occurs in the social quadrant (LR, the interobjective dimension, including forms of the techno-economic base and social systems), as well as the cultural quadrant (LL, the intersubjective dimension, including ethics, values and meaning). Both quadrants profoundly influence each other. But for Ken Wilber, it is not enough to say that organism and environment co-evolve; it is not enough to say that culture and consciousness co-evolve. All four of those 'tetra-evolve' together. That is, objective organism (the Upper-Right quadrant), with its DNA, its neuronal pathways, its brain systems, and its behavioral patterns, mutually interact with the objective environment, ecosystems and social realities (the Lower-Right), and all of those do indeed coevolve. Likewise, individual consciousness (Upper Left), with its intentionality, structures, and states, arises within and mutually interacts with, the intersubjective culture (Lower Left) in which it finds itself, and which it in turn helps to create, so that these, too, coevolve. But just as important, subjective intentionality and objective behavior, mutually interact (e.g., through will and response), and cultural worldviews mutually interact with social structures, as does individual consciousness and behavior. In other words, all four quadrants—organism, environment, consciousness, and culture—cause and are caused by the others: they 'tetraevolve.'"[54]

How does Ken Wilber look at a future spiritual culture which pays attention to all the four quadrants?

The individual's spiritual development will have its influence on the culture and social reality as a whole. Spirituality even has an inevitable political dimension. Human development is a process that points in the direction of a global consciousness. In the first stages of development, the ego is tied to the body (biocentric), but later on, it learns to adjust itself to the surrounding culture and becomes sociocentric; afterwards, it reaches a certain level of independence and develops a rational ego which is able to think in universal terms and becomes worldcentric. When the rational stages of the ego are succeeded by the spiritual stages, then the transpersonal stages will use this global consciousness as its platform. For Ken Wilber, a spiritual culture is based on a future oriented progressive spirituality in which the biosphere, as well as the noosphere, are taken up in the wider whole of the mystical theosphere. Nevertheless, Ken Wilber also knows that sociocultural evolution itself has been variously criticised by liberal social theorists, traditionalists, and idealists. In his integral worldview, he honors the truth of the premodern, modern and postmodern insights. In order to reunite humanity with the rest of the Kosmos, Ken Wilber is aware that notwithstanding the availability of certain aspects of spirituality in the higher stages of development, we also need to be alert to the problems in the higher stages which are not present in the lower stages, i.e., new tautologies, repressions, and oppressions that each new evolutionary advance makes possible.

SRI AUROBINDO'S VIEWS ON RELIGION

For Sri Aurobindo, a religion which is most in consonance with the preparation and furtherance of the spiritual evolution, is a religion which is itself a congeries of religions and which simultaneously provides each individual with one's own inner experience. The inmost essence of religion is the search for God; it is the idea, activity and discipline in man which aims directly at the Divine. As a first attempt of man to go beyond oneself and beyond the material facts of existence, the seeker discovers that he or she is not only a body but also a soul, and one's earthly life is a means by which one determines the future conditions of one's soul.

When religion entrenches itself in some narrow exaltation of its members or exclusively emphasises intellectual dogmas and ceremonies or insists on some fixed moral code or some religio-political or religio-social system, then such a religion becomes a retarding force. As long as the prominent aim of religion remains caught in the observation of a socioreligious system with its rites and forms, it leaves out the spiritual element of religion as well as the spiritual growth of the individual and the race.

Religions themselves have not changed human life and society; they could insist only on an adherence to and acceptance of its ethical standards and on conformity to institution and ritual, but they could not instigate the inner change of the whole being. As such, religion has not transformed the race and has not been able to create a new principle of human existence. Integral Yoga meets the religious ideal at several points but goes beyond it in the sense of a greater wideness. According to Sri Aurobindo, "the religious ideal looks, not only beyond this earth, but away from it to a heaven or even beyond all heavens to some kind of Nirvana. ... Its ordinary idea of perfection is a religio-ethical change, a drastic purification of the active and the emotional being ... and in any case a supraterrestrial motive and reward or result of a life of piety and right conduct. In so far as it admits a change of knowledge, will, aesthesis, it is in the sense of the turning of them to another object than the aims of human life and eventually brings a rejection of all earthly objects of aesthesis, will and knowledge. The method, whether it lays stress on personal effort or upon divine influence, on works and knowledge or upon grace, is not like the mundane a development, but rather a conversion; but in the end the aim is not a conversion of our mental and physical nature, but the putting on of a pure spiritual nature and being, and since that is not possible here on earth, it looks for its consummation by a transference to another world or a shuffling off of all cosmic existence. But the integral Yoga founds itself on a conception of the spiritual being as an omnipresent existence, the fullness of which comes not essentially by a transference to other worlds or a cosmic self-extinction, but by a growth out of what we now are phenomenally into the consciousness of the omnipresent reality which we always are in the essence of our being. It substitutes for the form of religious piety its completer spiritual seeking of a divine union."[55]

For Sri Aurobindo religion cannot be the solution to the present crisis of humanity, as humanity's future development does not lie in reverting to religion, but in moving forward towards an all-embracing spirituality. In fact, religion and spirituality are too intimately connected to be divided from each other. Religion founds itself on the immediate reality of the Infinite, it sees the Infinite as the secret highest Self or God, and it sees man as a soul and power of this being of God in Nature. Religion "must address its appeal to the whole of our being, not only to the suprarational and the rational parts, but to all the others. The imagination, the emotions, the aesthetic sense, even the very instincts of the half-subconscient parts must be taken into the influence. Religion must lead man towards the suprarational, the spiritual truth and it must take the aid of the illumined reason on the way, but it cannot afford to neglect to call Godwards the rest of our complex nature. And it must take too each man where he stands and spiritualise him through what he can feel and not at once force on him something which he cannot yet grasp as a true and living power."[56] This truth is not a mere intellectual or theological conception to be indulged in, but has to be lived and to be made the governing idea of life and action, i.e., the sole thing needful is to attain the truth by inner experience.

The illuminating faculties of religion are the revelations, intuitions and inspirations that come down to the seeker from the higher planes of supramental light and not by rational judgement or logical analysis. Reason does play a part in relation to this highest field of religious experience, but this comes only secondarily and subordinately. It can explain in its own language and to the rational parts of man the laws, truths and experiences of our spiritual existence. However, aspiration, surrender to and faith in God do not admit any rational limitations, it passes all understanding and practical reason.

For Sri Aurobindo true religion is spiritual, beyond the intellect, the aesthetic, ethical and practical being of man. A religion of humanity may be an intellectual or sentimental ideal or a spiritual aspiration, and partly the cause of a change of the soul in humanity. The sentimental humanitarian religion assumes that respect, service and progress of the human being and human life are the chief aims of the human spirit. Mankind is the godhead to be worshipped, and the life of man is to be held sacred, strengthened and uplifted. However, its present intellectual form does not seem sufficient to bring about and guarantee a great change in our psychology, in the principle of freedom and in human oneness, for it has to concede too much to the egoistic side of human nature and it leans principally on reason which turns too readily to mechanical solutions. A religion of humanity can only be made real if it spiritualises itself and becomes the general inner law of human life.

According to Sri Aurobindo, "A religion of humanity means the growing realisation that there is a secret Spirit, a divine Reality, in which we are all one, that humanity is its highest present vehicle on earth, that the human race and the human being are the means by which it will progressively reveal itself here. It implies a growing attempt to live out this knowledge and bring about a kingdom of this divine Spirit upon earth. By its growth within us oneness with our fellow-men will become the leading principle of all our life ... There must be the realisation by the individual that only in the life of his fellow-men is his own life complete. There must be the realisation by the race that only on the free and full life of the individual can its own perfection and permanent happiness be founded. There must be too a discipline and a way of salvation in accordance with this religion, that is to say, a means by which it can be developed by each man within himself, so that it may be developed in the life of the race ... No doubt, if this is only an idea like the rest, it will go the way of all ideas. But if it is at all a truth of our being, then it must be the truth to which all is moving and in it must be found the means of a fundamental, an inner, a complete, a real human unity which would be the one secure base of a unification of human life. A spiritual oneness which would create a psychological oneness not dependent upon any intellectual or outward uniformity and compel a oneness of life not bound up with its mechanical means of unification, but ready always to enrich its secure unity, by a free inner variation and a freely varied outer self-expression, this would be the basis for a higher type of human existence. Could such a realisation develop rapidly in mankind, we might then solve the problem of unification in a deeper and truer way from the inner truth to the outer forms. Until then, the attempt to bring it about by mechanical means must proceed."[57]

For Sri Aurobindo, "the religious life may be the first approach to the spiritual, but very often it is only a turning about in a round of rites, ceremonies and practices or set ideas and forms without any issue. The spiritual life, on the contrary, proceeds directly by a change of consciousness, a change from the ordinary consciousness, ignorant and separated from its true self and from God, to a greater consciousness in which one finds one's true being and comes first into direct and living contact and then into union with the Divine."[58]

A spiritual life cannot be founded on a moral basis but must be formed on a spiritual foundation, because morality belongs.to the lower mental and vital plane whereas spirituality belongs to the higher Divine Consciousness.

The spiritual life, however, is not something that can be formulated in a rigid definition, "it is an immense kingdom potentially larger than other kingdoms below it, with a hundred provinces, a thousand types, stages, forms, paths, variations of the spiritual ideal, degrees of Spiritual advancement."[59]

Ken Wilber's ideas on science and religion are found specifically in *The Marriage of Sense and'Soul,* where he uses an integral approach to integrate science and religion. Where science offers us a solid method for the discovery of truth (empirical, experimental and evidence-based), it does not offer depth, value or anything about how to use that truth wisely. Religion, on the other hand, generates a basic meaning of life and genuine wisdom. However, in order to reach a common grounding in experimental data that finds the existence of matter and Spirit equally demonstrable, religion has to engage itself, like science, in the three strands of knowledge and open its truth 'claims' to direct verification by experiential evidence. In this way, religion has to give up its pseudo claims and move from its dogmatic proclamations to direct, authentic spiritual experiences. As described already in *One Taste,* Ken Wilber makes a meaningful distinction between the translative function of religion (prayers, rituals, dogmas), where the self is given a new approach to reality and learns to translate its world in terms of the new approach, and the transformative function of religion (contemplative practices), where the self itself is analysed and the world gets transformed, rather than only translated. Both these functions are important, even indispensable, but at a certain point in our development, the translative function of religion ceases to console. However, Ken Wilber assumes that most religions will continue to offer translative comfort in addition to transformative practices of vertical contemplation. He hopes that true religion will become the vanguard of a progressive evolutionary force and adds, "this idea is likewise behind the extraordinary integral yoga of Sri Aurobindo, arguably the greatest spiritual evolutionary theorist." [60]

How does Ken Wilber integrate religion in his all-level, all-quadrant model? The all-level, all-quadrant approach integrates deep religion with broad science. The interior experiences of deep religion (the Upper Left quadrant) can be investigated by broad science—the contemplative phenomenological sciences of the interior—but it also has correlates in the Upper Right quadrant, which can be investigated by narrow science. The empirical claims of narrow religion can be put to test by empirical (narrow) science. In other words, "an integral model—namely all-quadrant, all-level model—attempts to provide a framework in which all those 'facts' [spiritual and empirical realities], if you will, can be accommodated. The facts, that is, of both interior realities and exterior realities, 'spiritual' experiences and 'scientific' experiences, subjective realities and objective realities." [61]

SRI AUROBINDO'S VIEWS ON ETHICS

Most of the works of life seem to be actuated by ethical and religious motivations with threads of altruism, philanthropy and self-sacrifice woven through it. But Sri Aurobindo assumes that when we are not limited by the human standpoint, "we do not live in an ethical world." To force an ethical meaning into the whole of Nature is an act of self-confusion, as material or vital Nature is not ethical. But nonetheless in the process of man's self-development man needs ethics as a stage in one's urge for Sachchidananda. According to Sri Aurobindo, "The ethical impulse and attitude, so all-important to humanity, is a means by which it struggles out of the lower harmony and universality based upon inconscience and broken up by Life into individual discords towards a higher harmony and universality based upon conscient oneness with all existences."[62] This middle truth of consciousness awakens us to the values of good and evil and the appreciation of their importance. This ethical awakening is, therefore, one of the indispensable steps in the process of evolutionary nature.

On the human level, a standard of conduct may be temporary yet necessary for its time, until it can be replaced by a better divine standard. For Sri Aurobindo, "all standards by which we may seek to govern our conduct are only our temporary, imperfect and evolutive attempts to represent to ourselves our stumbling mental progress in the universal self-realisation towards which Nature moves. But the divine manifestation cannot be bound by our little rules and fragile sanctities. Once we have grasped this fact, we shall better be able to put in their right place in regard to each other the successive standards that govern the different stages in the growth of the individual and the collective march of mankind."[63] All these temporary constructions have a relative imperativeness only as one rests content with the physical and vital life or remains fixed in the ranges of the mental plane. But in the supramental ranges, all these temporary structures cease. It seems, therefore, that the ethical notions, as a means to control the lower nature, are necessary at present for our spiritual evolution, but in the supramental stage the seeker arrives at a universal, action of the dynamic spiritual force in which one's own force and will are turned into pure instruments of a greater divine working. The true inmost aim and meaning of ethics is described by Sri Aurobindo as "to lessen and tame, purify and prepare to be fit instruments the vital and physical and lower mental life so that they may be transformed into notes of the higher mental and eventually the supramental harmony, but not to mutilate and destroy them."[64]

Ethics, as a transitional stage, is able to control the difficult parts of our Nature, but it has no power to transform Nature. At best its method is able to lay down limits and put a relative safety around us. This device of self-protection may be necessary for a time in ordinary life, but in integral Yoga it can only be a mark of transition. Integral Yoga aims at a fundamental transformation and a pure wideness of spiritual life, and an ethical solution is insufficient to reach that aim; it needs a surer supra-ethical dynamic principle. For Sri Aurobindo the development of "a nature of light, understanding, balance, harmony, sympathy, good-will, kindness, fellow-feeling, self-control, rightly ordered and harmonised action, is the best we can do in the limits of the mental formation, but it is a stage and not the goal of our growth of being. These are solutions by the way, palliatives, necessary means for a partial dealing with this root difficulty, provisional standards and devices given us as a temporary help and guidance because the true and total solution is beyond our present capacity and can only come when we have sufficiently evolved to see it and make it our main endeavour.

The true solution can intervene only when by our spiritual growth we can become one self with all beings, know them as part of our self, and deal with them as if they were our other selves. ... But even oneness with others is not enough by itself, if it is a oneness with their ignorance. Our oneness with others must be fundamental, not a oneness with their minds, hearts, vital selves, egos—even though these come to be included in our universalised consciousness,—but a oneness in the soul and spirit, and that can only come by our liberation into soul-awareness and self-knowledge."[65]

Altruism, humanitarianism, service for the well-being of mankind are all inspiring movements of the mental consciousness, but are only a pale imitation of the spiritual flame of universal Divine Consciousness. The religious, ethical and cultural ideals are able to modify and palliate the ego-sense, but are impotent in practice to change man's vital life and nature. Thus Sri Aurobindo observes that, "Intellectual, volitional, ethical, emotional, aesthetic and physical training and improvement are all so much to the good, but they are only in the end a constant movement in a circle without any last delivering and illumining aim, unless they arrive at a point when they can open themselves to the power and presence of the Spirit and admit its direct workings. ... So long as there is only an intellectual, ethical and other selftraining for the now normal purposes of life which does not travel beyond the ordinary circle of working of mind, life and body, we are still only in the obscure and yet unillumined preparatory yoga of Nature."[66]

Sri Aurobindo's object of integral Yoga is based on living a divine life, and the greatest service of man is to prepare or find the way by which the individual and the collective man can transcend the ego and live in its true self, no longer bound by ignorance, disharmony and sorrow. It seems that for Sri Aurobindo all sorts of social and moral standards or is to ethical ideals as empirical means are either too narrow, complex, confused and uncertain, as they have no vision of the cause and origin of the malady it attempts to cure.

It is held by the intellect and the mind that "the spiritual tendency in humanity has come to very little; it has not solved the problem of life nor any of the problems with which humanity is at grips. ... But this is not the standpoint from which the true significance of the spiritual evolution in man or the value of spirituality can be judged or assessed; for its real work is not to solve human problems on the past or present mental basis, but to create a new foundation of our being and our life and knowledge ... the solution of the problem which spirituality offers is not a solution by external means, though these also have to be used, .but by an inner change, a transformation of the consciousness and nature.... Only a spiritual change, an evolution of his being from the superficial mental towards the deeper spiritual consciousness, can make a real and effective difference. To discover the spiritual being in himself is the main business of the spiritual man and to help others towards the same evolution is his real service to the race; till that is done, an outward help can succour and alleviate, but nothing or very little more is possible."[67]

In integral Yoga the sadhak refuses to rely only upon fragile moral ideals but puts his or her whole emphasis on the elevation of the mental consciousness into the supramental consciousness. Until the soul finds the secret of divine oneness, man's altruism remains essentially egoistic. For Sri Aurobindo, "All or most of the works of life seem to be actuated by this soul of desire [ego]; even those that are ethical or religious, even those that wear the guise of altruism, philanthropy, self-sacrifice, self-denial, are shot through and through with the threads of its making. This soul of desire is a separate soul of ego and all its instincts are for a separative self-affirmation; it pushes always for its own growth, for possession, for enjoyment, for conquest and empire."[68] But beyond the mental and moral being in us is a greater divine being that is spiritual and supramental. Ultimately, what accepts and rejects is not the mind, vital will of desire, or the ethical sense, but the insistence of the psychic being, the Divine Guide of the Yoga. However, he points out that "There alone [in the supramental spirit] is there any possibility of an absolute justice, love and right. ... There alone the unification of the transformed vital and physical and the illumined mental man becomes possible in that supramental spirit which is at once the secret source and goal of our mind and life and body."69

The spiritual and supramental life cannot be turned into a mental idea or an external rule, it has its own lines and forces which can lead to individual and collective perfection. According to Sri Aurobindo, "the perfect supramental action will not follow any single principle or limited rule. ... It will, proceed by a spontaneous outflowing from the summits in the totality of an illumined and uplifted being, will and knowledge and not by the selected, calculated and standardised action which is all that the intellectual reason or ethical will can achieve. Its sole aim will be the expression of the divine in us and the keeping together of the world and its progress towards the Manifestation that is to be."[70]

For Sri Aurobindo it is only the full emergence of the soul and the descent of the power of the Spirit and the consequent transformation and replacement of one's insufficient mental and vital nature by a spiritual and supramental Supernature that can effect this evolutionary miracle. The soul's perception of good and evil may not coincide with the mind's artificial standards as it has a deeper sense, which points to the higher Light. It is the soul in us which turns always towards Truth, Good and Beauty; the rest, their opposites are a necessary part of experience, but have to be outgrown in the enlarged spiritual being. When the higher law of being intervenes, there is no longer any utility for moral values. The self-law of supreme Truth is above all standards.

Sri Aurobindo assumes that a theory of Maya, in the sense of the unreality of a cosmic existence, creates more difficulties than it solves. The ultimate effects of the theory carry in them a devastating simplicity, as in Maya's thesis world-acceptance and world-refusal are the two sides of an illusion. "An -uncompromising theory of Illusion solves no problem of our existence ... in its extreme form and effect, our being and its action become null and without sanction, its experience, aspiration, endeavour lose their significance. God and ourselves and the universe become myths of Maya."[71] Sri Aurobindo does not deny the reality of the individual and the cosmos, and for him the theory of illusion functions merely as an escape but not a solution. It may seem that the thinking mind arrives at the conclusion that there is an illusion behind all human effort and terrestrial endeavour, the illusion of political, social and ethical efforts at perfection, the illusion of all achievement. For Shankara's theory of Maya, "Human, social and political endeavour turns always in a circle and leads nowhere; and neither laws nor institutions nor education nor philosophy nor morality nor religious teachings have succeeded in producing the perfect man, still less a perfect humanity. ... Altruism, philanthropy and service, Christian love or Buddhist compassion have not made the world a whit happier, they only give infinitesimal bits of momentary relief here and there, throw drops on the fire of the world's suffering."[72]

But Sri Aurobindo disagrees with this aimless cosmic illusion as an explanation of suffering. Religious, ethical, political, social, economic, cultural utilitarian or hedonistic thoughts and actions are not illusions, though they are also not the essence or object of life. These thoughts and actions are only activities of the surface powers of the mind which try to create mental solutions and may, at their best, function only as palliatives as they leave the roots of the human problem untouched.

Moral, social and religious laws have an immense significance in the unfolding of the soul and inspire human development to a high degree of excellence, yet they are relative to a certain stage of evolution, and when over-emphasised these laws become a stagnation on the march of evolution beyond mental development. True harmony is attained in the wideness of the supramental consciousness where all temporary mental constructions cease and where the free soul spontaneously wells out in works of a supreme truth and love that replaces human virtue. Ordinary man needs some noble principles to guide one's thoughts and actions, but once the individual soul realises its essential nature and becomes one with the Spirit, the seeker goes beyond all mental laws.

The essence of spiritual activity is related to inward activity, beyond ethical activity. But beyond does not mean anti-ethical but supra-ethical. As mentioned before, in the supra-ethical mode of action, the truth of morality is not negated but transformed beyond itself and enriched in the supranormal mode of activity.

Although Sri Aurobindo emphasises the Divine, he does not reject everything human; the sadhaks who enter the yoga need the human approach at the beginning and long after. "Divinisation itself does not mean the destruction of the human elements; it means taking them up, showing them the way to their own perfection, raising them by purification and perfection to their full power and that means the raising of the whole of earthly life to its full power."[73]

SRI AUROBINDO'S FUTURE VISION AND KEN WILBER'S WORLD-VIEW

Sri Aurobindo's concept of the divinisation of man and nature through a collective perfection and a general integral transformation of mankind are his unique contributions to the coming of a Divine Life. The concrete realisation of the divine community will lead to the perfection of man. The spiritualised man in *The Human Cycle* and the gnostic man in *The Life Divine* are based on man's persistent aspiration for perfection and oneness with the Divine.

Sri Aurobindo is aware that "at present mankind is undergoing an evolutionary crisis in which is concealed a choice of its destiny; for a stage has been reached in which the human mind has achieved in certain directions an enormous development while in others it stands arrested and bewildered and can no longer find its way. ... Man has created a system of civilisation which has become too big for his limited mental capacity and understanding and his still more limited spiritual and moral capacity to utilise and manage, a too dangerous servant of his blundering ego and its appetites."[74]

It seems that the destiny of the race is dangerously heading into a prolonged confusion and crisis, a darkness of chaotic incertitudes, because the burden which is laid on mankind is too heavy for his present limited mind and moral capacity. The inferior lower instrument is not able to use the divine potentialities of existence and incorporate them within himself and within society.

Our current secularism and liberal humanism is unprecedented in human history, and it seems that the present crisis is not so much in the extraordinary external events themselves, but more in the unprecedented secular ethical indigence and spiritual instability which they reveal. For Sri Aurobindo, no adequate answer to the principle questions of politics, economics and social reforms is possible without first finding an adequate answer to the larger questions of life itself. These secular processes may be used as palliatives which may relieve human discomfort and which may lead to partial happiness but not to radical changes.

Sri Aurobindo is not sure if the present change will take place by a destruction or a new construction on the basis of a greater Truth. If humanity fails to overcome the obstacles that have been persistently preventing the realisation of human unity, then it may create a too prolonged chaos and confusion and render a solution impossible. It depends upon the readiness of humanity to receive the supramental Truth; evolutionary development will work itself out harmoniously when humanity willingly agrees to change its consciousness and rise to a new state. But if its present egoistic consciousness persists in refusing to collaborate with this change, then it will not be able to avert destruction, and man may even be annihilated in its very existence as a race. True harmony and unity can be realised only by a rejection of the individual and collective ego consciousness, transforming our present ego-bound nature by the supramental Power and consciously establishing the supramental unity in human life. "For a supramentalised consciousness it would be utterly possible to embrace all contacts with men and the world in a purified flame-force and with a transfigured significance."[75] The evolutionary crisis can be resolved only when a radical transformation of human nature has its effect in the outward world in the form of a new creation.

Intuitions of the future city of God "have lacked a basis of assured knowledge and the mind of man has remained swinging between a bright future hope and a grey present certitude. But the grey certitude is not so certain as it looks and a divine life evolving or preparing in earth-Nature need not be a chimera "76 For Sri Aurobindo the supramental change is inevitable in the evolution of earth-consciousness, and "the dynamic side of the spiritual urge has not been absent ... there has even been the dream or a psychic prevision of a fulfilment exceeding the individual transformation, a new earth and heaven, a city of God, a divine descent upon earth, a kingdom of God not only within us but outside, in a collective human life."[77] Such a future divine life for the individual and the collective man cannot be reached by the machinery of reason but needs an inner change in human nature, "a change too difficult to be ever effected except by the few. This is not certain; but in any case, if this is not the solution, then there is no solution; if this is not the way, then there is no way for the human kind. Then the terrestrial evolution must pass beyond man as it has passed beyond the animal and a greater race must come that will be capable of the spiritual change, a form of life that must be born that is nearer to the' divine."[78]

A psycho-spiritual transformation, as a radical change of consciousness, alone can free men from their present darkness. This transformation is beyond the ability of any modern science, or psychology, philosophy, politics, economics, ethics, sociology, etc.

For Ken Wilber, like Sri Aurobindo, the real problem of the present global crisis is not exterior but interior, and needs first of all a mutual understanding and mutual agreement on the noosphere. He assumes that "the most radical, pervasive, and earth-shaking transformation would occur simply if everybody truly evolved to a mature, rational and responsible ego. ... There would be the *real* New Age. We are nowhere near the stage 'beyond reason', simply because we are nowhere yet near universal reason itself."[79] Along with engaging in exterior, economic and technological development, Ken Wilber encourages the interior development of our moral and spiritual depths.

However, Ken Wilber also maintains that future development may take place at the integrative vision-logic level, where world citizens are united on the basis of an existential planetary vision. Individuals on that level "create 'a cognitive potential' in the form of *new worldviews* (in this case centauric-planetary) that in turn feed back into the ongoing mainstream of *social institutions.*[80]

Ken Wilber estimates that one per cent of the population has arrived at the vision-logic level and that its emergence has to face a lot of resistance from the lower levels. But even with the emergence of the cognitive vision-logic level, it is not possible to overcome the problems of our fragmented world. Like Sri Aurobindo, Ken Wilber is of the opinion that external changes might be a beginning on the spiritual path, but real growth occurs through sustained practice, which is able to actualise deeper and higher individual and global stages of consciousness.

Sri Aurobindo and Ken Wilber agree that the solution to the present global crisis does not need human efforts merely on the biomaterial and economic-financial front which is where most efforts are now being concentrated: "none of those physical and material and economic components *can be secured* in the long run without a *corresponding change in consciousness* among the citizens of the nations."[81] Ken Wilber does not deny "the crucial importance of ecological and economic and financial factors in the world-demanding transformation, let us not forget that they all rest ultimately on a correlative transformation in human consciousness."[82]

The global embrace can be implemented by those individuals with a universal vision-logic where the new resources are related to the resources of a 'meaning-in-life' that is found in a worldcentric embrace of a common humanity rather than the involvement of only material-economic changes. At the vision-logic level nature is not just a collection of 'its' but includes 'I's' and 'we's', which are all integral expressions of Spirit, and the individual can integrate them because one is a vehicle of Spirit. Ken Wilber believes that, "at this point, aside from the inner work that each of us individually can do, I personally see no obvious collective bearers of the new and deeper within [centauric visionlogic]."[83]

Integration at the vision-logic level is possible but

is not guaranteed, "extinction seems to be a genuine possibility for humans". He does not see "the emergence of the 'aperspectival world-centric structure as being a sure thing, as being somehow guaranteed. ... Evolution, we have amply seen, is not predictable, only reconstructable. Nor does the fact that the integral structure is integral guarantee that the necessary integration will in fact occur ... the integral structure *can* integrate the physiosphere, the biosphere, and the noosphere—it has the *potential* for that integration. Whether that potential becomes actual is up to you and me; it depends on the concrete actions that each of us takes."[84]

A solution lies in the marriages of tomorrow, not in the syncretism (attempt to reconcile different systems of belief) of yesterday, and Ken Wilber, like Sri Aurobindo, maintains that man's greatness is not what one is at present, but what man makes possible in the future.

Nevertheless, Ken Wilber also believes that "the world is in the midst of the torturous birth throes of a collective emergence of an entirely new structure of consciousness, the centaur in vision-logic, the integral-aperspectival mind." [all perspectives are interrelated and no perspective is final].[85] This crucial change of consciousness has already been accomplished by many, "and whereas they were, in their times, the rare and isolated, the average mode is now catching up with them: their paths can be ours, collectively, now."[86]

In *A Theory of Everything,* however, Ken Wilber is a little bit more cautious about the future development of the middle and late vision-logic levels. What is hidden in contemporary philosophy as narcissism and nihilism is, for him, one of the greatest obstacles for an adult spirituality in Western society. But he is also aware that the most important reforms at present are related to the improvement of the lower and more fundamental stages, and an integral vision is one of the least pressing issues on earth. He now believes that a genuine universal integralism implies simple fundamental changes in the magic, mythic and rational waves of existence, rather than a collective move into transpersonal domains. He prefers the health of the lower waves in their own terms, i.e., "The major reforms do not involve how to get a handful of boomers into second-tier, but how to feed the starving millions at the most basic waves; how to house the homeless millions at the simplest of levels; how to bring health care to the millions who do not possess it... The health of the entire spiral, and particularly its earlier waves, screams out to us as the major ethical demand."[87] However, for Sri Aurobindo, unlike Ken Wilber, "The true spiritual significance of the spiritual evolution in man is not to solve human problems on the past or present mental basis but to create a new foundation of our being and our life and knowledge. The solution of the problem which spirituality offers is not a solution by external means, though these also have to be used, but by an inner change, a transformation of the consciousness and nature. ... Spirituality cannot attempt to cure its ills [of life] by the panaceas, the political, social or other mechanical remedies which the mind is constantly attempting. The most drastic changes made by these means change nothing."[88] The main business of the spiritual seeker is to discover the spiritual being in onself, and his or her real service to humanity is to help others towards the same evolution. An outward help may alleviate but does not solve the problems which humanity is facing.

Ken Wilber's more encompassing future, instead of aiming at third-tier constructions to find a solution 'for a world gone slightly mad', aims at a better understanding of the interior development of the second-tier constructions. In Ken Wilber's own words, "But second-tier constructions are everywhere making impressive gains—in more integral views and more, holistic perspectives—and thus I am cautiously optimistic that postgreen constructions will continue to blossom." [89]

CONCLUSION

A rational and scientific formula of materialistic and vital human beings and their life, and a perfected economic, democratic society with religious-ethical tendencies seems to be the solution that modern mind presents us in this crisis. But for Sri Aurobindo such a solution does not transform the individual and the race; it does not create a new principle of human existence. It is by the possession of the Divine only that all discords of life can be resolved, and the one effective way of helping mankind is to raise men towards the Divine. All other activities of our self-experience have their use and power, they may create a mental, moral and social unity, but the true unity is spiritual. Human qualities such as love, sympathy, compassion, brotherhood, loyalty, etc., will not be destroyed but perfected and enlarged to their widest capacity. In the *initial* stages of sadhana the development of these qualities support the seeker's growth process, but *ultimately* these qualities have to be transcended.

For Ken Wilber, however, the root of all longing is based on the divine verities of higher values such as Truth, Good and Beauty. Qualities like virtue, justice, duty, compassion, love, etc., have intrinsic value though they should be seen in a larger context. In themselves they do not constitute the fully human life, but to degrade them as secondary aims only is to deny the integrality of these qualities for the full life of man.

Ken Wilber, like most transpersonal psychologists, maintains that the fulfilment of the Divine realisation needs not only a spiritual force, but simultaneously the actualisation of these higher human qualities which function as instruments to bring about a desired change within oneself and in the world.

Could it be that Sri Aurobindo, interpreting the longings for these pure and natural human characteristics as inferior (a means only) to the ways of the Divine, subordinating the former to the dynamic supra-ethical principles, fails to emphasise the underlying identity between them? They are mutually supportive processes and co-dependent. In spirituality, emphasis on detachment from desires and transcendence (Infinite) is counter-balanced by emphasis on embodiment and descent (Finite). In the exploration of the unknown both illumine the essential nature of the individual's soul and one's world with a fresh vision. Ken Wilber considers these universal, benevolent qualities and contemplative tendencies as equally real and therefore equally important. In the higher stages of contemplative development these human excellences are granted a legitimate life of their own; they are not merely temporary palliatives but often man's only route to Godhead and can therefore never be dismissed as a mark of transition.

For Sri Aurobindo, as mentioned above, qualities like sympathy, compassion and love are ultimately transitional values and, therefore, apparent and not real, as "we do not live in an ethical world", i.e., in the supra-ethical realm there is no need for ethics. But for Ken Wilber and transpersonal psychologists in general, if the Absolute creates human life, it also creates an ethical, cultural, social and economic life, and in order to maintain that man is real, man's higher human qualities and actions must be as real and cannot be ultimately denied as ineffectual. To affirm the Absolute implies the affirmation of man's life and one's activities in that life, otherwise man becomes deprived of his or her significance. After all, an integrated worldview starts from man in order to arrive at the ultimate principles of the universal and transcendental Absolute. To characterise common civilisation, culture, science, religion, social laws, etc., as ineffective means of changing human life, because they have no power to transform human psychology and the human race, may be arguable and not easily accepted by Ken Wilber and other transpersonal psychologists.

Ken Wilber's ethical imperative is related to the health

of the overall spiral and not to any one privileged domain, i.e., its purpose is to help each level develop its healthy and not its pathological dimensions, and thus allowing each level to be as healthy as it can be within its own domain. An increase of love and compassion on the level of egocentric consciousness is not something to be recommended, only by shifting our attention to the interior of the sociocultural quadrants is the individual able to move to post-conventional universal love and compassion for humanity.

Ken Wilber uses the emergence of complex subtler emotions, such as universal love, care and compassion ('vertical affects') as motivational currents for higher growth, in contrast to the horizontal emotions such as anger, desire, hatred, etc., in the lower stages of development, which must be conquered so that the enduring change and continual development may occur. In the transpersonal waves, these emotions expand into universal compassion for all sentient beings. For Ken Wilber, we are never without these vertical affects in the realm of manifestation. Moral actions, in addition to whatever relative value they may have in their own right, are in their ultimate value conductive to the direct realisation of Spirit itself. These higher emotions and affects take the seeker closer and closer to the Divine, and Ken Wilber assumes that in the realm of manifestation we are never without these higher vertical affects, although in the nondual formless Emptiness there are no affects.

Sri Aurobindo maintains that at the human level, the standard of conduct may be temporary yet necessary for its time until it can be replaced by a better standard. It is in God alone, by the possession of the Divine only that all the divisions of life can be restored and the one effective way of helping mankind is by the growth and surrender of oneself towards the Divine. For Sri Aurobindo, human tendencies and human values need a metaphysical justification. Sri Aurobindo moves to the divine origin of these human potentials, beyond the transpersonal experience in the spiritual mind of man, to the source of them, i.e., God. Man is not a self-sufficient being but a being supported from within and above by the divine spiritual principle. These human tendencies have ultimate value only in this wider spiritual context and cannot be separated from God.

Ken Wilber, in his integral approach to transformation, attempts to integrate matter, mind, soul and spirit which includes physics, biology, psychology, theology and mysticism. Each of these levels has four aspects or dimensions— the objective and subjective side as well as the individual and collective forms. Ken Wilber's integral view is not merely matter, body, mind and soul; each of these levels has a dimension of it, we' and 'I', which needs to be included in all of them.

Each of the vertical levels from Matter to Spirit needs to be differentiated into four horizontal dimensions, i.e., the four quadrants. According to Ken Wilber, "the great traditions rarely understood that states of consciousness (Upper Left) have correlates in the organic brain (Upper Right), a fact that has revolutionized our understanding of psychopharmacology, psychiatry, and consciousness studies. Likewise, the traditions evidenced little understanding that individual awareness (Upper Left) is profoundly molded by both its background cultural worldviews (Lower Left) and the modes of techno-economic production (Lower Right) in which it finds itself. This left the Great Nest [The Great Chain of Being] open to devastating critiques from modem biological science, from Marxists, and from cultural and historical studies, among others, all of which demonstrated that consciousness is not merely a disembodied, transcendental noumenon, but is deeply embedded in contexts of objective facts, cultural backgrounds, and social structures."[90]

This integral approach, integrating the empirical with the transcendental, can be used in education, scientific research, politics, medicine, business and spirituality. All these levels (twelve) with their (four) quadrants are present not only in the higher spiritual levels of each quadrant, but also cover the lower 'ordinary' levels of each quadrant. The quadrants themselves are useful, "because they give a simple, easily understood way to fight the flatland reductionism so prevalent in the modem and postmodern world."[91] It is for this reason why Ken Wilber claims that this integral approach is now being applied in many different areas, theoretical as well as practical.

In all his books Ken Wilber distinguishes the absolute from the relative, and he assumes that the person who has a direct recognition of the absolute need not have mastered all the details of the relative. According to Ken Wilber, "My books deal more with all these relative details, some of which are not covered by any of the world's wisdom traditions."[92]

Examples of relative truth are the scientific and philosophical teachings of the West (the eye of the flesh and the eye of the mind), whereas the recognition of formless Witness or pure Emptiness is more an example of absolute truth (the eye of contemplation). Each relative realm has its own truth, yet they are all illumined by the wisdom of the absolute. The relative truth and its conventional reality are changing ceaselessly, and in the relative world new truths are constantly emerging. For Ken Wilber, "The West has its relative truths, the East has its relative truths. And mostly in the East we further get a clear understanding of absolute truth, ... my theme is that a judicious blend of relative truths, East and West, set in the primordial context of radical Emptiness, is a very sane approach to the human situation."[93]

A comprehensive worldview in general includes both absolute and relative truths, and psycho-spiritual development can best proceed by an integration of Eastern contemplative approaches with Western psychodynamic approaches. Ken Wilber's integral approach honours and incorporates all sorts of relative truths—covering the physical, vital, mental, cultural and communal aspects of the human being— in preparation for the realisation of the ultimate truth.

Sri Aurobindo, like Ken Wilber, maintains that the highest spiritual realisations have been unconnected with the bodily life and life of the mind, and most spiritually realised souls remain content with their own realisations. For Ken Wilber, however, those seekers who did not remain content with their own realisations and have mixed with humanity succeeded in establishing an ethical and religious temperament (I, we, it), whereas for Sri Aurobindo the discovery and effort to make mind, life (emotions and actions) and physical substance perfect vehicles for the Divine Force and the transformation of Nature is of primary importance.

What is new in Ken Wilber's integral approach is not so much his metaphysical vision of the ultimate Truth, but his emphasis on the relative truth as expressed in his all-quadrant, all-level model. This comprehensive endeavour to integrate the various relative truths ultimately aims at the Absolute Truth.

Sri Aurobindo is aware that spiritual development is not exclusively an individual, subjective matter but also has social, cultural and biochemical correlates, however in his vision he emphasises the Ultimate Truth through the mystical experience, and pays less attention to relative truths.

NOTES

1. Ken Wilber, *The Eye of Spirit*, p. 303.
2. Ken Wilber, *Integral Psychology*, p. 84.
3. Sri Aurobindo, *The Human Cycle*, p.lll.

4. Ibid., p. 472 - 473.
5. Ibid., p. 729.
6. Sri Aurobindo, *The Synthesis of Yoga,* p. 133.
7. Sri Aurobindo, *Letters on Yoga,* p. 189.
8. Ibid., p. 201.
9. Sri Aurobindo, *The Life Divine,* p. 650.
10. Ken Wilber, *Eye to Eye,* p.6.
11. Sri Aurobindo, *The Life Divine,* p.773-774
12. Ibid., p. 772.
13. Ibid., p. 15-16.
14. Sri Aurobindo, *Letters on Yoga,* p. 205.
15. Sri Aurobindo, *The Human Cycle,* p.70.
16. Sri Aurobindo, *Letters on Yoga,* p.176.
17. Ibid., p.188.
18. Ken Wilber, *Eye to Eye,* p.135.
19. Ibid., p.153.
20. Sri Aurobindo, *The Life Divine,* p.13-14.
21. Ken Wilber, *Sex, Ecology, Spirituality,* p.336.
22. Ibid p 512
23. D. Rothberg, *Re-Vision,* Vol.18. No 4:1996, p.7.
24. R Walsh and F. Vaughan, *Paths Beyond Ego,* p.265.
25. Ken Wilber, *Sex, Ecology, Spirituality,* p. 496.
26. Ibid., p. 497
27. Ibid., p. 497
28. SriAurobindo, *The Synthesis of Yoga, p.* 44.
29. Sri Aurobindo, *The Life Divine* p. 1050
30. Sri Aurobindo, *The Human Cycle,* p. 231- 232.
31. Sri Aurobindo, *The Ideal of Human Unity,* p. 267.
32. Sri Aurobindo, *The Human Cycle,* p. 202.
33. Ibid., p. 206.

34. Sri Aurobindo, *The Life Divine*, p. 1030.
35. Ibid., p. 1068.
36. Ibid., p. 694.
37. Ibid., p. 1034.
38. Ibid., p. 1031.
39. Ibid., p. 1035.
40. Sri Aurobindo, *The Human Cycle*, p. 232.
41. Ibid., p. 66.
42. D.P. Chattopadhyaya, *Sri Aurobindo and K. Marx*, p. 67 - 68
43. Sri Aurobindo, *The Ideal of Human Unity*, p. 261 - 262.
44. Ibid., p. 263.
45. Sri Aurobindo, *The Human Cycle*, p. 238.
46. Ibid., p. 241.
47. Ibid., p. 238.
48. Sri Aurobindo, *The Foundations of Indian Culture*, p. 51-52.
49. Sri Aurobindo, *The Human Cycle*, p. 77.
50. Sri Aurobindo, *The Foundations of Indian Culture*, p. 323.
51. Sri Aurobindo, *The Human Cycle*, p. 76.
52. Ibid., p. 162.
53. Sri Aurobindo, *The Foundations of Indian Culture*, p. 140.
54. Ken Wilber, *Integral Psychology*, p.183-184.
55. Sri Aurobindo, *The Synthesis of Yoga*, p. 594-595.
56. Sri Aurobindo, *The Foundations of Indian Culture*, p. 90.
57. Sri Aurobindo, *The Ideal of Human Unity*, p. 554-555.
58. Sri Aurobindo, *Letters on Yoga*, p. 137.
59. Ibid., p. 1668.
60. Ken Wilber, *The Marriage of Sense and Soul*, p.208.
61. Ken Wilber, *A Bief History of Everything*, p. 66.
62. Sri Aurobindo, *The Life Divine*, p. 97.
63. Sri Aurobindo, *The Synthesis of Yoga*, p. 181.

64. Sri Aurobindo, *The Life Divine*, p. 714-715.
65. Ibid., p. 629-630.
66. Sri Aurobindo, *The Synthesis of Yoga*, p. 592.
67. Sri Aurobindo, *The Life Divine*, p. 883-884.
68. Sri Aurobindo, *The Synthesis of Yoga*, p. 164.
69. Ibid., p. 190.
70. Ibid., p. 194-195.
71. Sri Aurobindo, *The Life Divine*, p. 467- 468.
72. Ibid., p. 416.
73. Sri Aurobindo, *Letters on Yoga*, p. 125.
74. Sri Aurobindo, *The Life Divine*, p.1053.
75. Sri Aurobindo, *The Synthesis of Yoga*, p.159.
76. Sri Aurobindo, *The Life Divine*, p.486.
77. Sri Aurobindo, *The Life Divine*, p.846.
78. Sri Aurobindo, *The Human Cycle*, p.207.
79. Ken Wilber, *Up from Eden*,p.328.
80. Ken Wilber, *Sex, Ecology,Spirituality*, p.197.
81. Ibid., p.200.
82. Ibid., p.201.
83. Ibid., p.197.
84. Ibid., p.191.
85. Ken Wilber, *Sex, Ecology,Spirituality*, p.188.
86. Ibid., p. 522.
87. Ken Wilber, *A Brief History of Everything*, p. 57.
88. Sri Aurobindo, *the Life Divine*, p.' 884.
89. Ken Wilber, *Collective Works*, Volume 8, Introduction, p.47.
90. Ken Wilber, *One Taste*, p. 114.
91. Ibid., p. 251.
92. Ibid., p. 350.
93. Ibid., p. 364.

Chapter Eleven

Ken Wilber's Critical Interpretations of Various Aspects of Sri Aurobindo's Metaphysical Vision

Ken Wilber has clearly stated that he does not criticise Sri Aurobindo's vision, though he claims to offer a 'refinement' of Sri Aurobindo's metaphysical vision. He updates Sri Aurobindo's integral views by incorporating the latest research developments in the various fields of science.

This chapter looks at the critical commentaries that Ken Wilber has made on Sri Aurobindo's views, but it also raises questions about the possibility of a misunderstanding or occasional misrepresentation of Sri Aurobindo's metaphysical vision by Ken Wilber.

KEN WILBER ON SRI AUROBINDO'S ULTIMATE REALISATION

As mentioned in *Up front Eden,* Ken Wilber is not sure if Sri Aurobindo actually realised the *Turiya* or *Svabhavikakaya* level of consciousness. In a footnote Ken Wilber mentions that "a complete understanding of the *Svabhavikakaya,* reached perhaps as early as eighth century A.D. in Buddhism, but which likewise is peaking with certain *modern-day* sages, especially Sri Ramana Maharshi, Bubba Free John, perhaps Aurobindo."[1]

He equates the *Svabhavikakaya* with the *Dharmakaya* or higher causal realm; the former is the Source of all levels, the latter is the Suchness of all levels, where the soul no longer communes with oneness but becomes oneness; in this unification of Creator and creature, both disappear as separate entities.

Ken Wilber describes the *Svabhavikakaya* level as "perfect and radical transcendence into and as ultimate Consciousness as Such, or absolute Brahman-Atman."[2] This level in the superconscious sphere is the ground or condition of every level of the Spectrum. For Ken Wilber "Consciousness as Such is released in Perfect Transcendence, which is not a transcendence from the world but a final transcendence as the World. Consciousness henceforth *operates,* not on the world, but only as the entire World Process, integrating and interpenetrating all levels, realms, and planes, high or low, sacred or profane."[3] In the ultimate Unity all things and events are only One, and this radically perfect integration of all prior levels is the final differentiation of Consciousness from all forms in Consciousness.

In *Sex, Ecology, Spirituality,* Ken Wilber is more outspoken in his evaluation of Sri Aurobindo's realisations when he writes, "This is not to imply that Plotinus or Aurobindo were ultimate Realizers in a permanent or perfected sense, but rather that they are superb representatives of a full-spectrum approach to human growth and development based on their own experiential disclosures of the higher domains."[4]

For Sri Aurobindo, Ken Wilber's ultimate Unity is only a static unity. Ken Wilber may not be sure about Sri Aurobindo's static realisation, but Sri Aurobindo wrote about his own first concrete realisation as follows: "a realisation of the personal Divine or of the impersonal Brahman or of the Self does not usually come at the beginning of a Sadhana or in the first years or for many years. It comes so to a very few; mine came fifteen years after my first pre- experience in London and in the fifth year after I started Yoga."[5] This

Nirvanic realisation was in Sri Aurobindo's case "the first positive spiritual experience and it made possible all the rest of the Sadhana."[6]

Sri Aurobindo was exploring greater realisations beyond the static Brahman consciousness. Self-realisation is the goal of any traditional Yoga, but Sri Aurobindo points out that such a spiritual realisation is mostly concerned with the individual rather than with humanity as a whole, and the lower nature and the world are neglected or given up as incorrigible. For him realisation of the true eternal Self beyond the manifested world is not the primary aim, but only a first step. The realisation of the pure quiescent Self is the basis for a dynamic realisation which is characterised by the establishment of the true relations between the eternal Self and the mutable world. The realisation of the Self or Atman is not the final goal but only a means towards the Divine transformation. Sri Aurobindo developed his dynamic Brahman realisation in the course of his sadhana in Pondicherry from 1910 to 1926. This realisation of the supreme Reality is the experience of the multiform Unity, the integral Spirit which expresses itself, on one hand, as the profound peace of timeless perfection and, on the other hand, as the creative joy of spiritual self-expression.

About the dynamic Brahman realisation, Sri Aurobindo wrote in 1934, "As an experience [a pantheistic experience], it is a very common thing to have this feeling or realisation in the Vedantic Sadhana. I have had it myself on various levels of consciousness and in numerous forms, and I have met scores of people who have had it very genuinely—not as an intellectual theory or perception, but as a spiritual reality."[7] These two realisations, the static and the dynamic, were still marked by the absence of integrality, an integral change of consciousness and nature. Sri Aurobindo's final crowning realisation in the higher planes of consciousness revealed to him the whole of existence, including being and becoming, spirit and matter as an integral and undivided whole. The vision of the Supramental created the possibility of a transformation of matter into a medium of the Spirit, of a potentiality of a divine life here on this earth and in the earthly existence. About this integral realisation *[annam-brahman]* Sri Aurobindo wrote in 1935, "24th [November 1926] was the descent of Krishna into the physical. Krishna is not the supramental Light. The descent of Krishna would mean the descent of the Overmind Godhead preparing, though not itself actually, the descent of Supermind and Ananda. Krishna is the Anandamaya; he supports the evolution through the Overmind leading it towards the Ananda."[8] For Sri Aurobindo there must be a descent of the light not merely into the mind, but into all the various parts of the being down to the physical and below before a real transformation can take place.

These quotations of Sri Aurobindo's realisations indicate that Ken Wilber is rather rash in his judgements regarding Sri Aurobindo's spiritual realisations and perhaps he could have been a bit more cautious and reserved about interpreting and classifying the spiritual realisations and development of modern-day sages.

Sri Aurobindo's realisation of the superconscient state was initially experienced in a state of meditative trance (samadhi), but afterwards these realisations were constant in his waking state, then established themselves as a permanent basis and were able to function as a condition for the spiritual transformation of his nature. To use his own words, "The only real difficulty which took decades of spiritual effort to work out towards completeness was to apply the spiritual knowledge utterly to the world and to the surface psychological and outer life and to effect its transformation both on the higher levels of Nature and on the ordinary mental, vital and physical levels."[9]

Sri Aurobindo seeks a physical transformation on earth while "neither Buddha nor Shankara nor Ramakrishna had any idea of transforming the body. Their aim was spiritual *mukti* [liberation] and nothing else."[10] In attempting to bring down the Supermind he wrote; "If greater men than myself have not had this vision and this ideal before them, that is no reason why I should not follow my Truth-sense and Truth-vision. If human reason regards me as a fool for trying to do what Krishna did not try, I do not in the least care."[11]

Sri Aurobindo does not want to stand up on a high and distant Supermind level and change the world from there, but to bring some principles of inner Truth, Light and Power into the earth-consciousness. In a note written in 1947 he explains that, "at the present stage the progressive supramentalisation of the Overmind is the first immediate preoccupation [as mentioned above, Sri Aurobindo realised the descent of the Overmind Godhead into the physical realm on the 24th of November 1926] and a second is the lightening of the heavy resistance of the Inconscient and the support it gives to human ignorance which is always the main obstacle in any attempt to change the world or even to change oneself."[12]

Ken Wilber's classification of Sri Aurobindo's spiritual realisations ignores this fact, and also the fact that Sri Aurobindo did not try to rise individually to the supramental plane and pass away into a Superconscient moksha, but rather to bring it down and make it a permanent part of earth-consciousness. Sri Aurobindo's spiritual realisations aim at the integrality of the Divine in this world and not only beyond it. Are Ken Wilber'S insights into Sri Aurobindo's integral realisations limited by certain confusions regarding the results of Sri Aurobindo's actual yogic practice? It seems that Ken Wilber has the tendency now and then to use inaccurate language while expressing his sympathetic views in relation to Sri Aurobindo's spiritual realisations.

When Ken Wilber explores the implications of an evolutionary view of the Kosmos in the Introduction to the

4th volume of *The Collective Works,* he describes the general stages through which worldviews develop. Each next-to-highest stage of development involves the double process of differentiation and integration. It is the vision-logic level, with its capacity for systems thinking that is able to create an opening to the higher stages of transrational or transpersonal development. As already explained in the section on *Integral Psychology,* Ken Wilber divides vision-logic into three major substages. Early vision-logic (the greenmeme) recognises and differentiates systems and begins to relate them, whereas middle (yellow, integrative) and late (turquoise, holistic) vision-logic integrates these disparate and pluralistic systems, contexts and cultures into dynamic, holistic structures. When early vision-logic matures into its middle and late phases, it develops more holistic modes of awareness, and pluralistic relativism gives way to universal integralism. The difference between early vision-logic and middle/late vision-logic is the difference between first- and second-tier thinking. With second-tier thinking, the individual can think both vertically and horizontally; second-tier awareness is used in terms of the overall spiral of existence and not merely in terms of any one level. Ken Wilber adds three higher or transpersonal levels beyond the highest *mental* realms of mature vision-logic, i.e., the psychic (Coral) as the beginning of the truly transpersonal levels, the subtle and causal. He indicates these higher levels as third-tier thinking.

In explaining the details of the mature vision-logic as the highest of the mental realms, Ken Wilber again evaluates Sri Aurobindo's realisations and assumes that Sri Aurobindo has written all his main works through this mature vision-logic. He notes that "this mature vision-logic with its dynamic/dialectical/developmental worldview, is the level *through which,* most of the great modem philosopher-sages (such as Hegel, Whitehead, Gebser, and Aurobindo) have written, even though they are often expressing insights seen at even higher, transpersonal, transmental levels—and for the simple reason that, in order to mentally communicate at all, the mental realms must be used. These great philosopher-sages speak through the highest of the mental realms the vision-logic mind—even as they are trying to communicate even higher transmental truths and realities."[13] Ken Wilber then claims that he has attempted to write most of his works on the 'late' or 'high' vision-logic level. He defines himself as a 'constructive postmodernist, in contrast to the merely 'early' or 'low' vision-logic level, which he relates to deconstructive postmodernism. According to Ken Wilber, "*Constructive postmodernism* (as I use the term) takes up the multiple contexts freed by dynamic relativism, and then integrates them into mutually interrelated networks, as opposed to deconstructive and extreme postmodernism."[14]

Does Ken Wilber imply that his later works, written through the vision-logic mind, can be equated with Sri Aurobindo's *The Life Divine, The Synthesis of Yoga* and his other main works, which were written through the silent mind or direct Knowledge? In order to clarify this question, we have to refer to Sri Aurobindo's *Letters on Yoga* and *On Himself,* where he describes the progress of his integral sadhana and his spiritual realisations in greater detail. Sri Aurobindo's main works are not a product of mental reasoning or speculation, but something that has grown out of his own authentic permanent yogic realisations, i.e., he worked from a yogic state or 'action-in-yoga'. Sri Aurobindo was not an abstract theoretician and he did not arrive at his philosophical views by a sudden revelation, but through a steady growth of consciousness. Supra-intellectual thinking "is not an expression of ideas arrived at by speculative thinking. One has to arrive at spiritual knowledge through experience and a consciousness of things which arises directly out of that experience or else underlies or is involved in it. This kind of knowledge, then, is fundamentally a consciousness and not a thought or formulated idea." [15] Sri

Aurobindo's philosophy is not an intellectual exercise and there are not many logical arguments in his philosophy, though the explanations of his yogic viewpoint do not lack a logical basis. When he wrote *The Arya* (the vehicle for his main works, including *The Life Divine, The Synthesis of Yoga, The Human Cycle,* and *The Ideal of Human Unity),* "I Sri Aurobindo was setting forth an overmind view of things to the mind and putting it in mental terms, that was why I had sometimes to use logic. For in such a work—mediating between the intellect and supra-intellectual—logic has a place, though it cannot have the chief place it occupies in purely mental philosophies." [16] *The Life Divine,* presenting his metaphysical vision of a divine life for man, is based on supramental facts and presented to us in terms of the intellect. When he used intellectual abstractions, he did so in order to explain his philosophy and to justify it to the intellect of others. While writing *The Life Divine,* Sri Aurobindo began ascending into the higher planes of the mind, where he was guided by direct Knowledge, always translating itself into experience. As described in his own words, "The mental being in me became a free Intelligence, a universal Mind, not limited to the narrow circle of personal thought as a labourer in a thought factory, but a receiver of knowledge from all the hundred realms of being and free to choose what it willed in this vast sight-empire and thought-empire. I mention this only to emphasise that the possibilities of the mental being are not limited and that it can be the free Witness and Master in its own house. It is not to say that everybody can do it in the way I did it and with the same rapidity of the decisive movement." [17] In other words, his main works were produced without the aid of thought, as his mind remained always in a state of silence. It seemed that, for Sri Aurobindo, words came from somewhere else than the thinking mind, and thoughts occurred to him generally in the wideness above the head. In a letter to a disciple, Sri Aurobindo wrote "I have made no endeavour in writing, I have simply left the higher Power to work and when it did not work I made no effort at all. ... Let me remind you also that when I was writing The Arya I never think ... It is out of a silent mind that I write whatever comes ready-shaped from above."[18] This mental silence remained unimpaired for several months and to this inner passivity (passive Brahman realisation) Sri Aurobindo gradually added an outer action (active Brahman realisation), each independent of the other. Sri Aurobindo distinguishes these spiritual realisations from spiritual experiences, i.e., an experience only comes in flashes and is the beginning of a realisation. "Repetition of the experience leads to a fuller and more permanent realisation."[19] "They are spoken of as full realisations only when they become very positive or frequent or continuous or normal."[20]

While being guided by direct Knowledge from the higher planes, Sri Aurobindo was able to write for six years without interruptions all his main works, almost 5000 pages, not just one book after another but "four and even six books currently, on the most varied subjects, such as *The Life Divine,* his fundamental 'philosophical' work and spiritual vision of evolution, *The Synthesis of Yoga,* in which he describes the various stages and experiences of the integral yoga and surveys all the past and present yogic disciplines, *Essays on the Gita,* which expounds his philosophy of action, *The Secret of the Veda,* with a study on the origins of language, and *The Ideal of Human Unity* and *The Human Cycle,* which approach evolution from its sociological and psychological standpoint and examine the future possibilities of human societies."[21] Though Sri Aurobindo has written philosophy, he claimed that he was never a philosopher but a poet and a politician. He managed to write philosophy because "My theory was that a Yogi ought to be able to turn his hand to anything ... Secondly, because I had only to write down in terms of the intellect all that I had observed and come to know in practising Yoga daily and the philosophy was there automatically. But that is not being a philosopher!"[22]

Some reviews of Ken Wilber's *Sex, Ecology, Spirituality* were "very positive (along with Aurobindo's Life Divine, Heidegger's Being and Time, and Whitehead's Process and Reality, Wilber's Sex, Ecology, Spirituality is one of the four great books of this century)."[23] That's fine, as far as it goes, and this author does not want to argue in favour of or against the correctness of this quote from Michael Murphy. However, it is one thing to compare or evaluate and criticise the contents of the vision of various system thinkers in order to find out the objective truth, but it is quite another thing to evaluate the actual realisations of these system thinkers and thereafter equate—in this case, subtly denigrate—Sri Aurobindo's direct Knowledge on the Overmind level with his own vision-logic level. Ken Wilber cannot equate the two-tier thinking through which he attempted to write his later works with Sri Aurobindo's third-tier consciousness, through which he wrote all his main works. For Sri Aurobindo, the third-tier transpersonal states were not merely altered or passing states of consciousness but, became permanent traits.

SRI AUROBINDO'S AND KEN WILBER'S CONCEPT OF INTEGRATION AND TRANSFORMATION

For Sri Aurobindo, each form that emerges in evolution is assumed to exist implicitly in the form from which it emerges, i.e., matter contains life but in veiled form while life is a form of veiled mind. The urge towards growth implies the pressure of the Consciousness-Force of the Cosmic Spirit (the Energy of consciousness that creates the universe) from the higher planes to manifest itself in the lower planes, i.e., the self-manifestation of the higher in the lower. The principles in the lower realms are subordinate powers of those in the higher realms, but the upsurging of the Consciousness-Force from its descent implies the presence of the Divine in the lower planes, including the physical, vital and mental levels. Because of the higher divine presence in the lower, the latter has the inherent potency to change into divine elements and transcend their limitations. This is the basis of Sri Aurobindo's concept of transformation and a divine life on earth.

The term transformation should not be confused with mere change. Change is related to altering something and placing it somewhere else or moving from one state to another, whereas transformation is related to an inner modification which uplifts the individual to a higher or deeper grade of being. Transformation enables the seeker to get in touch with one's inward likeness to the Divine, by changing all that is not divine in him or her into something divine. This power of self-transformation urges the seeker to complete one's divine destiny. Transformation for Sri Aurobindo is not a moral or spiritual purification, but a *radical change of consciousness and being,* or a radical conversion of the natural parts into their spiritual equivalents so that the whole of human nature can be transfigured into the divine Supernature. It enables the seeker to live in the Divine, not only in the absorbed state of trance, but at all times and in all the parts of our being; it enables mankind, through sadhana, to live the Life Divine on earth—physically, vitally, mentally and spiritually.

Transformation of the lower nature and its evolution to the higher Nature is a complex process involving an ascension to a higher stage of development, and the descent of the powers of the higher stage into the lower, so that the lower gets purified and converted upwards, and finally there is a simultaneous widening of the faculties of the previously achieved higher level, which is again preparatory to the next still higher stage of development. This long process, a moving upwards and downwards proceeds from stage to stage until our whole human nature is divinised. As described by Sri Aurobindo, "First there must be a conversion inwards, a going within to find the inmost psychic being and bring it out to the front, disclosing at the same time the inner mind, inner vital, inner physical parts of the nature. Next there must be an ascension, a series of conversions upward and a turning down to convert the lower parts. When one has made the inward conversion, one 'psychicises' the whole lower nature so as to make it ready for the divine change. Going upwards, one passes beyond the human mind and at each stage of the ascent, there is a conversion into a new consciousness and an infusion of this new consciousness into the whole of the nature."[24]

Sri Aurobindo's concept of integral transformation aims at the alteration of the very structure of the being, i.e., the higher structure is not merely integrated into the lower and acted upon, but the lower needs to be simultaneously purified through psychic transformation in order to allow any descent of the higher. Ken Wilber leaves out this process of the psychicisation of the whole lower nature in preparation for the divine change.

The purpose of integral transformation is to manifest the divine in our life. This manifestation of the Divine in life implies the realisation of the Divine consciousness in all the different parts of the being and not only in the soul. All parts of the being—mind, life, body and soul—must be equally filled with the Divine Presence and be effective centres for the outpouring of the Divine Power in the universe. For Sri Aurobindo diverse principles do not unite on their original level, but are first transformed and then enter into a greater synthesis. Within this view of integration through transformation what appears diverse is transformed and then integrated in order to arrive at unity in diversity.

Unlike Ken Wilber, Sri Aurobindo maintains that an entire transformation of the lower instrumentation needs not only the action of the higher principle helping to transform the lower, but also the full emergence of the law of the Spirit or the power of the Supermind. Mental man cannot make an ascent to the Supermind and bring down its powers into the terrestrial existence in a single leap, and the gulf between mind and Supermind can be bridged only by the process of triple transformation.

For the transpersonal psychotherapist the lower cannot explain the higher, but the higher can be described in terms of the lower by contrasting them with ordinary psychological functions of consciousness. As such, the transpersonal movement includes a detailed view and study of the lower realms of experience within their own terms. These lower realms may act either as an obstruction or as an entrance to the realisation of one's true being or existence. The higher foundation does include and transcend the lower, but the lower exercises its right of recognition as long as it is in need of it. The higher levels can exert control over the lower levels, but they can also dominate or even repress and alienate the lower levels, which leads to a whole host of pathological difficulties in both the individual and society at large.

In his earlier works, *the Atman Project* and *Up from Eden*, Ken Wilber does refer to the process of involution, where the higher levels are already present in the lower levels though obscured, i.e., all the higher levels are already, though unconsciously, present in the lower levels. According to Ken Wilber, "in the ground unconscious, the Ursprung, there exist all the higher structures in a *potential* form, ready to unfold into actuality, or emerge in consciousness. Involution, then, is the *unfolding* or in-turning of the higher structures into successively lower ones, and evolution is the subsequent *unfolding* into actuality of this enfolded potential. In short, once involution is complete, evolution can begin. As involution was the enfolding of the higher in the lower, evolution is the unfolding of the higher from the lower. But 'from' is the wrong word: it is not that the higher actually *comes from* the lower as a cause from an effect. The lower can never produce the higher. It is rather that the higher comes *from* the Ursprung, where it already exists as potential. But when the higher emerges it does indeed pass *through* the lower."[25] In the process of evolution, each higher level contains all the capacities of the lower ones, but not vice versa, not all of the higher levels are in the lower. The transpersonal realm has a higher level of integration from where the lower levels are being viewed in a different perspective and from where the lower levels can be inferred. However, the lower levels are not destroyed and never disappear from consciousness; developmental stages proceed by disowning the previous stage and moving on to the next stage. The disowned stage is retained though not necessarily in any conscious way, i.e., the lower levels no longer comprise the essential focus of consciousness. This process of evolution (ascent) and involution (descent) is described by Ken Wilber as, "where involution proceeded by successive separations and dismemberments, evolution, as the reverse, proceeds by successive unifications and higher-order wholes. ... Evolution is the remembering, or putting back together, of that which was separated and alienated during involution. And evolution, as a successive remembering or joining together in higher unity, simply continues until there is *only* Unity and *everything* has been remembered as Spirit by Spirit." [26]

Sri Aurobindo would agree with Ken Wilber that the preceding lower levels with which the individual has disidentified oneself are integrated in the higher, but for Sri Aurobindo the lower in its transformed state becomes a conscious instrument for the higher. *This integration is not a mere logical harmony or non-contradiction, nor unification through eliminating the opposition; this unifying character involves the psychic being.* The realisation of the psychic being leads to integration in which the outer instrument is purified and integrated with the inner and higher levels of being.

In Ken Wilber's later work, *Sex, Ecology, Spirituality,*

he explains and refines, in great detail, the process of ascent and descent in relation to the concept of integration. Growth occurs in stages, which necessitates a chronological order or hierarchy. In any developmental sequence, the higher or deeper level includes the capacities of the previous levels, which function as building blocks in subsequent development and then adds its own more encompassing capacities. The new level includes the development of the previous stage, plus something extra, i.e., more integrative capacities. In transcendence the lower, when it functions adequately, sets the foundation and prepares the possibilities for, but does not determine the emergent higher; it preserves or incorporates some of the fundamental features of the previous level but negates its partialness or separateness. Each development involves a greater degree of consciousness or a new emergence, a new transcendence, a new differentiation/integration. As expressed by Ken Wilber, "each new and emergent interior holon transcends but includes, and thus *operates upon,* the information presented by its junior holons, and thus it fashions something *novel* in the ongoing cognitive or interior stream. Hence, each new growth in consciousness is not just the 'discovery' of more of a pregiven world, but the co-creation of new worlds themselves, ... a discovery/ creation of higher and wider worlds."[27] "Integration produces a new level, a new deep structure—it is a transformation."[28]

In summary, at every stage of development, the process of evolution unfolds/enfolds its predecessors; there is "a profound integration of Spirit descending into even the lowest state [involution] and ascending back to itself [evolution], with Spirit nonetheless *fully present at each and every stage* as *the process* of its own self-unfolding and self-enfolding development, a divine play of Spirit present in every single movement of the Kosmos."29

"The higher stages are implicit in the lower, and as they develop they envelop."[30] As described later on by

Ken Wilber "All things and events, of whatever nature, are perfect manifestations of Spirit. No holon, whether conventionally considered high or low, sacred or profane, simple or complex, primitive or advanced, is closer or farther from Ground, and thus all holons have equal ultimate value or equal *Ground-value*."[31]

Ken Wilber agrees with Sri Aurobindo's involutionary view, in which the depth of the higher potentials is already present in the lower levels, but these potentials are not yet actualised and realised.

The manifest All-Unity evolves as All-Form, and the pure unmanifest Spirit is the Source of all other levels and their ultimate goal. This manifest All is as fully present in the lowest level as well as in the highest level. The lower itself possesses equal Ground-value (ultimate value) and its own degree of intrinsic value. "The involutionary theories are all attempts to take into account that the depth of the higher structural potentials are already present but not seen."[32]

For Ken Wilber the lower realms are merely connecting links, but cannot have an integrative function, as the integrative process is to be found in the higher realms only. He claims that his developmental model is not a rigid model, "the various stages not only spiral, meander, wobble and regress, they are themselves simply mileposts in the winding road of growth. This is so taken for granted by developmentalists that I assumed I would not have to keep repeating it."[33] But if the higher includes, embraces and incorporates the lower, and each ascent brings in a new and higher integration, then the lower itself, controlled and influenced by the higher, seems to remain unchanged and cannot become a *fit* instrument for the higher.

Inclusion of the lower in the higher need not be the same as integration of the lower into the higher. It seems to Ken Wilber that when the achievements of the lower are included in the higher we speak of integration, but this appears to be a partial integration. Conceptual emphasis on a 'higher' level need not ensure the completion of the lower level task. If the lower is not transformed and is unduly and illegitimately dominated by the higher, then the lower is not granted its proper autonomy, which may result in distortions of the lower itself, but also of the higher.

In *The Eye of Spirit,* however, Ken Wilber explains that any basic structure that remains in existence can be further developed and trained because as a basic structure it is also its own line, i.e., the vertical transformative development has also a horizontal or translative development. "Once major transformations come to rest for any individual there remains only translative growth. These translative unfoldings are both enduring and transitional."[34]

In *Sex, Ecology, Spirituality,* Ken Wilber also modifies his "linear" developmental model as previously described in *Eye to Eye* and *Transformations of Consciousness.* He assumes that the ladder metaphor partially fails as "each higher stage does not actually sit on top of the lower stage but rather *enfolds* in its own being."[35]

Development is now a series of concentric circles with each higher level transcending and including its predecessor. In the actualisation holarchy each stage unfolds and then enfolds its predecessors in a concentric way. The self as the climber of the ladder—the ladder itself is selfless—identifies itself with a particular rung of the ladder and this generates various self-stages. The overall development of enduring structures (waves), transitionary structures (streams), and self-system takes place.as follows:

(1) "the proximate self (at whatever level) is the *locus of identification;* (2) the proximate self successively identifies with each emerging basic structure (or level of consciousness) and thus becomes embedded at that level (or at that wave); (3) which generates a stream of transitional

self-stages (selfsense, self-needs, morals) supported by the *exclusiveness* of the proximate identification; (4) these exclusivity structures can develop in a quasi-independent fashion, though they tend to be held together in a bundle by the self; these remain in place until (5) the self de-embeds or dis-identifies with that level, (6) embeds at the next level, (7). which *integrates* the previous *enduring* structures but negates the previous exclusivity/transitional structures—and so on."[36]

In its development the self can choose which way to go; it has to negotiate the developmental rungs of expanding awareness. It is obvious that things can go wrong when the self climbs the rungs of the ladder at any stage. In the developmental unfolding aspects of the self may be repressed, dissociated or alienated, ranging from psychosis to spiritual crisis depending upon where the distortion occurred.

In Ken Wilber's latest refinement on integration, he uses Fred Kofman's four basic entities in existence—individual and social holons, artifacts and heaps—in order to explain that for each of those four entities, 'whole', 'part', and 'hierarchy' mean something completely different. It seems that all attempted 'integral' approaches confuse all four of these. For Ken Wilber, in individual holons, "the senior elements subsume the junior elements and exercise some sort of control over them. But social holons are composed of members or partners, not elements. So this remains a copartnership at all levels" (Ken Wilber Online. A Shambhala Interview with Ken Wilber). Social holons transcend and include the previous social holons in their own line of development but do not transcend and include the previous individual holons. It is the membership of the social holon which enacts laws that are accepted by all members, and not the individual who controls another individual. Trying to treat the social holon as if it were an individual holon ends up in totalitarian oppression, or trying to reduce individual holons to mere parts ends up reducing all holons to parts of the physical Cosmos. In constructing nested hierarchies, an ontological division must be made between these four entities. Social holons are not sitting on top of individual holons, but rather both are correlative aspects of sentient holons at each level of development. This is exactly like the four quadrants model, where the two upper quadrants and the two lower quadrants are correlative social forms of individuals at each stage of evolution. In a nested hierarchy, each higher wave of development is more inclusive and has more consciousness, more care and more compassion.

For Sri Aurobindo integration, as a process of widening and heightening, widens, opens and adapts lower principles so that they are able to ascend to higher stages. In the process of widening, evolution increases organisation and differentiation in order to be capable of evolving to higher principles. The process of heightening can be described as the ascent from grade to grade upwards, and once the higher stage is reached the process of integration takes place. In this integral process there is a mode of making further complex the less complex. As explained by Sri Aurobindo: "an ascent to a new level and a taking up of the lower levels, a new integration of the existence by a superior power of Being which imposes its own way of action and its character and force of substance-energy on as much as it can reach of the previously evolved parts of nature."[37]

For Sri Aurobindo integration means the harmonisation of the different parts of the being into an organic whole. Each successive movement of the evolutionary psychology of the being is an ascent to a wider consciousness, and the progressive freedom from subjection to the lower determinism. Each evolving gradation contains in it the potentiality of the next higher stage. The ascent of consciousness towards freedom implies a greater development of the lower parts of Nature and a progressive integration of them all into an organic unity.

SRI AUROBINDO'S COSMIC EVOLUTION IN TERRESTRIAL NATURE

For Sri Aurobindo and Ken Wilber, evolution is preceded by involution, and what was original and primal in involution is in evolution the Supreme emergence. The movement of evolution towards a progressive self-manifestation of the Spirit in a material universe has to square at every step with the fact of the involution of the Spirit in matter. The threefold movement of the integral process of evolution is described by Sri Aurobindo: "The principle of the process of evolution is a foundation, from that foundation an ascent, in that ascent a reversal of consciousness and, from the greater height and wideness gained, an action of change and new integration of the whole nature."[38]

Through the process of evolution, the lower levels of being are brought to such a point that it comes under pressure from some superior plane where the new power is dominant. This is how a decisive transition takes place from the lower level to the higher one. But it must be clear that a mere isolated lifting of a part of the nature of a being by dissociating it from the other parts, without any attempt to keep in touch with the rest of the being, has not much significance from the evolutionary point of view.

Ken Wilber agrees with this triple process of evolution. Many mystics who have obtained liberation by detaching themselves from the world have failed to transform the world into any higher status. For what is wanted is the emergence of a divine life on earth, and not the isolated realisation by a few individuals of their true inner life. Ken Wilber is aware of this when he refers to Sri Aurobindo's overall view as, "Sri Aurobindo, India's great modern sage, has written extensively on just this viewpoint [the union of evolution and involution]—Brahman getting lost in involution and then evolving back ... and he sees it occurring cosmologically as well as psychologically."[43] Spirit, as the creative power, can bring about the entire transformation of the material universe. As a result of this transformation the law of supramental consciousness will be established in our whole evolutionary being and nature.

In order to understand the nature of reality it is essential to. consider the levels of Creation of Being as conceived by Sri Aurobindo. Reality is essentially one; nevertheless, creation is the expression of the essential unity of reality which expresses itself in terms of multiplicity. The eight levels of Being are the expression of reality seen in the context of creation. The first four, Pure Being, Pure Consciousness-Force, Pure Bliss (these three levels form the concept of Sachchidananda) and the Supermind belong to the higher hemisphere, and to the lower hemisphere belong Mind, Psyche, Life and Matter. The two hemispheres are not opposite in nature, as aspects of the lower correspond to those of the higher sphere. According to Sri Aurobindo, "The Divine descends from pure existence through the play of Consciousness-Force and Bliss and the creative medium of Supermind into cosmic being; we ascend from Matter through a developing life, soul and mind and the illuminating medium of Supermind towards the divine being. The knot of the two, the higher and the lower hemisphere, is where mind and Supermind meet with a veil between them. The rending of the veil is the condition of the divine life in humanity. ... And if there be any goal to the evolution other than an aimless circling and an individual escape from the circling, if the infinite potentiality of this creature, who alone here stands between Spirit and Matter with the power to mediate between them, has any meaning other than an ultimate awakening from the delusion of life by despair and disgust of the cosmic effort and its complete rejection, then even such a luminous and puissant transfiguration and emergence of the Divine in the creature must be that high-uplifted goal and that supreme significance."[39]

These eight principles are essential to all cosmic

creation, the higher Trinity is the source and the basis of all existence, and all cosmos must be the expression and action of its essential reality. This cosmic action needs the play of the infinite Force of Existence, which produces and regulates all these forms and movements. Sri Aurobindo maintains that the infinite Consciousness, as a vast universal self-delight, is the cause, essence and object of cosmic existence. "This self-bliss may become subconscient, seemingly lost on the surface, but not only must it be there at our roots, all existence must be essentially a seeking and reaching out to discover and possess it, and in proportion as the creature in the cosmos finds himself, he must awaken to something of the secret ecstasy. ... Wherever, then, cosmic existence manifests itself, these three must be behind and within it. ... There must be in every cosmos a power of Knowledge and Will which out of infinite potentiality fixes determined relations, rolls out the mighty rhythms of cosmic Law. This power indeed is nothing else than Sachchidananda Himself; it creates nothing which is not in its own self-existence, and for that reason all cosmic and real Law is a thing not imposed from outside, but from within."[40] Sri Aurobindo's triple process of widening, heightening and integration is therefore not only related to the evolution of the individual, but it is also related to cosmic evolution. The movement of evolution, as the progressive self-manifestation of the Spirit in a material universe, proceeds by an awakening of the involved consciousness and force, and its ascent from grade to grade. To each grade in this series belongs its appropriate class of existence; each new advance of formation takes up what was before. Thus it can be said that there are two principle factors at work in the emergence of a new principle in terrestrial nature; firstly, the heightening and intensification of consciousness from below, and secondly the pressure from a plane above that of the material nature. All the principles that are to evolve in the terrestrial nature are already present in a latent form in matter, but their existence is not felt. In the evolution of nature it is the Spirit which is the guiding principle, but in its outward form it assumes the appearance of Inconscience. Though nature is still in the state of inconscience, it does not stop here. The Consciousness-Force present in nature develops itself in the form of a higher vital or life force, and this emergence of life gives the old status of the world a new life-value. The next upward movement of the Consciousness-Force develops a new principle of existence, the mental principle or mind-world. Once the course of evolution reaches the stage of man, the universal Spirit in man transforms the lower grades of existence according to the higher universal laws and values, and man moves upward towards what is above mind. In the scheme of cosmic evolution man is a stage, a transitional being and not a goal. Man cannot be considered as the consummation of the cosmic evolutionary process, the individual's glory consists in his or her ceaseless aspiration to transcend oneself. The object of our terrestrial existence is the perfect self-expression of the Spirit, which includes an initial involution of Sachchidananda in the inconscience, thereafter an evolution of ignorance into the possibilities of a partial developed knowledge, and finally the culmination and a fulfilment of Sachchidananda in manifestation.

Evolution is, therefore, not an isolated phenomenon unrelated to the universal Being, and this evolutionary develpoment, as pointed out by Sri Aurobindo "has a universal as well as an individual aspect: the Universal develops the grades of its being and the ordered variation of the universality of itself in the series of its evolved forms of being; the individual soul follows the line of this cosmic series and manifests what is prepared in the universality of the Spirit. The universal Man, the cosmic Purusha in humanity, is developing in the human race the power that has grown into humanity from below it and shall yet grow to Supermind and Spirit. ... The individual must have followed this line of development. ... He now appears as a human soul, the Spirit accepting the inner and outer form of humanity, but he is not limited by this form any more than he was limited by the plant or animal forms previously assumed by him; he can pass on from it to a greater self-expression in a higher scale of Nature." 41

This cosmic evolution is accompanied by the evolution of the individual. The individual life has the same rhythm and law of progression as the cosmic life, because human life is a term in a series through which Brahman in the universe gradually works out, through the individual, its purpose.

Earth is not a material world alone though it is fundamentally based on matter; it is a centre of progressive evolution constantly trying to evolve the principles involved in itself and to manifest the higher truth-principles here on earth. This process is not limited on the macrocosmic scale but is reproduced in the microcosmic scheme as well. Man as a miniature universe in himself has the capacity to evolve from one's present status of mental being into a spiritual being. "The cosmic self-expression and the individual selfexpression are the two aspects of the evolutionary process. The individual soul-experience and self-development follows the process of cosmic evolution. It means that as the Spirit hidden in the cosmos has revealed itself through the various grades and sub-grades of matter, life, mind and intellect, so the individual soul also must have presided over the lower forms of life before it took up the human evolution."[42]

It is the individual who first actualises higher states of consciousness within oneself and afterwards radiates them in the world, gradually producing an uplifting in the environment. For Sri Aurobindo universal nature comes to its self-consciousness only through individuals, and it is the individual who gives higher values to nature or the universe. After all, it is the individual that is the medium through which the Spirit reveals and discloses itself.

SEQUENCE: KEN WILBER'S AND SRI AUROBINDO'S DEVELOPMENTAL MODELS

Ken Wilber maintains that the individual doesn't have to develop perfect mastery of a lower stage before moving to a higher stage, though a certain competency of the lower is required. One can arrive at some very high stages of development, but still have all sorts of problems at various lower stages. According to Ken Wilber, "Human growth and development generally unfolds from body to mind to soul to spirit not as a linear ladder, but as nested waves, with each wave enveloping its predecessor(s)—if all goes well."[44]

In his later books, development no longer occurs in a stepladder-like fashion where one rung has to be completed before the next rung can occur. Ken Wilber refers now to some aspects of development which are related to higher stages of a particular line, and some aspects of development which are themselves a separate distinct line. In other words, psychological and spiritual development do not occur only in stages but also in lines, and when psychological and spiritual development are seen as two separate lines of development, then a spiritual stage of development in one line may occur simultaneously with a psychological stage of development in another line.

Various lines develop relatively independently, and a higher stage of development in one line can occur alongside a lower stage in another line. In this way, "spiritual and psychological growth, in the various developmental lines, are occurring alongside of each other and not stacked on top of each other like so many bricks. The idea that any of these lines must be fully completed before another can begin is silly."[45] As spiritual lines themselves they usually have their own invariant developmental sequence and unfold hierarchically, but overall spiritual development will not follow a stage-like course and does not develop in a specific sequence. So whether spirituality develops in stages depends completely on the way one defines spirituality; is it a separate developmental line, the highest level of the developmental line, the sum total of the highest levels of the developmental line, an attitude one can have at whatever stage one is, or is it the involvement of peak-experiences in spirituality?

Ken Wilber concludes that many aspects of spirituality show a stage-like development, but this does not mean that the overall psychological development has to be completed before spiritual development can take place. It again depends on how one defines these terms; when using psychological and spiritual development as personal and transpersonal stages respectively and "when looking at *any one developmental line,* the psychological must generally be completed before the spiritual can stably emerge. ... However, because the developmental lines themselves can unfold independently, an individual can be at a very high spiritual stage in one line and still be at a very low personal or psychological stage in others. ... Thus, even though, with these definitions, the spiritual comes only after the psychological in any given line, nonetheless all sorts of spiritual developments can occur before, alongside, or after, all sorts of psychological developments, precisely because the lines themselves are relatively independent."[46]

So it can be said that even though various lines can progress relatively independently through the levels, a fully integral development still involves a hierarchical unfolding of all of the major levels in a conscious fashion; a basic competence in each level is required in order for an overall development of consciousness to move permanently into higher realms. Though many of the developmental lines proceed through the levels in a stage-like manner, yet development in the sum total of all these different lines is a massively complex affair which follows no sequential development.

Like Sri Aurobindo, Ken Wilber admits that development is not an easy affair and there is nothing linear about the various levels; each level infinitely grades into each other, like the colours of a rainbow. He agrees with Sri Aurobindo that all sorts of regressions, dissociations, fixations, and temporary leaps forward are possible in the process of development, but "the empirical fact remains as Aurobindo said; individual streams obey the law of successive unfolding (undulating through the waves of the Great Nest itself)."[47] Nevertheless, he repeats again that the overall mixture of lines do hot follow their own stages, as the overall self juggles through all the various developmental lines which makes each individual's unfolding a unique affair.

When Ken Wilber refers to Sri Aurobindo's hierarchical developmental model, he claims to have improved his own model by adding the concept of lines that develop and unfold their own trajectory. It is the Self in the causal realm which is ultimately responsible for the overall integration of all the other lines; "it is the Self supreme that prevents the three realms—gross, subtle and causal—from flying apart in the first place. For, even though the three domains can show relatively independent development, they are still held together, and drawn together, by the radiant Self."[48]

While almost mercilessly criticising B. Cortright for his assumed misreporting of Sri Aurobindo's non-specific sequence of spiritual development, Ken Wilber quotes again (also in *Sex, Ecology, Spirituality*, p. 609, and *Eye of the Spirit*, p. 245), Sri Aurobindo's passage in *The Life Divine*, "The spiritual evolution obeys the logic of a successive unfolding; it can take a new decisive main step only when the previous main step has been sufficiently conquered: even if certain minor stages can be swallowed up or leaped over by a rapid and brusque ascension, the consciousness has to turn back to assure itself that the ground passed over is securely annexed to the new condition."[49]

However, Ken Wilber takes this passage as a general rule but he omits the part in the next page where Sri Aurobindo elaborates on the exceptions to this rule. "The necessary turn or change can also be brought about by an occult descent of the spiritual force from above, in which the influx, the influence, the spiritual consequence is felt, but the higher source is unknown and the actual feeling of a descent is not there. A consciousness so touched may be so much uplifted that the being turns to an immediate union with the Self or with the Divine by departure from the evolution and no question of graduality or steps or method intervenes ... for the law of departure, once it is made possible, is not or need not be the same as the law of the evolutionary transformation and perfection."[50]

Actually although Ken Wilber uses this quotation of Sn Aurobindo in order to defend himself against B. Cortright's arguments, in *A Brief History of Everything,* he had already admitted that Sri Aurobindo does not enunciate a successive unfolding or a specific sequence of spiritual development. In Ken Wilber's words, "And please, for both of them [Plotinus and Sri Aurobindo], this holarchy is not actually a step ladder, but a series of nested and enfolded dimensions."[51]

Sri Aurobindo never proposed a mere linear level of consciousness in his evolutionary model. Chapter six describesin detail the triple path of transformation and evotution which is based on parallel lines of development

In which manner does Ken Wilber improve Sri Aurobindo's hierarchal developmental model? Sri Aurobindo never proposed a mere linear model of consciousness in his evolutionary model. Chapter six describes the triple path of transformation and evolution which are based on parallel lines of development.

For Sri Aurobindo, evolutionary Nature is not a logical series of separate segments; "there is not actually a series of simple clear-cut and successive stages in the individual's evolution; there is instead a complexity and a partly determinate, partly confused comprehensiveness of the movement."[52]

In the rhythm of progress there are two traditional notions, the linear and the cyclical. Sri Aurobindo rejects the idea of a slow and gradual progression in a straight line and he assumes that evolution is cyclical rather than linear. However, in order to make progress possible he assumes that the result of one cycle may well carry over to the other.

Sri Aurobindo differentiates the cyclic evolution from the circular; in the latter everything is repeated as it is, whereas in the former there is repetition but nothing is exactly the same as it was in the previous order. There is a forward movement in the broad round that gives the impression of a circle, i.e., the spiral has something of the circular as well as the linear movements. Progress and development does not continuously advance in a straight line but in a series of cycles in which periods of progress alternate with periods of decline, but eventually the curve of progress resumes at a higher level. According to Sri Aurobindo; "Progress admittedly does not march on securely in a straight line like a man sure of his familiar way. ... Human progress is very much an adventure through the unknown, an unknown full of surprises and baffling obstacles; it stumbles often, it misses its way at many points."[53]

The series of cycles is the result of a series of zigzags caused by the conflict of forces arriving by a continual struggle at a continual compromise. The periods of decline can be used as fruitful periods in which the previous gains are combined in the new curve of progress. In other words, "the cycles of evolution tend always upward, but they are cycles and do not ascend in a straight line ... but what is essential in the gains of the evolution is kept or, even if eclipsed for a time, re-emerges in new forms suitable to the new ages."[54]

In *A Brief History of Everything,* Ken Wilber questions Samuel Huntington's evolutionary versus circular models of history and he agrees with Sri Aurobindo's sequential pattern of development. According to Ken Wilber, "There are evolutionary waves of development, within which there are cycles, seasons or phases of development. The former refers to transformational development, the latter to translational development. In many cases, the completion of a cycle opens a system (individual or collective) to a transformation, which may be either transcendental and progressive or disintegrative and regressive." [55]

The gradations of planes are a great, connected complex movement; the higher planes precipitate their influences on the lower, and the lower develop in themselves within their own formula something that corresponds to the higher power and its action. But according to Sri Aurobindo, "all this must not be taken in too rigid and mechanical a sense. It is an immense plastic movement full of the play of possibilities and must be seized by a flexible and subtle tact or sense in the seeing consciousness. It cannot be reduced to a too rigorous logical or mathematical formula ... each plane, in spite of its connection with others above and below it, is yet a world in itself, with its own movements, forces, beings, types, forms existing as if for its and their own sake, under its own laws, for its own manifestation without apparent regard for the other members of the great series ... only a limited part of the action of the higher plane is concerned with the earth-existence. But even this creates a mass of possibilities; all these possibilities do not realise themselves."[56]

Sri Aurobindo maintains that in integral Yoga the rigidity of a strict and precise mental rule is seldom applicable, "because no two natures proceed on exactly the same lines, in the same series of steps or with quite identical stages of their progress. It may yet be said that a logical succession of the states of progress would be very much in this order."[57]

Ken Wilber assumes that, "following Aurobindo's lead we can treat gross (frontal), subtle (psychic), and causal (higher and superconscient) development as three broadly distinct lines, which means that, within certain limits, they can each develop quasi-independently. This means that individuals (ontogenetically and phylogenetically) might make strides in psychic/subtle development while still being relatively undeveloped in frontal structures (ego, rationality, conventional verbal, etc.). This further points up why I believe these various streams are not stacked linearly on top of each other like bricks, but rather alongside each other like columns— and further, why progress in some lines might run ahead, or lag behind, others."[58]

Sri Aurobindo would certainly not disagree with Ken Wilber's developmental sequence of lines and stages, as far as it goes. According to Sri Aurobindo, "The various planes of evolution do not always follow each other in quite the same order; for in things psychological the Spirit in the World varies his movements more freely than in things physical. There, besides, he can anticipate the motives of a higher stratum of psychological development while yet he lives the life of a lower stratum; so too when he has got on to a higher level of development he may go strongly back to a past and inferior motive and see how it works out when altered by the motives and powers of the superior medium."[59]

For Ken Wilber, the different developmental lines are not necessarily coherently unified. One's spiritual development, as a separate line, may forge ahead or lag behind one's development in other lines. It is not clear from his writings how the developmental lines relate and are connected to each other. But his developmental sequence of lines and stages seems to overlook the influence of the higher and inner descending spiritual Forces on the surface levels. The higher and psychic as lines may indeed develop quasi-independently, but making strides in psychic development includes the annihilation of the surface frontal ego. For Sri Aurobindo, increased development of the psychic being as a separate line implies an increased annihilation in the other lines (affective, cognitive, ego, etc.). As such, the frontal and the psychic are not developing quasi-independently. Sri Aurobindo is unable to believe in absolute generalisations in the field of development. The development of spiritual consciousness is an exceedingly vast and complex affair in which all sorts of things can happen and for each seeker it differs according to one's nature.

KEN WILBER'S HIGHER VISION-LOGIC AND SRI AUROBINDO'S SPIRITUALISED MIND

Ken Wilber would like a unification of the Finite and the Infinite, without reducing one to the other. This needs an individual psycho-spiritual transformation which can reintegrate the Big Three of person, culture and nature (which were differentiated and separated in modernity). In his earlier works, Ken Wilber maintains that this integration will take place at the vision-logic stage, "the highest integrative structure in the *personal realm.*"[60] Because humanity is not yet prepared to enter the transpersonal stage, "it will take a vision-logic movement of tremendous integrative power (integral-aperspectival as universal-integral) in order to unite world citizens on the *centauric* [the highest of the personal realms] basis that we all share matter *and* bodies *and* minds in common (not to mention a Spirit and a Self prior to *all* that). ... As for the coming transformation itself, it is being built, as all past transformations have been, in the hearts and minds of those *individuals* who themselves evolve to centauric planetary vision. ... The revolution, as always, will come from the within and be embedded in the without."[61]

Ken Wilber emphasises the need for an ascent into the higher vision-logic level, yet at the same time he assumes that the individual has to regress, in the service of the ego, to recontact the lower structure that has been previously dissociated, alienated or distorted, in order to heal the split. Initially, this appears confusing as, for Ken Wilber, "*recontacting the lower* is not at all the same as discovering the higher; and it is *only* in the higher that the true healing and the true integration can occur; it is only in the higher that global consciousness, global conceptions, and global solutions can even be entertained in the first place."[62] However, a primary concentration on ascent may overlook the integrative capacities of the present rational mental-egoic level. Ken Wilber is aware of this and for him the greatest world transformation is the global embrace of intersubjective egoic- rationality on the way to centauric vision-logic. From a healthy rationality, at the final personal level, the vision-logic can emerge. When Ken Wilber assumes that the individual has to regress in order to recontact the lower structures that have been previously dissociated, he most probably refers to some psychopathological defects at the lower levels which need to be healed (recontacted) before an ascent to the higher vision-logic level can take place.

Whenever vision-logic, as a dialectical mode of consciousness begins to integrate and transcend the biosphere and noosphere it is not driven by the individualistic needs of a separate self but includes "the other". The integrated self at this vision-logic level is not the egocentric self but a self integrated in its character of service. It is the higher vision-logic realm which is able to integrate the 'I' 'we' and 'it' domains, "they are all integral expressions and moments of Spirit; none can claim isolated authority; each is honored in its respective task."[63] The individual at the vision-logic level is able to grasp the whole, the multiple contexts within contexts that endlessly disclose the Kosmos. In its cognitive capacity, the vision-logic level "can be applied to any of the four quadrants." Vision-logic can spot massive interrelationships and is itself an intrinsic part of the interrelated Kosmos. Ken Wilber assumes that only when a mature vision-logic becomes a permanent capacity will then higher transpersonal llevels themselves become permanent, and competence in vision-logic is therefore necessary for stable growth into higher levels.

The integrative power of the vision-logic level is needed on a global scale, because this late vision-logic with its centauric worldview is a new structure of consciousness which is lying in our collective future. The centauric vision-logic level opens the way for transpersonal stages, which connect us with the purpose of life on earth. Although Ken Wilber hopes for the development of transpersonal awareness, he does not guarantee that such awareness will happen on this earth.

The integrative potentials of the vision-logic level will have to be actualised first, before the transpersonal awareness can integrate nature, humanity and Spirit. The actualisation of the vision-logic potentials depends upon the concrete actions of the individual, as without these concrete actions "there is the ever-lurking possibility that the whole thing might simply blow up, that evolution will take a wrong turn."[64]

Later on, in *The Eye of Spirit,* Ken Wilber answers the question whether the development of the vision-logic level is a necessary prerequisite for higher or transpersonal development. For him, vision-logic is the gateway through which stable transpersonal stages of spirituality must pass, but one can also have spiritual development without vision-logic when the latter is seen as a quasi-independent line of development. This means that the individual can have various kinds of higher or spiritual development without the prior achievement of the necessary prerequisite of the integrative vision-logic capacities. But a global spirituality, which honours the perspectives of all sentient beings, needs the integrative capacities of vision-logic first, and from there could proceed to postconventional spirituality.

Ken Wilber's vision-logic is the upcoming level of a new cognitive integration that is struggling to emerge. In describing this vision-logic level he also refers to Sri Aurobindo's truth-vision, "which can freely express itself in single ideas, but its most characteristic movement is a mass ideation, a system or totality of truth-seeing at a single view; the relations of idea with idea, of truth with truth, self-seen in the integral whole."[65] But it seems that Ken Wilber confuses Sri Aurobindo's truth-vision of the (transpersonal) spiritual mind with his basic vision-logic level between the personal and transpersonal realm. For Ken Wilber the integrative power of the vision-logic level is able to unify opposites, and see identity-in-difference; although it is the first stage of going beyond rationality, this level is still partially embedded in the personal domain.

The world-view of vision-logic is related to the centauric integral structure, which has the potential of integrating the physiosphere, the biosphere and the noosphere in its own compound individuality. Unfortunately, Ken Wilber leaves out the theosphere on this level; not only mind and body are experiences of an integrated self, the latter includes Spirit.

Sri Aurobindo's spiritual mind is beyond ordinary mentality, above the realm of mental constructions and closer to the individual's spiritual nature. In its cognitive aspects it functions as an instrument of cosmic truth-cognition, which is beyond the conceptual and ratiocinative mind. Through the realisation of this spiritual mind the individual becomes less bound to the automatism of the lower vital nature, mastering it by a greater enlightened thought, sight and will which is in touch with the Infinite.

Like Ken Wilber, Sri Aurobindo affirms that "in becoming more perfect mental beings we get the possibility of a subtler, higher and wider existence, consciousness, force, happiness and delight of being; in proportion as we rise in the scale of mind, a greater power of these things comes to us: our mental consciousness acquires for itself at the same time more vision and power and more subtlety and plasticity, and we are able to embrace more of the vital and physical existence itself. ... The mind liberated from a lower control and preoccupation introduces into life a government, an uplifting, a refinement, a finer balance and harmony; the vital and physical movements are directed and put in order, transformed even as far as they can be by a mental agency; they are taught to be the instruments of reason and obedient to an enlightened will, an ethical perception and an aesthetic intelligence: the more this can be accomplished, the more the race becomes truly human, a race of mental beings."[66]

But for Sri Aurobindo the pure mental being itself is not enough, for we are not merely pure embodied minds, there is a spiritual plane of nature into which we have to heighten our force of consciousness. Our labour of mind cannot come to any solution until we go beyond our inferior nature and learn to utilise our natural instruments by the force of the Spirit. In the words of Sri Aurobindo, "Mind, though it imposes a certain, a considerable mentalised harmony, cannot integrate the whole being and nature. These harmonisations by an inferior control are, besides, inconclusive, because it is one part of the nature which dominates and fulfils itself while the others are coerced and denied their fullness. They can be steps on the way but not final... Mental representations, emotional and dynamic figures have their use and value; Truth, Good and Beauty are in themselves primary and potent figures of the Reality, and even in their forms as seen by the mind, as felt by the heart, as realised in the life can be lines of an ascent: but it is in a spiritual substance and being of them and of itself that That which they represent has to come into our experience."[67]

For Sri Aurobindo, the higher spiritual mind, (confused by Ken Wilber as the cognitive vision-logic level) far beyond one's present mentality, may come close to a mental translation, but it still acts in its nature by division; "it takes the aspects of the Eternal and treats each aspect as if it were the whole truth of the Eternal Being and can find in each its own perfect fulfilment."[68]

Mental spirituality has something one-sided and exclusive as it is marred by its imperfect power of self-expression in life. "The mental being can develop a spiritual interest or preoccupation and may evolve perhaps in consequence a spiritual as well as an intellectual mentality ... but there can be no such thing as a spiritual being taking up and transforming the mental into the spiritual nature. There is no evolution of the spiritual man; there is only an evolution of a new and possibly a finer and rarer element in a mental being. This then is what' has to be brought out,—a clear distinction between the spiritual and the mental."[69] Spirituality is not merely a high activity of the embodied mental being; the emergence of the Spirit should not remain a dominating feature of one's mentality; it also has to define itself as a new power beyond the mental part of our being. Spirituality is something other than mentality, and the truth of Spirit is a truth of being and consciousness rather than a truth of thoughts. A mentalised spirituality can formulate some aspects of the truth, but to know it one has to grow into it and *be* it. There is a spiritual consciousness which is other than mental, and the spiritual being can develop in mind higher states of being, bringing down the Supramental force and transforming the ordinary mental instrumentation. The spiritualised mind can certainly establish a preliminary change in some parts of the being by calling in the spiritual force, but this change is limited as it is not able to bring in a new and higher dynamic principle for the integral transformation of all the lower parts of the being.

Until it disengages itself from the preliminary mental approaches and opens the door to inner realisations by a transmutation of the consciousness, the spiritualised mind cannot create in mental man the spiritual being; for Sri Aurobindo it can exercise an influence on earth-life but not bring about a transformation of that life.

KEN WILBER'S PSYCHIC LEVEL AND SRI AUROBINDO'S PSYCHIC BEING

In order to get a better understanding of the difference between Ken Wilber's psychic level and Sri Aurobindo's psychic being, it may be useful first to explain Ken Wilber's views on the transcendence of the ego and Sri Aurobindo's views on the annihilation of the ego.

Ken Wilber regards the development and strengthening of the ego as a constructive therapeutic goal towards an integrated personality and, for Sri Aurobindo, ego-development is a necessary stage in the evolution of consciousness and the attainment of the true Self. Once a strong ego has been created and here both approaches agree—only then is one able to overcome the sense of a separate ego, as expressed by Ken Wilber: "a strong ego before a transcendence of the ego" and by Sri Aurobindo: "Ego was the helper, Ego is the bar."[70]

Ken Wilber presupposes a more or less "normal" ego development or an integrated and cohesive self-sense as a precondition for ego transcendence. Without such a developed self a clear sequence of pathological consequences may arise. For Ken Wilber, "you have to be somebody before you can be nobody." Although his Wilber-IV model extends this view, and includes the All or everybody in the 'we' quadrants (LL and LR) to form a complete wholeness of Being, he leaves out the sense of individuality without ego- ness, i.e., the psychic being.

In Ken Wilber's first book, *The Spectrum of Consciousness,* he affiliates himself with the insights of Shankara as the expounder of the Advait Vedanta (Level of Mind) and he assumes that "the level of Mind (Ultimate Reality as nondual consciousness) is in some way more real, more basic and more meaningful than the others ... he [the seeker] may now feel that the other levels of consciousness (such as the ego and the existential levels) are completely unreal, illusory and dreamlike."[71] On this level of Mind-consciousness man is identified with the Superconscious All, and this level is the only real state of consciousness, all other levels are essentially illusions. Ken Wilber concludes, "At any rate let us simply note that this Wholeness [Infinite Eternal] according to the perennial psychology is what is real and all that is real."[72]

In his later works, however, he relates egolessness, not to the non-existence of a functional self, but by now the individual is no longer exclusively identified with that self. The ego can exist alongside the soul and the Self and transcending the ego does not mean the annihilation of the ego: it means to transcend but include the ego. The ego is being negated but also preserved as a functional centre of activity in the lower realm. The small ego, as a vehicle of the physical, emotional and mental dimensions of humanness, is used as the necessary instrument through which the inner and higher realm expresses itself. The presence of the ego as a strong personality is no hindrance as long as the individual is also in touch with the inner and higher dimensions of his being. In Ken Wilber's view the soul and the Spirit include body and mind, they are not erased by them, i.e., the ego is not an alienation from Spirit, "but a radiant manifestation of the Divine" and only the exuberance of the attachment of the small ego has to be overcome.

Ken Wilber clearly describes the place of the ego in *One Taste,* where the ego is not annihilated but simply used as a manifestation of Spirit itself, rather than that which obstructs Spirit. All Forms include the form of the ego, and it is only the ego that wants to get rid of the ego. In the words of Ken Wilber, "The ego itself is a perfect manifestation of the Divine, and it is best handled by resting in Freedom, not by trying to get rid of it, which simply increases the effort of ego itself... When you feel the selfcontraction [the ego] you are already free of it—you are looking at it, instead of identifying with it... The Witness is not the self-contraction—it is aware of it. The Witness is free of the self-contraction—and you are the Witness."[73] When he refers to the notion of transcending the ego he writes, "it doesn't mean destroy the ego, it means plug it into something bigger. ... The small ego does not evaporate; it remains as the functional center of activity in the conventional realm. As I said, to lose that ego is to become a psychotic, not a sage. 'Transcending the ego' thus actually means to transcend but include the ego in a deeper and higher embrace, first in the soul or deeper psychic, then with the Witness or primordial Self, then with each previous stage taken up, enfolded, included, and embraced in the radiance of One Taste. And that means we do not 'get rid' of the small ego, but rather, use it as the necessary vehicle through which higher truths are communicated. Soul and Spirit include body, emotions, and mind, they do not erase them."74 The ego as the functional vehicle of the gross realm exists alongside the soul and the Self; the true Self is not the small ego and to the extent that one is stuck in one's small ego a transcendence is required.

For Sri Aurobindo the ego is only a result and a circumstance of our mode of world-existence and not the cause of our world-existence. Sri Aurobindo describes the ego as "not a lasting truth, much less our essential part; it is only a formation of Nature, a mental form of thought-centralisation in the perceiving and discriminating mind, a vital form of the centralisation of feeling and sensation in our parts of life, a form of physical conscious reception centralising substance and function of substance in our bodies. All that we internally are is not ego, but consciousness, soul or spirit. All that we extenally and superficially are and do is not ego but Nature."[75]

The ego, constituted by nature, is meant to aid in centralising and individualising the outer consciousness and action. It serves to separate and sharply differentiate and is indispensable to the evolution of the lower life. In the course of its development, the ego made possible all sorts of things the individual might never have experienced otherwise, such as ambition, vanity, power, possession, etc. It became the means to bind together the individual's experiences and relations in the midst of the complex contacts in which one lives. In the evolution of consciousness, ego is a necessity; as long as the higher consciousness does not descend, ego remains essential even in aspiring and surrendering to the Divine. It is the ego that initiates this surrender and self-offering through personal effort.

Sri Aurobindo meaningfully describes the function of the ego as follows: "Until he has thus developed his individuality, his personality, his separate capacity, he cannot be fit for the greater work before him or successfully turn his faculties to higher, larger and more divine ends ... it is only when he has found himself that he can become spiritually one with all; if he tries to achieve that oneness in the mind, in the vital, in the physical and has not yet a sufficiently strong individuality, he may be overpowered by the mass-consciousness and lose his soul-fulfilment; he has to find himself as the mental and vital ego before he can find himself as the soul or spirit."[76]

Nevertheless, the ego has its limits, it is only an instrument, an image, and at every moment the slave of countless forces and influences in universal Nature. The ego principle has created separate individualities in human beings, but no divine centres of luminous self-awareness. This ego is not one's real self but an instrumentation of nature, and by this instrumentation the individual acts as if one were a separate being having a separate existence in the material universe. The ego is a pragmatic and effective fiction, a subjective substitute for the true self. The dissolution of this limited ego is the necessary means for cosmic Life to arrive at its divine fruition. The disappearance of the ego does not bring with it the destruction of one's true individuality, one's spiritual existence; the separate ego is replaced by the true spiritual Person and the sadhak can become a pure instrument of the Divine.

In Sri Aurobindo's integral Yoga, the ego is only necessary for the development of the lower levels but not for the inner and higher levels. Once the inner and higher levels are sufficiently developed, the ego is replaced by the inner or psychic being and by the higher illumined or intuitive mind. Sri Aurobindo seems to relate the ego to the processes of individuation and attachment, rather than to various regulatory and integrative functions of the self-system, as Ken Wilber does.

In his attempt to integrate Sri Aurobindo's model with his own model, Ken Wilber has had to face some criticism regarding some inaccurate details in his comparative model, which were pointed out to him by this author in *The Quest for the Inner Man,* but later denied by Ken Wilber. In focusing on discriminative wisdom and the engagement in polemic discourse, Ken Wilber at times has the tendency to cynically assault his opponents or critics when responding to their criticism. In *The Eye of Spirit* and *Integral Psychology* he accepts the three systems of Sri Aurobindo's overall model of consciousness; (1) the outer surface consciousness, (2) the inner psychic depth system, and (3) the vertical ascending/ descending system. But he is aware that he is sometimes accused of omitting Sri Aurobindo's concentric inner psychic system, i.e., the inner and the psychic being. He rejects this accusation because the entire last chapter of *The Atman Project* deals with the Tibetan Buddhist concept of the bardo realm, the intermediate stage between death and rebirth. Described in Ken Wilber's own words; "Nonetheless, I [Wilber] can certainly understand why a few Aurobindo followers believed [what] I had, in that *Atman Project* is a simple outline of Wilber II (and does not dwell on too many details, but everywhere clearly implies them), and in other outlines, such as *Transformations*, I do not mention it for space considerations. ... I return to this topic yet again in *Sex, Ecology, Spirituality*, and discuss it at length, (pp. 691-708). Thus, this topic has been addressed in my books over the last sixteen years; hardly a new interest."[77]

These remarks of Ken Wilber seem rather strange to this author and, as described by B. Cortright, it looks like "in Wilber's encyclopedic chronicles of various spiritual traditions and experiences there are very few phenomena that are not noted somewhere in his writings. (This has been a source of frustration for Wilber's critics who, when pointing out gaps in his model, find Wilber replying that he actually does refer to this area at some point in one of his books). However, it is one thing to enumerate the details of various spiritual systems and quite another to adequately account for those details when constructing a theoretical model. The spectrum model does not do this." [78] Could it be that Ken Wilber himself, within the context of the psychic realm, confuses his Tibetan/Aurobindo II model *(Atman Project)* with Wilber-III *(Transformations of Consciousness)* and Wilber- IV *(Sex, Ecology, Spirituality*—the four quadrant model)? It may be worthwhile to go into a more detailed analysis of Ken Wilber's views of the psychic level. If the soul is the psychic/subtle to the low causal level, then let us see how he describes this level in Ken Wilber -II, -III and -IV.

Wilber-II

In *The Atman Project,* Ken Wilber holds open the possibility that there are past life realms, and he devotes the entire last chapter of this book to the Tibetan Buddhist concept of the bardo realm. This Tibetan Buddhist model considers that in the heart centre of every human being there exists the essence of consciousness, which is divided into a 'lifetime indestructible drop' which develops during the individual's life but ceases to be upon biological death, and an 'eternal indestructible drop', which transmigrates from life to life until Buddhahood is reached. Ken Wilber equates this distinction between the frontal consciousness which develops during this lifetime, and the interior essence which transmigrates with Sri Aurobindo's surface system (made up of the physical, vital and mental levels of consciousness) and the deeper concentric system consisting of the inner and psychic being respectively. In Wilber's II model Sri Aurobindo would affirm that, "the highest level of stable evolution reached in any given life permeates the eternal indestructible drop and thus is carried, not usually as specific memories but as a mood of adaptation, to the next life."[79] Ken Wilber has an excuse for not integrating the bardo stages more extensively into *The Atman Project,* because he had literally thousands of pages of notes, summarising the works of several hundred theorists, East and West, and he preferred to present a brief outline rather than publishing all of this material.

The *Bardo Thodol,* or *The Tibetan Book of the Death,* "as an epitomized exposition of the cardinal doctrines of the Mahayana School of Buddhism", symbolically describes the Bardo existence as an intermediate state of forty-nine days between death and rebirth. The aim of the *Bardo Thodol* is to restore to the soul the divinity it lost at birth, i.e., it prepares the soul for a descent into physical being. Life in the Bardo existence brings a descent into a new life which guides the individual nearer to one's final goal, i.e., to the innermost recesses of the human mind, through one's own decisive effort and the spiritual path of liberation.

The soul in Buddhistic belief is an ephemeral illusion, which therefore has no real existence. One of the main teachings of the Mahayana doctrines is the realisation of voidness, which leads to liberation or Buddhahood. The *Bardo Thodol* teaches that the individual should be freed from all the obscurations of karmic or phenomenal illusions in a supramundane (nirvanic) state. Liberation results from the realisation of the unreality of the phenomenal universe, which leads to one's emancipation from it; the Supreme Nirvana is beyond heaven and hell, the end of sorrow, and the Absolute Reality is beyond all existence.

Tibetan tantrism bases its interpretation of the universe on two fundamental dogmas of Buddhism: impermanence and non-ego. The only reality is the undifferentiated Absolute or Nirvana. The Buddhists, unlike Sri Aurobindo, do not distinguish the ego and the real individual self or Soul. The state in which the ego is dissolved is called Nirvana, but for Sri Aurobindo there is a state in which the true individual self, the Jivatman, persists after the annihilation of the ego; the true individual self is as real as the universal Self. "The individual soul is the true spiritual individual which appears in its complete truth when we get rid of the ego and our false separative sense of individuality, realise our oneness with the transcendent and cosmic Divine and with all beings."[80]

For Sri Aurobindo, Nirvana or liberation, although of great value, cannot be Brahman's motive for manifestation. Brahman does not undertake a cosmic process only to return to its native state. The Self and the world are real, they evolve in cooperation with the divine purpose, and rebirth is a ladder of the soul's ascension and a succession of mighty spiritual opportunities. The human soul and the cosmic spirit look into each other's eyes with a noble and divine meaning.

In Buddhism there is no soul that reincarnates, it is karma that incarnates. "The Nihilistic Buddhistic teaching is plain and comprehensible that there is no soul, only a bundle of Sanskaras [fundamental tendencies of old habits and associations] continuing or a stream of them renewing themselves without dissolution (Nirvana). But this Mahayanist affair seems a sort of loose and curt compromise with Vedanta."[81]

Buddhism does not pay proper attention to rebirth and according to Sri Aurobindo, "It views the recurrence of birth as a prolonged mechanical chain; it sees, with a sense of suffering and distaste, the eternal revolving of an immense cosmic wheel of energy with no divine sense in its revolutions, its beginning an affirmation of ignorant desire, its end. a nullifying bliss of escape. The wheel turns uselessly for ever disturbing the peace of Non-being and creating souls whose one difficult chance and whole ideal business is to cease ... the Buddhistic statement admits no self, spirit or eternal Being in its rigorously mechanical economy of existence. It takes only the phenomenon of a constant becoming and elevates that from the physical to the psychical level ... the system of soul rebirth too is a constant prolongation of the principle of the soul-life by a continued creation through Karma ... so the cause of continued soul birth is an ignorant desire or will to be in the universal energy of Karma. ... An extinction of the embodied consciousness is our apparent material end; for soul too the end is extinction, the blank satisfaction of Nothingness or some ineffable bliss of a superconscient Non-Being."[82]

In *Tantra,* Sri Aurobindo finds a meaningful consequence in rebirth: "The Tantric solution shows us a supreme superconscient Energy ... and the soul rises from birth to birth and follows its million forms, till in a last human series it opens to the consciousness and powers of its. own divinity and returns through them by a rapid illumination to the eternal superconscience."[83] But the Tantric tradition more or less ignores the soul's divine possibilities, as if the soul were in a hurry to escape into a superconscient Spirit. Sri Aurobindo gives a wider view of our spiritual potentialities, and points out that "The Tantric system makes liberation the final, but not the only aim; it takes on its way a full perfection and enjoyment of the spiritual power, light and joy in the human existence ... but we add another stress which brings in a completer significance. We regard the spirit in man not as solely an individual being travelling to a transcendent unity with the Divine, but as a universal being capable of oneness with the Divine in all souls and all Nature and we give this extended view its entire practical consequence. The human soul's individual liberation and enjoyment of union with the Divine in spiritual being, consciousness and delight must always be the first object of the Yoga; its free enjoyment of the cosmic unity of the Divine becomes a second object; but out of that a third appears, the effectuation of the meaning of the divine unity with all beings by a sympathy and participation in the spiritual purpose of the Divine in humanity."[84]

When the soul or psychic entity, which is at first an undistinguishable power of the divine Consciousness, develops its individuality in nature, it is called the psychic being. The soul's descent into material birth effects a dynamic union between Spirit and Matter in which Matter functions as a medium of the Spirit's multiple self-expression. The nature that emerges from Matter and develops through life and mind needs to be refined and purified of its ignorance before it can be lifted up to the divine stature. Such preparation cannot be done in a single birth of the individual soul, it needs a series of births in which each birth marks a step forward in working out some of the complex potentialities of the evolving individual. Moreover, rebirth does not come to an end as soon as the mental consciousness of the individual abolishes itself in the spiritual. Sri Aurobindo regards rebirth as an evolutionary necessity and not a mere mechanism of karma from which the soul has to escape into the immutable eternity of its non-existence.

Wilber-III

In *Eye to Eye,* Ken Wilber refers to the psychic as a *higher* level of development than the rational mind. In the higher levels of consciousness, he distinguishes the "high-subtle" (an extraordinary high-order transcendence, differentiation and integration) from the "low-subtle", which includes psychic events and lower forms of mystic-like experiences. "We call it 'psychic' simply as a reminder that even if paranormal events might more easily occur here, they are said to reach *no higher* than this, the lowest of the transcendental realms."[85] In its cognitive structure he calls the psychic 'vision-logic', which he correlates with Maslow's self-actualisation needs. This vision-logic "is thus the beginning of truly higher-order synthesizing capacity, of making connections, relating truths, coordinating ideas, integrating concepts. It culminates in what Sri Aurobindo called 'the higher mind ... in my opinion it is the highest integrative structure in the personal realm; beyond it lie more transpersonal developments."[86]

In *Transformations of Consciousness,* Ken Wilber refers to the psychic as the beginning of the transcendence of the mind's cognitive and perceptual capacities and now the psychic is related to Sri Aurobindo's 'illumined mind' (see Figure 1). He quotes Sri Aurobindo as follows: "As the higher mind [i.e., vision-logic] brings a greater consciousness into the being than the idea and its power of truth, so the illumined mind [psychic level] brings a still greater consciousness through a Truth sight and Truth Light and its seeing and seizing power."[87] Notice that the brackets are added by Ken Wilber himself, and though by now the psychic has been moved from the personal to the transpersonal domain, it seems that he mixes up Sri Aurobindo's higher spiritual level (the Illumined mind) with

Ken Wilber's basic structures of development

1. Sensoriphysical	Pre-personal stages
2. Phantasmic-emotional	
3. Rep-mind	
4. Rule/Role mind	Personal stages
5. Formal-reflexive	
6. Vison-logic	
7. Psychic	Transpersonal stages
8. Subtle	
9. Causal	
10. Ultimate	

Sri Aurobindo's levels of consciousness

Physical subconscient	Conventional stages
Vital-emotional	
Will-mind	
Sense-mind	
Reasoning mind	
Higher mind	Contemplative stages
Illumined mind	
Intuitive mind	
Overmind	
Supermind	

Figure 1

his inner psychic structure. Moreover, it may be questioned whether or not Ken Wilber's *structures* of development can be equated with Sri Aurobindo's *levels* of consciousness. In this comparison of Sri Aurobindo's model with his own model, he has to face some other occasional inaccuracies regarding the actual details of his comparative model.

For Sri Aurobindo the Higher mind is related to the transpersonal or spiritual realm, unlike Ken Wilber's vision-logic, which is a transitional stage between the personal and transpersonal, and thus not "what Aurobindo called the higher mind". For Sri Aurobindo, unlike Ken Wilber, it is the subliminal and not the psychic being that possesses powers of telepathy, clairvoyance and other supernormal faculties. It is the inner subliminal being which achieves an immediate accurate knowledge of the occult energies of the World-Nature that surrounds us; and it is the subliminal which has the power to enter into a direct contact with other beings or with objects, to act without other instrumentation, by a direct mental vision, by a direct feeling of things. According to Sri Aurobindo, "These emergent operations of the subliminal being or some of them are now fragmentally studied under the name of psychic phenomena,—although they have ordinarily nothing to do with the *psyche,* the soul, but only with the inner mind, the inner vital, the subtle-physical parts of our subliminal being. [88]

Wilber-IV

In *Sex, Ecology, Spirituality,* Ken Wilber claims to have some preliminary evidence that suggests four stages of transpersonal development, which he refers to as the psychic, the subtle, the causal, and the ultimate stages.

In the vertical scale of the transpersonal development he does not differentiate the level of depth from the level of height, he uses the two words interchangeably even though he is aware that Huston Smith (like Sri Aurobindo) relates height to Kosmos and depth to individuals. Later on, in *Integral Psychology,* he adjusts his integral approach by admitting Huston Smith's reference to greater levels of reality as higher, and greater levels of the self as deeper. The depth dimension indicates that, for Ken Wilber, the soul is experienced as being within the mind, and yet also far beyond it. In the vertical height dimension the Spirit descends from above into each of us.

The domain of the psychic and the subtle are the domains of the soul, the transpersonal, and though the soul is grounded in God, the personal dimension is not completely negated; it is transcended but included. Though the psychic level involves the beginning transcendence of the ordinary body, mind and culture, "what all of the psychic-level developments have in common is that they have one foot in the gross ordinary personal realm and one foot in the transpersonal realm."[89] When the self no longer identifies itself exclusively with the individual personality then the soul-force is able to flow through one's personality.

According to Ken Wilber, "the Soul is tied to no individual, no culture, no tradition, but rises fresh in every person, beyond every person,"[90] but for Sri Aurobindo the psychic being is a spark of the Divine within and tied to the individual person. The difference between the Self or Atman and the psychic being or *Chaitya Purusha* is that one is felt like universal and the other as individual, and one-psychic being can be in sympathy with the other but cannot unite. According to Sri Aurobindo, "The psychic being cannot take up more than one body; there is only one psychic being for each human being."[91] Nevertheless, though the psychic being is related to the depth dimension of the inner reality of the individual, it also opens and unites the individual with the cosmic existence, but due to the ego's actions it appears to be deprived of its universality.

When Ken Wilber mentions the commonality of the soul in all beings, he refers to Emmerson's 'Over-

Soul', which is the same in all individuals. Individuality does not disappear in the Over-Soul or World-Soul but is preserved in a deeper and wider ground. In this Over-Soul the individual experiences a conscious union with all of manifestation itself, not just with all humans, but with all nature, and with all the physical cosmos, with all beings, great and small."[92] In the Over-Soul, there is a oneness with the physiosphere, biosphere and noosphere; it includes all of nature but also culture and morality. However, for Sri Aurobindo the psychic is an expression of the Divine, while Ken Wilber leaves out this primary oneness with the Divine, and it seems therefore that the Over-Soul becomes more a psychological soul than a divine Soul. Moreover, Sri Aurobindo describes the Oversoul not in terms of the psychic being but as the highest superconscient Self, "a supreme highest Reality sustaining and exceeding them all, which humanity speaks of vaguely as Spirit, God, the Oversoul... with the extension of our knowledge we discover what this Spirit or Oversoul is: it is ultimately our own highest deepest vastest Self, it is apparent on its summits or by reflection in ourselves as Sachchidananda creating us and the world by the power of His divine Knowledge-Will, spiritual, supramental, truthconscious, infinite. That is the real Being, who, as the Cosmic Self has descended into that which we call the Inconscient and has ascended out of the Inconscient."[93]

When describing the ethics in the Over-Soul, Ken Wilber gives a quotation of Schopenhauer in which he attempts to compare the experience of the psychic soul with human love, "the sort of act that I am here discussing is ... compassion, which is to say, immediate participation released from all other considerations ... which alone is the true ground of all autonomous righteousness and of all true human love."[94] But Sri Aurobindo relates psychic love to divine love; such love is not dependent upon external satisfactions, not moved by disappointments, strife or anger, but is pressing always straight towards the inner union. The 'outer parts' of the being are used as a means of expression and share in the whole meaning of love, provided they have the right and not the wrong movement, i.e., as long as they are used in the right spirit and for the true purpose. According to Sri Aurobindo, "The psychic love is pure and full of self-giving without egoistic demands, but it is not usually left pure in the attraction of human beings to one another."[95] For Sri Aurobindo conscience is a mental and moral construction of the mind, but to reach the psychic being the sadhak has to go deep within oneself, beyond the mind and its ideas. "It is this secret psychic entity which is the true original Conscience in us deeper than the constructed and conventional conscience of the moralist, for it is this which points always towards Truth and Right and Beauty, towards Love and Harmony and all that is a divine possibility in us.[96] It is the psychic being as soul personality whose soul's perception of good and evil may not coincide with the mind's artificial standards, because it has a deeper sense of what points to the higher Truth and what points away from it. In the words of Sri Aurobindo, "This voice of the soul is not what we call conscience—for that is only a mental and often conventional erring substitute ... it is better to wander at the call of one's soul than to go apparently straight with the reason and the outward moral mentor."[97] It is not the mental ethical sense which must accept or reject. Sri Aurobindo insists on the subjection to the psychic being, which, is the Divine Guide in integral Yoga.

In a full-spectrum approach to human growth, Ken Wilber compares Sri Aurobindo's developmental holarchy with Plotinus' stages of development. The following figure shows Ken Wilber's comparison between the hierarchies of Plotinus and Sri Aurobindo.

PLOTINUS	SRI AUROBINDO
Absolute One (Godhead)	Sachchidananda/ Supermind (God head)
Nous (Intuitive Mind) [subtle]	Intuitive Mind/Overmind
Soul/ World-soul [psychic]	Illumined World-Mind
Creative Reason [vision-logic]	Higher-mind /Network-mind
Logical Faculty [formop]	Logical mind
Concepts and Opinions	Concrete mind (canop)
Images	Lower mind (preop)
Pleasure/ pain (emotions)	Vital-emotional; impulse
Perception	Perception
Sensation	Sensation
Vegetative life function	Vegetative
Matter	Matter (physical)

Figure 2

It seems Ken Wilber equates Sachchidanada and Supermind, but for Sri Aurobindo the Supermind allows the multiplicity of creation and diversity as its premise, whereas Sachchidananda is Unitarian, invisible and as such it does not partake in the play of creation.

Ken Wilber adds the concept of 'concentric spheres' to his linear representation; he compares the concentric spheres with "a spiral staircase with all sorts of ups and downs, but an overall unmistakable direction; transcend and embrace."[98] But Plotinus' psychic, as a developmental process of inferiority (inwardness), is not like Sri Aurobindo's psychic being which is a representative of Jivatman. The personal is indeed transcended but not included; on the contrary, when the ego is annihilated there are no traces left of the empirical ego (desire-soul) and the latter is replaced by the psychic being which is an expression of the Divine. As long as the desire-soul is not annihilated and replaced by the true psychic being, it will remain difficult for the Divine Force to flow through that personality.

Besides, in this comparison, Ken Wilber again omits Sri Aurobindo's depth system and equates Plotinus' Soul/ Worldsoul [psychic] with Sri Aurobindo's higher Illumined World- Mind but, as mentioned before, Sri Aurobindo's concentric sphere is made up of the inner individual being, and it seems that Ken Wilber again confuses the latter with Sri Aurobindo's higher Illumined Mind, in which there is an opening of the limited personal being into the Cosmic Existence.

In one of the notes in *Sex, Ecology, Spirituality,* Ken Wilber does refer once more to Tibetan, tantric Buddhism, which divides the overall Buddhist teachings into nine levels. The last three levels are centred on the higher and inner states of consciousness. Tantric Buddhism divides consciousness into the gross, the subtle and the causal [very subtle] dimensions, and it is this causal nondual consciousness which the tantric Buddhists associate with the 'eternal indestructibly drop which partakes of the psychic subtle level' in the heart. In the words of Ken Wilber, "This, as we will see, is also quite similar to Aurobindo's distinction between the frontal consciousness, which develops in this lifetime, and the deeper psychic being, which transmigrates" (The Eye of Spirit, p 180.) "The Tibetans discribe this psychic being as the interior indestructible drop which partakes of the psychic/subtle level itself, and which Ken Wilber refers to as 'an essence that carries Karma from birth to birth" This interior drop is in Ken Wilber's terminology, the psychic subtle being, which he also deliberately refers to as "soul" since that too lasts until actual spiritual resurrection in the causal/non-dual Divine Domain of pure Emptiness. (The Eye of Spirit.p.207)

How this is all related to Sri Aurobindo's experience of the psychic being in the context of a divine life remains an open question. It is one thing to compare the evolving *bardo* realm with the psychic being, but it is quite another thing to place this comparison in the proper context of the developmental model of the Tibetan tantric Buddhist philosophy and Sri Aurobindo's integral Yoga philosophy. In other words, how far can the Tibetan Buddhist bardo *realm* be applied to the realisation of the psychic *being* in Sri Aurobindo's model?

To bring matters to a head, it must be clear that Ken Wilber's psychic level as a stage of transpersonal development and as the domain of the soul is not the same as Sri Aurobindo's inner psychic being. For Ken Wilber the psychic level, on the border between the gross and the subtle states, is the realm of initial transpersonal or mystical awareness, but these mystical experiences of the psychic level are still related to the gross/waking realm.

In *One Taste,* the soul is no longer only a basic level or wave of development, but the soul is also described in terms of a developmental line. Ken Wilber creates a general scheme of the three major lines of the self: the ego, the soul and the Self. The soul is now equated with deeper psychic development, a developmental line navigating in the psychic and subtle realms, but which cannot reach the causal realm. "The soul can see from afar, but never actually enter, the Promised Land."99 The soul, as a psychic/subtle self, unfolds its own holarchical stream and integrates consciousness in the subtle domain. The Self as Witness, beyond the soul, integrates consciousness in the causal domain, and it is this Self which is responsible for the overall integration of all other selves, waves, and streams. According to Ken Wilber, "the soul (for Aurobindo and myself) is not to be confused with pure Atman. The ego is that which evolves in this lifetime; the soul is that which evolves between lifetimes (or, if you prefer, evolves to the superconscient in this lifetime ... but the pure Atman does not evolve or involve at all. The *evolving soul* is superseded by the *Unborn Spirit* (pure Atman—Brahman). Technically, in my model, the soul is the psychic/subtle to low-causal, and thus, being of manifestation, it evolves; the pure Atman is high causal, and being unmanifest, does not evolve."[100]

But it seems that Ken Wilber confuses Sri Aurobindo's concept of the soul as *essence* or *entity* with the soul that evolves between lifetimes (Sri Aurobindo's psychic being). The soul as essence, like Jivatman, does not evolve and as such is not a stage, level or line of development between lifetimes; the soul is a spark of the Divine within man, and essentially one with the Divine. For Sri Aurobindo, Jivatman is "the Unborn who presides over the individual being and its developments, associated with it but above it and them and who by the very nature of his existence knows himself as universal and transcendent no less than individual and feels the Divine to be his origin, the truth of his being, the master of his nature, the very stuff of his existence."[101] The realisation of the Jivatman is the realisation of the Divine Individual, but the individual is a spiritual centre of action for the One, and feels no separation from all that is One, i.e., there is no separateness in this self-vision.

As Ken Wilber rightly assumes, this Jivatman in its essence does not change or evolve, its essence stands above the personal evolution. However, the soul or psychic as a representative of Jivatman, contains all the possibilities of the Divine within it and is in that sense immutable, but since it has to manifest itself it assumes the form of a psychic individual which is taking part in the evolution. The psychic entity, unlike the universalised Jivatman, is the individual soul supporting the mental, vital, physical and psychic evolution of the being in Nature. Sri Aurobindo points out that "the word 'psychic' is indeed used in English to indicate anything that is other or deeper than the external mind, life and body, anything occult or supraphysical, but that is a use which brings confusion and error and we entirely discard it when we speak or write about yoga."[102]

For Sri Aurobindo, "the Jivatma, spark-soul [soul-essence] and psychic being must not be mixed up together, as that confuses the clearness of the inner experience. The Jivatma is self-existent above the manifested or instrumental being, it is the individual Self or Atman; the eternal true being of the individual. The soul is a spark of the Divine in the heart of the living creatures of Nature. It is not seated above the manifested being; it enters into the manifestation of the self, consents to be a part of its natural phenomenal becoming, supports its evolution in the world of material Nature. It carries with it at first an undifferentiated power of the divine consciousness containing all possibilities which have not yet taken form but to which it is the function of evolution to give form. This spark of Divinity is there in all terrestrial living beings from the earth's highest to its lowest creatures."[103]

For Sri Aurobindo the Jivatman and the soul are both in different ways portions of the Divine, two aspects of the same entity, but the Jivatman is unevolving above Nature, whereas the soul evolves a psychic being in Nature.

He distinguishes the soul in its essence and the psychic being. "The soul is there before the development of an organised vital and mind. The soul is something of the Divine that descends into the evolution as a divine Principle within it to support the evolution of the individual out of the Ignorance into the Light. It develops in the course of the evolution a psychic individual or soul individuality which grows from life to life, using the evolving mind, vital and body as its instruments."[104]

The soul or psychic entity is a spark of the Divine present in all living beings, whereas the psychic being is formed by the soul only in the course of its evolution. This means that there is a soul, a spark of the Divine, in each and every being, also in those individuals who have not evolved a psychic being, i.e., "the psychic being is a spiritual personality put forward by the soul in its evolution."[105] In other words, the psychic has two aspects; the psychic essence, the soul behind or inmost entity which is fundamentally *the same always*, and in front the form of individuality it takes in its evolution in Nature, i.e., the inmost entity puts forward a psychic personality which *changes* and *develops* from life to life.

The soul supports the nature in its evolution through matter, life, mind, and Supermind, but the soul itself is not any of these things and is always pure. The soul, though an ever-pure flame of the divinity in things, is mostly veiled in its inner sanctum, and in order to reveal itself it needs the ignorant outer instrumentation of the mind, life force and physical consciousness. Nevertheless, this veiled psychic entity is always alight within any person, and this portion of the Divine is *permanent* from life to life, taking the experience of life through its outer instruments. It is a flame born out of the Divine, it is that which endures and is imperishable in us. This soul or psychic entity is not limited by what it manifests, nor tarnished by the imperfections and impurities of the surface being. It is aware of truth, good and beauty, but also of all that contradicts these things, falsehood- and evil, although it does not become these opposites of itself. It is the soul acting through the psychic being that influences mind and heart and vital, and turns their ideas, feelings, dynamisms in the direction of what is divine and luminous. When the psychic being grows stronger, it increases its communion with the psychic entity behind it and improves its communication with the surface being. By now the soul can transmit its intimations to the psychic being with a greater purity and force. But this natural evolution if left solely to the difficult automatic actions of the evolutionary Energy, will be slow and long; it is through some kind of yoga or sadhana—an awakening of the soul within—that a quicker conscious method of evolution intervenes.

When the psychic being becomes dominant through

the practice of sadhana and freely uses its instruments, then the transformation of mind, vital and body becomes possible and not merely their liberation. According to Sri Aurobindo, "the power of the psychic, however, can act upon the mind and vital and body, purifying thought and perception and emotion (which then becomes psychic feeling) and sensation and action and everything else in us and preparing them to be divine movements."[106] It is this purifying action which is one of the main contributions of the psychic being to the sadhana. The psychic development prepares the lower nature to receive the higher spiritual consciousness with a complete receptivity and right attitude. To explore spiritual experiences before purification often creates a dangerous situation, and it is for this reason that Sri Aurobindo advises the sadhak not to plunge into spiritual experiences in sadhana without a fairly long period of preparation and purification. When the psychic being is in front the sadhak gets the right guidance from within, which makes the descent of the higher consciousness safer and easier. It is the psychic being which is able to awake the spiritual force which must stamp itself upon heart, mind and life, and give them their upward orientation, purify and uplift their motions and suffuse them with a higher consciousness.

Ken Wilber places the soul in the psychic/subtle to low-causal realm where it evolves. Such a view explicates the essential difference between Ken Wilber's evolving soul in the psychic/subtle to low-causal realm and Sri Aurobindo's soul which evolves a psychic being in Nature. For Sri Aurobindo the psychic being is not a state of consciousness or a realm of transpersonal awareness, but a conscious form of the soul growing in the evolution. The psychic being and consciousness are therefore not identical, but when there is the full consciousness of the Jivatman and the psychic being they may join together.

Ken Wilber also omits the development and realisation of the transformative function of the psychic being, whereas for Sri Aurobindo the awakening, of the psychic being is indispensable for his integral Yoga. A supramental change can take place only if the psychic being has been awakened and made the leader of the physical, vital and mental being and the chief support of the descending supramental power.

KARMA AND REBIRTH

Ken Wilber does not fully integrate the supportive metaphysical context of rebirth, reincarnation and karmic principles in the process of spiritual development. For Sri Aurobindo faith in karma and rebirth are essential for metaphysical premises in one's present-day life. This creates a more adequate insight into the real nature of man and his world in relation to one's essential being and one's destiny. It seems that Ken Wilber focuses mainly on the psycho-spiritual development of the self within one single life and, although he is aware of the deeper psychic awareness that the individual brings to this life [reincarnation], he hardly elaborates on the spiritual development of the inmost Self that occurs over numerous lives.

Sri Aurobindo assigns an important place to the notion of rebirth in his scheme of evolution and ascent. Rebirth has never been proved or disproved by the methods of modem science, and its existence must be established by psychological rather than physical evidence. The body is not the whole of our being and the physical is not the whole secret of the world and existence. Life on earth is not the sole reality and its vicissitudes do not exhaust man s entire duration.

Birth is a vehicle through which the process of evolution can be moved ahead. Since the soul has not completed its task by merely developing into humanity, it needs to develop that humanity beyond the human level. The *individual*I is a medium through which creation discloses itself, and this individual must be re-born till the spiritual goal is attamed. The spiritual possibilities may not be exhausted in one bulb.

In the words of Sri Aurobindo, "if there is an evolution of consciousness in an evolutionary body and a soul inhabiting the body, a real and conscious individual, then it is evident that it is the progressive experience of that soul in Nature which takes the form of this evolution of consciousness: rebirth is self-evidently a necessary part, the sole possible machinery of such an evolution. It is as necessary as birth itself; for without it birth would be an initial step without a sequel, the starting of a journey without its farther steps and arrival. It is rebirth that gives to the birth of an incomplete being in a body its promise of completeness and its spiritual significance."[107]

Through rebirth each soul assimilates various growing experiences, which it holds together in an evolving intermediate psychological form of itself, between its pure spiritual essence and its expression in life. The true foundation of the theory of rebirth is the evolution of the soul or rather its gradual self-finding and its flowering out of the veil of Matter. According to Sri Aurobindo, "A past terrestrial soul evolution sufficiently accounting for these variations and degrees of our mixed being and a future soul evolution that helps us progressively to liberate the godhead of the Spirit, seem the only just and reasonable explanation of this labour of a matter-shackled soul which has attained a variable degree of humanity in the midst of a general progressive appearance of life, mind and spirit in a material universe. Rebirth is the only possible machinery for such a soul evolution."[108]

Rebirth as a means of spiritual evolution opens to us divine perspectives of a growing soul, and makes life a. significant ascension and not a mechanical recurrence. The circle of mechanical recurrence fails to explain God, man and existence to us with a sufficient wholeness, and misses the divine utility of the cosmic workings. Through constant rebirth we have developed into what we are; the past terms are contained in the present middle human term of the ascension but, once fulfilled, we exceed them. The present terms are not an unprofitable recurrence but an expanding series of powers of the Infinite, which are yet to be unfolded by the Spirit.

In future terms there are the greater potentialities and intended mightier manifestations.

The traditional view on rebirth emphasises an excessive individualism without the universality which is part of the light of spiritual perfection. For Sri Aurobindo the idea of universality - oneness with God and with all humanity - has to be taken more largely into account in any future idea of the significance of karma and rebirth.

Rebirth and Karma are the soul-side and the nature-side of one and the same cosmic sequence. For Sri Aurobindo, "Rebirth is meaningless without Karma, and Karma has no fount of inevitable origin and no rational and no moral justification if it is not an instrumentality for the sequences of the soul's continuous experience.... And on the other side of Karma, if we give to that its integral and not a truncated meaning, we must admit rebirth for the sufficient field of its action.'[109]

An account of the process of rebirth is therefore incomplete if it does not refer to the law of karma, which is usually conceived as a metaphysical and moral law. Sri Aurobindo accepts the importance of karma in both the metaphysical as well as the moral context, though he explains the limitations of the moral law in detail. It is impossible for the moral law to be the sole determinant of the working of the cosmos unless the whole process is comprehended as absolutely mechanical. The individual's true Self must be greater than its karma. According to Sri Aurobindo, "a law or chain of Karma is only an outward machinery and cannot be elevated to a greater position as the sole and absolute determinant of the life-workings of the cosmos. ... But all is not Law and Process, there is also Being and Consciousness; there is not only a machinery but a Spirit in things... if the fundamental truth of our being is spiritual and not mechanical, it must be ourself, our soul that fundamentally determines its own evolution, and the law of Karma can only be one of the processes it uses for that purpose: our Spirit, our Self must be greater than its Karma. There is a Law, but there is also spiritual freedom. ... It is not conceivable that the Spirit within is an automaton in the hands of Karma, a slave in this life of its past actions. If a certain amount of result of past Karma is formulated in the present life, it must be with the consent of the psychic being which presides over the new formation of its earth-experience and assents to a secret Will and Guidance. That secret Will is not mechanical, but spiritual. ... There must therefore be two elements, Karma as an instrument, but also the secret Consciousness and Will within working through the mind, life and body as the user."[110] As an all-pervading mental and moral law, karma supports the dictum that what 'I sow I shall assuredly reap', but this mechanical rebound is not the whole principle of karma. Such a view may satisfy the intellect, as it would resolve everything in the predestination of karma, i.e., all personal acts are chains of determination over which the individual has no control. The law of karma is not simply an extension of the human idea of practical justice into future births.

For Sri Aurobindo the whole law of cosmic action is not the measure of physical, mechanical and chemical energy, not the law of a life force or a moral one, these are all means to other laws in the Infinite. These means, however, have to be taken into account, but they are transitional and cannot be the whole law of karma. The moral approach of karma overlooks the complexity of the world and human nature. There is a more authentic and spiritual truth at the base of Nature's action, and a less mechanically, calculable movement, and according to Sri Aurobindo, "No rule imposed on him from outside, whether in the name of a supposed mechanical or impersonal law or of God or prophet, can be, as such, true or right or binding on man: it becomes that only when it answers to some demand or aids some evolution of his inner being. And when that inner being is revealed ... then we get the true, the inner and intuitive Law in its light of self-knowledge, its beauty of self-fulfilment, its intimate life significance."[111] The higher law of karma is for man a law of one's spiritual soul-evolution. The soul accepts difficulties and sufferings not as a punishment for its wrong doings, but as an opportunity for growth. The law of karma has its origin and greatness in the free spirit and ultimately when the seeker arrives there, he or she is able to exalt his or her state beyond all bondage of Karma to spiritual freedom.

Sri Aurobindo does not want to call Karma a Law, "but rather the many-sided dynamic truth of all action and life, the organic movement here of the Infinite.... Action of Karma follows and takes up many waves and streams of combining and disputing world-forces; it is the processus of the creative Infinite; it is the long and multiform way of the progression of the individual and the cosmic soul in Nature. Its complexities cannot be unravelled by our physical mind ever bound up in the superficial appearance, nor by our vital mind of desire. ... Nor can it be perfectly classified, accounted for by the precisions of our logical intelligence. ... The supramental eye can see a hundred meeting and diverging motions in one glance and envelop in the largeness of its harmonising vision of Truth all that to our minds is clash and opposition and the collision and interlocked strife of numberless contending truths and powers."[112]

He further observes, "The self-effectuation of the Spirit in the world is the truth on which we take our foundation, a great, a long self-weaving in time. Rebirth is the continuity of that self-effectuation in the individual, the persistence of the thread; Karma is the process, a force, a work of energy and consequence in the material world, an inner and an outer will, an action of mental, moral, dynamic consequence in the soul evolution of which the material world is a constant scene. That is the conception; the rest is a question of the general and particular laws, the way in which Karma works out and helps the purpose of the Spirit in birth and life. And whatever those laws and ways may be, they must be subservient to this spiritual self-effectuation. The law is a means a line of working for the Spirit, and does not exist for its own sake or for the service of any abstract idea.'[113]

Ken Wilber does not leave out the possibility of past life realms, the Tibetan Buddhist concept of the bardo realm, but this is not the same as having unconditional faith in the principle of Karma and Rebirth. Traditional contemplative systems maintain that the ego develops during this life, whereas the soul develops between lives. But in one of his later publications, *One Taste,* he writes that "it is not necessary to believe in either prenatal memory or past lives in order to acknowledge the deeper psychic self, which is *primarily* defined by its access to higher consciousness, not by its access to past lives."[114]

For Sri Aurobindo the evolutionary aim of reincarnation is not so much related to Ken Wilber's transcendence of the cycle of Karma and Rebirth, but to the transformation and perfection of life on earth. Every rebirth represents an advance of evolution towards a divine life on earth and a unique expression of the Divine.

A CRITICAL ESTIMATE OF KEN WILBER

Ken Wilber, as a leading philosopher and theoretical psychologist of the transpersonal movement, tries to give us insight into the fundamental questions about the deepest aspects of human nature, and as such his philosophical and psychological principles are of great value for any transpersonal psychologist/psychotherapist and enlivens and furthers the development of the transpersonal movement. Ken Wilber borrows extensively from Eastern thought and seems particularly indebted to Sri Aurobindo. His contributions, insights and achievements for the transpersonal movement have been appreciated all over the world. The scholarly adequacy of his discussion of the many texts, authors and fields he mentions and integrates within his work, however, may be questioned at times.

Representing the developmental phases of the transpersonal movement from its beginning, Ken Wilber attempts to establish a relationship between Western psychology and psychotherapy and the traditional contemplative psychologies. He claims to have produced an integrative model of both psychologies and to have identified, with some precision, the pros and cons of both modes of psychology.

For Ken Wilber, all evolution (matter, life, mind) aims at the self-realisation of Spirit, and his concept of individual development is based on a stage model. The four lower stages are similar to Piaget's cognitive development, up to the rational level, but Ken Wilber adds five higher integrative transpersonal levels: vision-logic (as a transitionary stage between the personal and transpersonal), psychic, subtle, causal, and nondual levels. In his earlier works he emphasised transcendence and the ascending path (evolution), but later on he attempted to integrate the ascending and descending paths (involution). In a similar way he emphasised in his earlier works the inner dimensions of psychological and spiritual transformation, but in his later works he used the four quadrant model, in which he assumed the interrelatedness of the inner and outer reality (individual, nature, culture and social system) in spiritual transformation. Ken Wilber's integral system may appear marginalizing but he does not try "to cram all differences into monological uniformitarianism. ... Rather, my 'big picture' is simply an explicit offer to take a larger view of things ... it is open-ended; it is not a 'foregone conclusion' nor a conceptual straightjacket."[115]

Ken Wilber's theory is just one of the many integral theories. His integral practice involves all the major levels and dimensions of the four quadrant model—the individual objective and subjective, the social interobjective and the cultural intersubjective. Though he mentions Sri Aurobindo's integral Yoga as a way to talk about integral practice, he nowhere mentions any of Sri Aurobindo's spiritual methods —aspiration for and faith in the Divine, self-opening, surrender and the paths of karma and bhakti —in each category.

His integral practice is an attempt to integrate Western 'depth-psychology' with the 'height psychology' of the great wisdom traditions, i.e., the integration of id and Spirit, or libido and Brahman. He wants the seeker to engage all the levels of one's own potentials, which helps the individual to discover one's deepest Self, the Ground and goal of the levels Such integral practice involves physical exercise with a nutritional programme, engagement in psychotherapy combined with meditative practice and engagement in community service. According to Ken Wilber, "practicing on only one level of your being will not enlighten all of you. If you *just* meditate, your psychodynamic "junk" will not automatically go away. If you *just* meditate, your job or your relationship with your spouse will not automatically get better. On the other hand, if you *only* do psychotherapy do not think that you will be relieved from the burden of death and terror. Render unto Freud what is Freud's, and render unto Buddha what is Buddha's. And best of all, render unto the Divine all of yourself, by engaging all that you are."[116]

For Ken Wilber, "the relation of spirituality to science in general and psychotherapy in particular, is the pressing issue for spirituality in the modern world, and most religions are not, it seems, handling them very well."[117]

Spiritual practice and psychological practice are different streams, and there are issues that either the spiritual practice or the psychological practice do not address; in the manifest world Freud and Buddha can help each other by a mutual fruitful dialogue. In Ken Wilber's words, "the West has contributed a thing or two to psychological and psychotherapeutic understanding, and these contributions are altogether beneficial and helpful, and they don't have many parallels in any of the ancient teachings."[118]

Ken Wilber, in trying to give psychology a philosophical and spiritual foundation creates a fascinating overview of the most divergent therapeutic approaches and spiritual wisdom. Human development becomes more comprehensible in his system, but it could be that this will never completely conform to such definition, as human beings are much less orderly than in Ken Wilber's system. Moreover, it is not always clear if his theoretical model is able to account for individual differences.

Ken Wilber's synthesis blends ideas drawn from developmental models offered by a variety of significant Eastern and Western schools, but is it possible to read a common underlying system into all these different explorations? His spiritual developmental model can function as a stepping stone, but to reach the Divine the seeker may have to abandon the model. According to S.K. Saksena, "each single philosophy of a particular culture has its own soul. It has an individual genius which creates, as well as reacts to, a problem in its own special way. We cannot afford to ignore this factor of individuality in a system of thought without effacing the special features of that philosophy. It is necessary, therefore, to try to discover—as a preliminary step for a perhaps later stage of synthesis—the distinctive and unique traits of each system of thought representative of a culture before an attempt is made towards a rapprochement of them."[119]

In his attempt to amalgamate various systems of thought, Ken Wilber uses terms from many schools of Eastern thought, such as Vedanta, Sufism, Kabbalah, Tibetan Buddhism, Yoga and Sri Aurobindo, and he borrows extensively from these thoughts. He is creative in the exploration of new terms, and his new terminology is initially difficult to grasp, though later on it facilitates the discussion. However, Ken Wilber gets into difficulty when he applies his new terminology to his comparative models. Without a more accurate representation of these systems—especially for his study on the formulation of Sri Aurobindo's model—his comparison, without fully explicating the context of integral Yoga, becomes too simplistic and does not always contribute to clearer formulations of his own model. In analysing the commonalties between overtly different Eastern and Western spiritual traditions and in comparing views from other cultures, Ken Wilber should not lose the context in which they originate, or use only parts of these views which suit his own ideas. For example, Ken Wilber accepts those passages of Sri Aurobindo's *The Life Divine* and *The Synthesis of Yoga* which support his own ideas, but in doing so he sometimes partially distorts the meaning of these passages so that he can harmonise them with his own views. A closer analysis of Ken Wilber's writings reveals that he sees Sri Aurobindo's concepts in the context of his own thoughts. When he compares and joins various elements of Sri Aurobindo's vision with his own model, Ken Wilber sometimes dissociates them from their overall perspective, so that these elements lose much of their significance and sometimes even assume a different meaning. When scarcely quoting relevant passages of Sri Aurobindo it is important to know that these passages are written in different contexts in different works and in certain places they present divergent views. Neglecting his complete view may create more problems, rather than contributing to a clear and synthetic idea of Sri Aurobindo's metaphysical vision.

It is useful to compare various aspects of Sri Aurobindo's vision with his own model and to explain that Sri Aurobindo means the same thing. This can be a fruitful attempt to provide a basis of understanding for those who are not familiar with Sri Aurobindo's thought. But are the similarities, when applied to life, used in the same way as in Sri Aurobindo's sadhana? Maybe Ken Wilber would understand Sri Aurobindo's vision better if he examined it more as a lived experience of sadhana.

Ken Wilber claims that his model is evidence-driven and not theory-driven. He does not merely describe what he theoretically thinks, but he formulates what he contemplatively sees on the vision-logic level. The methodology of an integral theory of consciousness includes "the simultaneous tracking of the various levels and lines in each of the four quadrants, and then noting their correlations, each to all the others, and the interior transformation of the researchers themselves."[120] Ken Wilber's model, though not based on philosophical assumptions, often depends on substantial amounts of the empirical, phenomenological, clinical and contemplative evidence of other researchers, which he scholarly combines with his own evidence on the integrative vision-logic level —the intersection between the personal and the transpersonal.

Sri Aurobindo's metaphysical works are representations of his consciousness and are conscious attempts to explain his experiences. Purely mental analysis and interpretation, even on a higher integrative vision-logic level, is not enough to understand Sri Aurobindo's writings. Only through a meditative reading of his works—

which creates an experience of the love for the Divine—is the reader able to understand Sri Aurobindo more deeply. As a theoretician, scholarship is very important, but it is not sufficient. Sri Aurobindo's metaphysical, universal and psychological views need not only an appropriate approach within the context of his vision; they simultaneously need the Divine Grace or the Guidance from within.

Sri Aurobindo does not mind when people find inconsistencies in his statements, often the same people have an inability to see more than their own personal view or experience of things and he adds that, "People do not understand what I write because the mind by itself cannot understand things that are beyond it. It constructs its own idea out of something that it catches or that it has caught and puts that idea as the whole meaning of what has been written. Each mind puts its own ideas in place of the Truth."[121]

It is interesting to note how Ken Wilber attempts to elaborate on some limitations he observes in Sri Aurobindo's vision, but unfortunately he does not always get the whole meaning of that which he sympathetically criticises. By omitting the essential significance and dynamic efforts of Sri Aurobindo's spiritual vision on life, Ken Wilber is sometimes led astray by the confusion of details and as a consequence he seems to miss the true significance of the matter.

Intellectual analysis on the vision logic-level may lead to a right arrangement of true concepts, but this is not the knowledge aimed at in integral Yoga. A greater intellectual illumination becomes effective only when the purified understanding is followed by the complete realisation of three successive movements: internal vision, complete internal experience and identity. Could it be that the difference between Ken Wilber, an intellectual thinker who mysticises, and Sri Aurobindo, an integral Yogi who philosophises, lies in the fact that Sri Aurobindo starts from his realisations which he tries to express in the inadequate language of the mind, whereas Ken Wilber starts from his mental abstractions of his vision-logic realisations and tries to reach the essential truths in flashes of mystical vision? There is no doubt that Ken Wilber's direct spiritual realisation of One Taste, as the ever-present nondual Divine Consciousness or the sense of oneness with the Ground of all creation and the simple Feeling of Being, created an entirely new motivation within the depth of his being. That constant consciousness or unbroken witnessing through all states—waking, dreaming and deep sleep—sometimes lasting for two or three days, occurred to Ken Wilber after many years of meditative practice. But are Ken Wilber's intuitions on the vision-logic level shadowy reflections which fall short of the flooding of the rays from the Centre of Light? Could it be that Ken Wilber's intellectual, theoretical and practical investigations on the integrative vision-logic level, when compared with Sri Aurobindo's intuitive vision on the Supramental level, need to be supplemented by the lived experience of more sadhana?

NOTES

1. Ken Wilber, *Up from Eden*, p.320.
2. Ibid., p.253.
3. Ken Wilber, *The Atman Project*, p.74.
4. Ken Wilber, *Sex, Ecology, Spirituality*, p.632.
5. Sri Aurobindo, *On Himself*, p.76.
6. Ibid., p.82.
7. Ibid., p.132.
8. Ibid., p.136.
9. Ibid., p.86.

10. Ibid., p.136.
11. Ibid., p.143.
12. Ibid., p.170
13. Ken Wilber, *Collective Works,* Volume 4, Introduction, p.4.
14. Ibid., p. 5.
15. Sri Aurobindo, *On Himself,* p.87.
16. Ibid., p. 100.
17. Ibid., p. 84.
18. Dilip Kumar Roy, *Sri Aurobindo came to me,* p.247.
19. Sri Aurobindo, *Letters on Yoga,* p.877.
20. Ibid., p. 885.
21. Satprem, *The Adventure of Consciousness,* p.294.
22. Sri Aurobindo, *On Hintself,* p.374.
23. Ken Wilber, *The Eye of Spirit,* p.viii.
24. Sri Aurobindo, *Letters on Yoga,* p.251.
25. Ken Wilber, *Up front Eden,* p.302.
26. Ibid., p.305.
27. Ken Wilber, *Sex, Ecology, Spirituality,* p.113.
28. Ibid., p.531.
29. Ibid., p.489.
30. Ibid., p.487.
31. Ibid., p.517.
32. Ibid., p.634.
33. Ibid., p.742.
34. Ken Wilber, *The Eye of Spirit,* p.341.

35. Ken Wilber, *A Brief History of Everything,* p.141.
36. Keri Wilber, *The Eye of Spirit,* p.351.
37. Sri Aurobindo, *The Life Divine,* p.934.-
38. Ibid., p.724.
39. Ken Wilber, *Up from Eden,* p.313.
40. Sri Aurobindo, The *Life Divine,* p.264-265.
41. Ibid., p.266-267.
42. Ibid., p.759-760.
43. R. S. Misra, *The Integral Advaitisnt of Sri Aurobindo,* p.346.
44. Ken Wilber, *One Taste,* p.215.
45. Ibid., p.285.
46. Ken Wilber, *Integral Psychology,* p.135.
47. Ken Wilber, *One Taste,* p.297.
48. Ken Wilber, *Integral Psychology,* p.127.
49. Sri Aurobindo, *The Life Divine,* p.931-932.
50. Ibid., p.933.
51. Ken Wilber, *A Brief History of Everything, p.* 247.
52. Sri Aurobindo, *The Life Divine,* p.956.
53. Sri Aurobindo, *The Foundations of Indian Culture,* p.26-27.
54. Sri Aurobindo, *Letters on Yoga,* p.l.
55. Ken Wilber, *A Theory of Everything,* p.176.
56. Sri Aurobindo, *Letters on 'Yoga,* p.253-254.
57. Sri Aurobindo, *The Synthesis of Yoga,* p.136.
58. Ken Wilber, *The Eye of Spirit,* p-340.
59. Sri Aurobindo, *The Future Poetry,* p.41-42.

60. Ken Wilber, *Eye to Eye*, p.288.
61. Ken Wilber, *Sex, Ecology, Spirituality*, p.196-197.
62. Ibid., p.609.
63. Ibid., p.507.
64. Ibid., p.191.
65. Ken Wilber, *Up from Eden*, p.328.
66. Sri Aurobindo, *The Life Divine*, p.730-731.
67. Ibid., p.900-901.
68. Ibid., p.228.
69. Ibid., p.852.
70. Sri Aurobindo, *The Supramental Manifestation*, p.347.
71. Ken Wilber, *The Spectrum of Consciousness*, p.214.
72. Ken Wilber, *The Atman Project*, p.102.
73. Ken Wilber, *One Taste*,, p.274-275.
74. Ibid., p. 300.
75. Sri Aurobindo, *The Synthesis of Yoga*, p. 203.
76. Sri Aurobindo, *The Life Divine*, p.692-694.
77. Ken Wilber, *The Eye of Spirit*, p.327-328.
78. B. Cortright, *Psychotherapy and Spirit*, p.79.
79. Ken Wilber, *The Eye of Spirit*, p.180.
80. Sri Aurobindo, *Letters on Yoga*, p.46.
81. Ibid J p. 68.
82. Sri Aurobindo, *The Problem of Rebirth*, p.38-39.
83. Ibid., p.42.
84. Sri Aurobindo, *The Synthesis of Yoga*, p.587.

85. Ken Wilber, *Eye to Eye,* p.288.
86. Ibid., p.288.
87. Ken Wilber, *Transformations of Consciousness,* p.72.
88. Sri Aurobindo, *The Life Divine,* p.537.
89. Ken Wilber, *A Brief History of Everything,* p.207.
90. Ken Wilber, *Sex, Ecology, Spirituality,* p.282.
91. Sri Aurobindo, *Letters on Yoga,* p.442.
92. Ken Wilber, *Sex, Ecology, Spirituality,* p.284.
93. Sri Aurobindo, *The Life Divine,* p.561.
94. Ken Wilber, *Sex, Ecology, Spirituality,* p.291.
95. Sri Aurobindo, *Letters on Yoga,* p.764.
96. Sri Aurobindo, *The Life Divine,* p.226.
97. Sri Aurobindo, *The Synthesis of Yoga,* p.145.
98. Ken Wilber, *Sex, Ecology, Spirituality,* p.334.
99. Ken Wilber, *Integral Psychology,* p.108.
100. Ken Wilber, *The Eye of Spirit,* p.328.
101. Sri Aurobindo, *Letters on Yoga,* p.274.
102. Ibid., p.294.
103. Ibid., p.280-281.
104. Ibid., p.295.
105. Ibid., p.281.
106. Ibid., p.289.
107. Sri Aurobindo, *The Life Divine,* p.764.
108. Sri Aurobindo, *The Problem of Rebirth,* p.34.
109. Ibid., p.89-99.

110. Sri Aurobindo, *The Life Divine,* pp.808-809.

111. Sri Aurobindo, *The Problem of Rebirth,* p.157.

112. Ibid., p. 168.

113. Ibid., p. 106.

114. Ken Wilber, *One Taste,* p.295.

115. Ken Wilber, *The Eye of Spirit,* p.276.

116. Ken Wilber, *One Taste,* p.213.

117. Ibid., p.348.

118. Ibid., p.353-354.

119. S. K. Saksena, *The Nature of Consciousness in Hindu Philosophy,* pp.7-8.

120. Ken Wilber, *The Eye of Spirit,* pp.375-376.

121. Sri Aurobindo, *On Himself,* p.378.

Chapter Twelve

Sri Aurobindo's Metaphysical Yoga Psychology

INTRODUCTION

Sri Aurobindo did not write a separate treatise on psychology, his psychology is based on his metaphysical vision and system of integral Yoga. He is not an academic or professional psychologist, but a yogi who takes psychology in his stride. Nevertheless, he gives the seeker plenty of psychological material on the unexplored inner regions of the subliminal, psychic and the superconscious levels of our being, as well as various levels of the surface consciousness, which will help the sadhak in the practice of yoga. Without a clear knowledge of these psycho-spiritual planes the seeker cannot comprehend the full meaning of the process of transformation which forms the centre of his integral Yoga.

For Sri Aurobindo all that exists in the universe can be rendered into terms of consciousness, because all is a creation of consciousness or of its forms. "All things are inhabited by this consciousness, even the things that seem to us inconscient, and the consciousness in one form can communicate or contact with the consciousness in another or else penetrate or contain or identify with it."[1] He describes psychology as "the science of consciousness and its states and operations in Nature and, if that can be glimpsed or experienced, its states and operations beyond what we know as Nature."[2] Observable consciousness is only the small visible part of our being, there are ranges of consciousness above and below the average human range, which support the surface nature. Although the inconscient, the subliminal, the circumconscient, universal Mind and universal Life are all unknown to us, they are all more original, more potent to shape and govern our being and actions. "The movements of this little surface nature cannot be understood, nor its true law discovered until we know all that is below or behind it, supplies it and know too all that is around it and above it."3 The knowledge of the external objective world outside and around man needs to be supplemented by the subjective world within, i.e., the awareness of the hidden ranges and forces of man's inner psychological being and its mastery over these forces. Mere mental knowledge of these hidden ranges and forces may be helpful as a preparation, but the concrete realisation of these planes needs the actual practice of integral Yoga. After all, "Yoga is nothing but practical psychology."[4]

Sri Aurobindo's psychology is related to the attainment of self-perfection leading to the divinisation of life. The beginning realisation of self-perfection requires authentic self-knowledge and effective self-control. For Sri Aurobindo self-knowledge implies the knowledge of our true self and the knowledge of the different parts of our total being with its complex functioning and movements. Man's conception of self-perfection varies according to the conceptions of one's true self at different stages of individual and collective evolution. During the development from a physical to a vital to a mental being, man is confined to the perfection of these parts. But man, on the way to discovering one's true self, has the capacity to rise into higher ranges and realise a spiritual self-perfection. Sri Aurobindo's metaphysical Yoga psychology aims at this spiritual self-perfection, in which the seeker raises oneself from the mental level to the Supramental level.

Sri Aurobindo's view of the psychological nature of man is intimately related to the metaphysical nature of the universe. Yoga psychology, as a scientific study that is concerned with the actual workings of the mind and consciousness, must be complemented by a metaphysical study that is related to the nature and the cause of ultimate reality. Although both metaphysics and yoga psychology constitute a unified body of knowledge, they differ in their provinces and nature of inquiry, and Sri Aurobindo describes the difference as follows: "Metaphysics deals with the ultimate cause of things and all that lies behind the world of phenomena. As regards mind and consciousness, it asks what they are, how they came into existence, what is their relation to Matter, Life, etc. Psychology deals with mind and consciousness and tries to find out not so much their ultimate nature and relations as their actual workings and the rule and law of these workings."[5] If both scientific study and metaphysical contemplation are united, the seeker gains a more complete knowledge of the whole, rather than just one aspect of the field of study. Sri Aurobindo wants to spiritualise rational psychology; he wants empirical science to widen its territory beyond the physical into the hidden ranges of the supraphysical Nature. It is a spiritual psychology and supraphysical science which create complete knowledge in all the realms of life.

The object of yoga psychology is to study and utilise the forms, forces and working movements of consciousness, just as physical science studies and utilises the forms, forces and working movements of matter. There is no difference of essential law in the physical and the psychological realms, as the Supreme Existence expresses itself equally in consciousness and matter, but only a difference in energy, instrumentation and exact process.

Sri Aurobindo emphasises exact observation and scrupulous experimentation as the true method of a scientific psychology. Such a direct experimental and experiential psychology must replace the mass of elementary and superficial generalisations of the empirical system. According to Sri Aurobindo, "The field of psychology needs a direct inner psychological instrumentation by which we can arrive at sure data and sure results in ourselves verified by equally sure data and results in our observation of others and of the hidden psychological world and its play of unseen forces. The physical is the outwardly seen and sensed, and needs physical instruments for its exploration; the psychological is the physically unseen and unsensed, to be discovered only by an organisation of the inward senses and other now undeveloped and occult means. It is through consciousness, by an instrumentation of consciousness only that the nature and laws and movements of consciousness can be discovered—and this is the method of Yoga."[6] The observed data in scientific psychology should include the subjective, fluid, intermittent, repeated data of self-observation which is not subject to exact instruments and do not afford proof easily verifiable by everybody as happens in the physical sciences. Yoga psychology examines the nature and movement of consciousness as they are revealed to us by the process and results of our yogic practice, but unlike ordinary psychology it extends the range of observation and experimentation to a realm which exceeds the common surface range. It utilises intuitive perception for observing and evaluating the significance of the higher and deeper ranges of consciousness. The tests possible in yogic research are twofold: the tests of the normal everyday facts of our surface personality and the tests of another subtler order of truths. "The tests of this other subtler order of truths are the same, experience, experimental analysis and synthesis, reason and intuition. Only, since these things are truths of the soul and spirit, it must necessarily be a psychological and spiritual experience, a psychological and psychophysical experimentation, analysis and synthesis, a larger intuition which looks into higher realms, realities, possibilities of being, a reason which admits something beyond itself, looks upward to the suprarational; ... Yoga is itself nothing but a well-tested means of opening up these greater realms of experience."[7]

Sri Aurobindo's system of yogic psychological research, which continues in the Ashram and Auroville, is not of an academic nature and is not immediately directed towards producing rapid external results. The research work done by the sadhaks aims at a gradual change of their present consciousness through an exploration of the hidden ranges of their inner consciousness. From an academic viewpoint, it may seem that Sri Aurobindo's yogic psychological research work overemphasises the power and potentialities of the inner and higher realms, and their influence on the lower levels. However, Sri Aurobindo maintains that inner development must be effective in all spheres of outer life, i.e., the seeker's psychological research on one's inner development has to be applied to the processes of every aspect of one's outer life, including the most practical.

But can Sri Aurobindo's processes of applied yogic research assimilate the present-day research work done by clinical psychologists, and does he overlook the psychopathological obstacles of the lower realms during the practice of sadhana? Could it also be that his vision lacks some of modern psychology's explorations in areas such as childhood development, differential diagnosis and intrapsychic conflicts? Does his view of man's developmental process ommits part of the early biographical level—the level which contains material related to one's infancy, childhood and adulthood— i.e., the developmental period crucial for the formation of a cohesive self? Can progress in sadhana be made more reliable and smoother if the practitioners of integral Yoga adopt some of the methods and procedures of research from Ken Wilber's integral all-level, all-quadrant model?

As mentioned above, for Sri Aurobindo "a complete psychology cannot be a pure natural science but must be a compound of science and metaphysical knowledge."[8] Metaphysical knowledge of the ultimate nature of things and everything that lies behind the world of phenomena can be acquired only through spiritual experience and realisation. But are the followers of Sri Aurobindo's metaphysical views incorporating the latest inventions and applications of new discoveries and developments in psychology? It seems that metaphysics is becoming more and more a handmaid of physics, the metaphysics of outwardness, but this naturalistic metaphysics should not leave out the reality of the transcendental realm, the metaphysics of inwardness. The knowledge of new discoveries in various fields in present-day psychology can enrich the world when properly incorporated. It is true that human nature, as a psycho-physical complexity, has a mechanical side where research work is able to lead to fruitful results, but its experimental method of investigation certainly has its limitations. Sri Aurobindo would not challenge the results of science, but he opposes the universalisation of naturalistic methods of enquiry. Such methods do not do justice to the deeper aspects of being and reality.

By verification through experience and experiment, and by earnestly and patiently testing his results, Sri Aurobindo was able to arrive at spiritual knowledge and truth. The rigorousness of such a scientific approach made it possible to watch the process and lay hold of the rationale of the mystic truths he later described in detail. The followers of Sri Aurobindo should not neglect this demand for scientific rigorous substantiation, as such an attitude may easily degrade his spiritual vision into a dogmatic system of metaphysics or may even create a new cultural-religious sect.

The term "integral psychology" should be used with caution, as Sri Aurobindo nowhere claims to have developed a sound basis for an integral psychology. The author frequently used this term himself in his previous works, but afterwards he became aware that this term might cause quite some counterproductive results when used indiscriminately. Sri Aurobindo did not integrate much of the Western psychological models which dominated psychological thought during the first half of the twentieth century. For Sri Aurobindo the observations in these fields are of an initial character, they need to be supplemented by a direct inner psychological instrumentation, "which will drive large and wide roads into the psychological Unknown". He did not hide his critical views regarding the limitations of behaviourist psychology, humanistic psychology and psychoanalysis. As Sri Aurobindo puts it, "the instability in psychology passes from one theory to another before the first is well-founded; indeed, several conflicting theories hold the field together. No firm metaphysical building can be erected upon these shifting quicksands."[9]

Behaviourism bases the study of mind upon the study of the body, and leaves out any hidden profundities of one's subjective existence. Sri Aurobindo was aware that the mechanical repetitions of the physical consciousness create consistent bahaviour patterns, but the behaviourists ignore all the other aspects of consciousness. According to Sri Aurobindo, "Modern science, obsessed with the greatness of its physical discoveries and the idea of the sole existence of Matter, has long attempted to base upon physical data even its study of Soul and Mind and of those workings of Nature in man and animal in which a knowledge of psychology is as important as any of the physical sciences. Its very psychology founded itself upon physiology and the scrutiny of the brain and nervous system."[10] The behaviouristic psychologist studies man from outside rather than seeing his true field of knowledge and experimental laboratory of experiment in oneself. Moreover, the knowledge of one's superficial mentality and the laws of one's bodily life do not bring the seeker to the hidden and mysterious depth behind the surface consciousness. Sri Aurobindo claims that the seeker cannot be guided in the process of one's self-exploration by "a scientific psychology with a materialistic basis which assumes that the body and the biological and the physiological factors of our nature are not only the starting-point but the whole real foundation (of man) and regards human mind as only a subtle development from the life and the body. That may be the actual truth of the animal side of human nature and of the human mind in so far as it is limited and conditioned by the physical part of our being ... but in man mind reveals itself as a greater energy escaping from the restrictions of the vital and the physical formula of being. But even this is not all that man is or can be: he has in him the power to evolve and release a still greater ideal energy which in its turn escapes out of the restrictions of the mental formula of his nature and discloses the supramental form, the ideal power of a spiritual being. In Yoga we have to travel beyond the physical nature and the superficial man and to discover the workings of the whole nature of the real man. In other words, we must arrive at and use a psychophysical knowledge with a spiritual foundation."[11] In integral Yoga, behaviourism as a scientific psychology cannot be of much help; this superficial psychology has its value in the mental and vital realms, but in the spiritual realm it has to be turned to a higher end where the lower realms are transmuted and then become capable of linking the sadhak's consciousness with the Divine. Sri Aurobindo does not look upon life and mind as merely phenomena in Matter, but as energies other than the material with their own peculiar qualities, powers and workings. Only a limited range of the phenomena of life and mind can be satisfied by a purely biophysical or psychophysical explanation.

Humanistic psychology, like Sri Aurobindo's yoga psychology, emphasises the inherent principles of personal growth and the unity of consciousness rather than the sum total of separate instincts and perceptions. Each individual is responsible for one's own actions and own choices among the infinite number of possibilities for growth. The root cause of the problem lies within oneself, and it is only through a deeper understanding of oneself that the seeker becomes able to cope with the problems of life. For Sri Aurobindo, as well as for the humanist psychologist, man is a never-finished product of evolution with endless potentialities for inner growth. However, the humanist's unifying process is based on mechanical principles rather than spiritual ones. Humanists consider man primarily as a biological organism and in their vitalistic biological approach they give insufficient significance to the spiritual dimensions of human development, in contrast with Sri Aurobindo, who assumes the divine essence of man. To use Sri Aurobindo's own words, "The mundane ideal regards man always as a mental, vital and physical being and it aims at a human perfection well within these limits, a perfection of mind, life and body, an expansion and refinement of the intellect and knowledge, of the will and power, of ethical character, aim and conduct, of aesthetic sensibility and creativeness, of emotional balanced poise and enjoyment, of vital and physical soundness, regulated action and just efficiency. It is a wide and full aim, but not yet sufficiently full and wide, because it ignores that other greater element of our being which the mind vaguely conceives as the spiritual element and leaves it either undeveloped or insufficiently satisfied as merely some high occasional or added derivatory experience ... it does not aspire beyond mind to that of which our purest reason, our brightest mental intuition, our deepest mental sense and feeling, strongest mental will and power or ideal aim and purpose are only pale radiations. Its aim [the humanistic ideal of perfection], besides, is limited to a terrestrial perfection of the normal human life."[12]

SRI AUROBINDO'S INTERPRETATION OF FREUDIAN PSYCHOANALYSIS

Freud's pioneering work explored the very early stages of human development and the decisive role they play in subsequent growth. He codified some of the mysteries of the unconscious mind and their relation to psychopathology and psychotherapy. The ego can repress the body and instincts, and the will can overwhelm feelings, which often results in alienation and emotional disturbances. Freud's psychoanalysis may be considered in several ways: as a method of investigating unconscious thoughts and feelings, as a theory of human personality, and as a technique of psychotherapy. For Freud, the past has a real existence and is not merely an inference from the individual's immediate experience. He believed that psychological disorders resulted from constitutional factors, early childhood experiences, and precipitating factors later in life. The relative influence of these factors varies.

Freudian psychoanalytic therapy is based on hypothetical postulates of unconscious processes and personality development; it aims at the insight of understanding the underlying unconscious psychodynamics through a rational interpretation. This insight in itself, whether an intellectual perception or an emotionally charged corrective experience, does not always have a sufficient impact to produce needed, lasting changes in the individual's behaviour and needs to be supplemented by a long process of "working through", so as to translate the insights into new patterns of behaviour.

Freud's psychoanalytic approach concentrates on repressed traumatic childhood experiences and the various defence mechanisms which are used by the individual to push away these painful experiences into the unconscious so as to be able to cope with them. These defensive avoidances become later the source of conflicts and inner fragmentation.

Freud's psychoanalytic therapy attempts to actively bring unconscious material back into awareness, where it can be expressed, analysed, explored and interpreted. The therapeutic process, in other words, aims at facilitating the re-experiencing and working through old patterns of distress, by lifting the defences that keep them unconscious. Once the trauma is healed the authentic self can build up a new self-structure with greater freedom.

The therapy focuses on the psychopathological and emotional disturbances of the individual through a reconstruction of the traumatic past. In this process, repressed energies are released and afterwards used for constructive purposes. The individual can master conflicts by placing them in historical perspective and by understanding one's own responsibility in their unnecessary continuance. Thereafter, the future can be seen as a period with challenges and possibilities rather than as a prolongation of a stifling past. In his analytical and empirical approach, Freud seeks to resolve the problem by re-establishing a working harmony between the contents of the ego-consciousness and the instinctual unconscious. This harmony is a necessary precondition for self-development.

Though Sri Aurobindo seems to be aware of the contents of Freud's views, it is doubtful if he was textually familiar with the works of Freud. Sri Aurobindo, like Freud, maintains that true psychological knowledge reveals that our waking or surface consciousness is only a minute part of our being, and does not yield to us the truth of our character or our actions. The sources lie deeper. For Freud, a scientific psychology aims at discovering these sources and knowing the nature and process of the subconscious self. The lower subconscient is a very important part of the being. Its opening always takes a long time as it is an obscure, dark and ignorant region, a storehouse of the seeds of all the old lower, often rejected vital instincts which may rise up from time to time. Like the Freudians, Sri Aurobindo insists that it is essential to raise up the old lower movements and become conscious of them in order to know, elucidate and reject them. According to Sri Aurobindo, "It is a known psychological law that whatever is suppressed in the conscious mind remains in the subconscient being and recurs either in the waking state when the control is removed or else in sleep. ... In order to make a true and complete change, one has to make all these conscious, to see clearly what is still there and to reject them from one layer after another till they have been entirely thrown out of the personal existence."[13]

Sri Aurobindo agrees with Freud that the obscure currents in the dark areas of the subconscient cannot be ignored. The seeker or client cannot run away from them forever. These obscure energies may take control of us and should, therefore, not be allowed to master and enslave us. These destructive potentialities are to be faced, understood and transformed into creative purposive potentialities. Both Sri Aurobindo and Freud maintain that there can be no complete change if consciousness is not brought into the lower subconscient because the contents of the unconscious powerfully influence the workings of the conscious mind. As Sri Aurobindo describes it, "The animal in us has its lair of retreat in the dense jungle of the subconscience. To penetrate there to bring in light and establish a control, is indispensable for the completeness of any higher life, for any integral transformation of the nature."[14] In this quotation, however, Sri Aurobindo does not refer to Freud's concept of the ordinary conscious will, but to the higher Consciousness-Force and Truth-light that has to be brought down so that the subconscient can be enlightened by it and accustomed to obey its control.

Freud's unconscious refers to the individual's lack of awareness of his or her own mental functioning, or the unawareness of all things at a given moment. He does not differentiate the separate though interacting physical, vital and mental aspects which characterise ordinary waking consciousness, the subconscient and the subliminal. Sri Aurobindo prefers to call the unconscious the subconscient as he maintains that all things have some sort of a consciousness. He describes the different planes of the subconscient as: "When I use the word [subconscient] I mean always what is *below* the ordinary physical consciousness, not what is behind it. ... The subconscient is universal as well as individual like all the other main parts of the Nature. But there are different parts or planes of the subconscient. All upon earth is based on the Inconscient as it is called, though it is not really inconscient at all, but rather a complete 'sub'-conscience, a suppressed or involved consciousness, in which there is everything but nothing is formulated or expressed. The subconscient lies between this Inconscient and the conscious mind, life and body."[15]

For Sri Aurobindo, Freud's unconscious is that which lies outside the awareness of the seeker's personality, and there is nothing which is 'truly' unconscious. He relates Freud's unconscious to a part of the subconscious. In Sri Aurobindo's yoga psychology, the seeker is not only unconscious of that which lies below the surface consciousness, but one is also unconscious of that which lies behind the surface consciousness (the subliminal), around the surface consciousness (the environmental), and above the surface consciousness (the superconscient).

Sri Aurobindo agrees with Freud's basic views regarding the contents of the unconscious subconscient as a source of problems, but Freud employs a different language to describe the process of becoming aware of these inner states. According to Sri Aurobindo, the unconscious is "the submental base of the being and is made up of impressions, instincts, habitual movements that are stored there; it contains the potentiality of all primitive reactions of life ... it retains the impressions of all our past experiences of life and they can come up from there in dream forms ... but also all that is consciously experienced sinks down into the subconscient as obscure yet obstinate impressions of experience All too that is suppressed without being wholly got rid of sinks down there and remains as seed ready to surge up or sprout up at any moment. The action of he subconscient is irrational, mechanical, repetitive, ... the subconscient is a thing of habits and memories and repeats persistently or whenever it can old suppressed reactions, reflexes, mental, vital or physical responses ... the subconscient is the main cause why all things repeat themselves and nothing gets changed except in appearance."[16]

Recent developments and major changes in the psychoanalytical theory of pathology and treatment focus more on the urge toward and development of the wholeness of the self, rather than on Freud's innate biological drives, as the basis of personality development. In the process of healing, the concept of cognitive insight is supplemented by the process of emotional insight. For example, in Kohut's psychoanalytic object-relation therapy, which basically uses a structural and developmental model, the ego functions as a synthesiser of inner and outer experience, therefore it creates a sense of personal continuity, a self. This energetic self is constructed out of one's object experience, as there exists a mutuality between self and self-object, the I and the other (the mother). The sense of selfhood is best developed by responsive mothering. Thus, for Kohut, human relationships are of primary importance in human behaviour and development, as opposed to Freud's instinctual drive conflicts. The ego has its own energy, separate from the libido. Kohut's intersubjective approach to 'regrowing' a basic sense of self, unlike Freud's dualistic model of the isolated individual, aims at healing through empathy. Lack of empathy in early childhood often results in narcissistic character disorders and borderline personalities. To create a coherent self that resists fragmentation, empathy is paramount in order to affirm the best in the child's talents and one's sense of belongingness in the world. Psychopatholpgical problems are often due to a lack of the sense of the self or to its disintegration, and Kohut's psychoanalysis attempts to re-establish and reintegrate a basic and stable sense of self. Working towards the improvement in the ego-organisation and its reintegration may include the resolution of conflicts between the various components of the personality structure (where the ego controls the 'id' and the 'superego'), increased ego strength and the improvement of interpersonal relationships. With the development of healthier ego-controls the individual arrives at a more complete and deeper understanding of oneself and is gradually freed from the debilitating anxiety that keeps the person from living a fully human life.

Memories of the past can be one of the main obstacles to spiritual growth and the primary hindrance to psychological health. In the initial stages of sadhana or psychoanalysis repressed memories seem to surge- up within the individual and are cast out only with great difficulty and intense effort, as they refuse to leave. For both Sri Aurobindo and Freud, the inner reality grasped through insight forms the basis from which external reality may be known. They both insist on the exploration of consciousness, but psychoanalysis remains more or less obsessed with the deficiency states of the self and its unconscious, whereas Sri Aurobindo aims at the transcendence of this finite self. In contrast with Freud's exploration of past unconscious traumatic experiences, Sri Aurobindo immersed himself in the process of transformation to a divine existence. Sri Aurobindo's integral Yoga moves from ego development to Spirit development, whereas Freud moves from instinctual development to ego development. Freud seems to overemphasise the extrovert attitudes of rationality and he ignores the introvert attitudes of intuition. For Sri Aurobindo, on the other hand, rational and emotional faculties are not ends in themselves, but instruments for the realisation of man's true self. The substratum of all experience is not the body, the mind or any complex chemical or biological product, but the Self as a pure Consciousness-Force. It is this Self which is the source of all human psychological behaviour. This Self pervades the entire life and each and every part of our being. Without this conscious Self, mind, heart and body—working as instruments—have no power.

Sri Aurobindo does not deny the existence of subconscious emotional undercurrents and drives which control the mind, but by a conscious action of the will the seeker can withdraw from such processes and thus reduce the mind's emotional involvement in them by a deliberate and purposeful act of choice. He does not ask the seeker to fight instinctive reactions, but to withdraw one's life-force from its downward destructive flow and to redirect it, free from emotional involvement in desires and urges. The seeker becomes fully conscious of one's problems but, guided by the principle of self-control, the individual no longer acts them out in the world. That is, the seeker is asked to watch, but not get involved in the fluctuations of thoughts and feelings. By observing one's thoughts, the seeker learns to gain insight into the conditioned, repetitive processes of one's uncontrolled mind. When the mind is released from its conditioned ways, it can lead the seeker to some sort of spiritual rebirth. Through a conscious control of one's vital and mental activities and the development of faith in and love for the Divine, the seeker is able to move towards the goal of ego-transcendence and obtain the strength of the Spirit.

For Sri Aurobindo, in the process of transformation, mere cognition of subconscious processes is not sufficient and he does not aim at an analytic realisation. Mental analysis through psychoanalysis can give some insights into the workings of the subconscient, but to be aware of repressed mental conflicts does not mean that these unresolved conflicts are healed and transformed. For an integral transformation, the subconscient must be made conscious and ultimately completely conquered. Psychoanalysis uses mental analysis as its method of gaining insight into unconscious processes, but in Sri Aurobindo's view such an approach remains relatively fragmentary. Mind, as an instrument of analysis and synthesis, has inherent limitations; it views every phenomenon as a thing-in-itself, separating the part from the whole without arriving at the sense of true unity. Psychoanalysis describes the whole of a vast complexity in terms of a small part. The Freudian analysts look from down up and explain the higher lights in terms of the lower obscurities, while the foundation of these things is above and not below. Sri Aurobindo's synthetic realisation aims at the integration of all the parts of one's being with and under the guidance of the soul within. It is this inmost Self or psychic being which acts as the true harmoniser and leader of the different parts of the individual.

If the sadhak enters deep into oneself, he or she will also discover a higher Power, which is able to act—in certain given circumstances—within oneself. It is, therefore, safer to explore the contents of the subconscient once the seeker has established contact with this inner and higher Power. Then the inner and higher ranges of consciousness are able to withstand the obscure subconscious forces that are released when they are raised up to consciousness. This does not mean that unconscious, repressed and undesirable states of mind are eliminated, but these contents are purified, reorganised and absorbed into the greater and wider environmental consciousness (the circumconscient).

As the seeker has no knowledge and therefore no control over the hidden parts of the obscure subconscient, Sri Aurobindo advises the sadhak not to descend into this part of the subconscient when he or she is not yet sufficiently ready. Mental insight can give the seeker only some indirect insight into these hidden activities. Before the higher and inner consciousness can go down into the subconscient to face and transform all the difficulties of the lower nature, it has to be established first in the lower parts of the conscious waking self. Sri Aurobindo does not want the seeker to raise up the difficulties from below before the descending power from above is there to transform them. It is only by establishing contact with the subliminal or by ascending into, the supercoriscient and from there looking down into these obscure depths that the seeker can gain control over the dark areas of one's subconscious nature, the higher the seeker ascends, the greater capacity one acquires to work on the lower.

No doubt in sadhana the seeker can minimise the difficulty by putting the right will and right habit of reaction onto each resurgence of the subconscious but this will not make it yield to a deep-rooted change. However, as long as the seeker is not in constant contact with the action of the Force from above or of a deeper will within, while forces of unconscious impulses come to the surface, the mental will is necessary to develop an attitude of control and detachment; this corrective attitude of the mind should not be prematurely abandoned. Sri Aurobindo expresses this view in the following words: "in order to reject anything from the being one has first to become conscious of it, to have a clear inner experience of its action and to discover its actual place in the workings of its nature. One can then work upon it to eliminate it.... It is this or something like it that is attempted crudely and improperly with a rudimentary and insufficient knowledge in the system of psychoanalysis. The process of raising up the lower movements into the full light of consciousness in order to know and deal with them is inevitable; for there can be no complete change without it. But it can truly succeed only when a higher light and force are sufficiently at work to overcome, sooner or later, the force of the tendency that is held up for change. ... To raise it up [the lower ignorant subconscious nature] prematurely is to risk suffusing the conscious parts also with its dark and dirty stuff and thus poisoning the whole vital and even the mental nature. Always, therefore, one should begin by bringing down something of the divine nature, calm, light, equanimity, purity, divine strength into the parts of the conscious being that have to be changed; only when that has been sufficiently done and there is a firm positive basis, is it safe to raise up the concealed subconscious adverse elements in order to destroy and eliminate them by the strength of the divine calm, light, force and knowledge."[17] Only when the higher consciousness-Force and Truth-light are brought to the subconscient is it able to change and eliminate its adverse movements.

Sri Aurobindo would differ with the Freudian method of raising up and stressing psychological difficulties and accepting and approving their presence, as the only way to get rid of them. In integral Yoga it is a mistake to dwell too much on the lower nature and its obstacles. They are not to be evaded, but preoccupation with them is not very helpful. It is well to see what the dark side of the obscure lower nature is, and how it acts in order to reject and change it, but to dwell solely on the dark areas of the subconscient and its aspects of imperfection creates depression and should, therefore, be avoided. Certainly, the more the lower nature is purified the easier is the descent of the higher Nature; but for Sri Aurobindo it is truer that the more the higher Nature descends the more the lower is purified. In the course of sadhana, a descent of the higher and a purification of the lower do not come all at once but go on progressing side by side.

Sri Aurobindo's views regarding Freud's psychoanalysis is best expressed in his own words; "The psycho-analysis of Freud is the last thing that one should associate with yoga. It takes up a certain part, the darkest, the most perilous, the unhealthiest part of the nature, the lower vital subconscious layer, isolates some of its most morbid phenomena and attributes to it and them an action out of all proportion to its true role in nature. ... Moreover, the exaggeration of the importance of suppressed sexual complexes is a dangerous falsehood and it can have a nasty influence and tend to make the mind and vital more and not less fundamentally impure than before. It is true that the subliminal in man is the largest part of his nature and has in it the secret of the unseen dynamisms which explain his surface activities. But the lower vital subconscious which is all that this psycho-analysis of Freud seems to know and even of that it knows only a few ill-lit corners,— is no more than a restricted and very inferior portion of the subliminal whole. ... If one wishes to purify and transform the nature, it is the power of these higher ranges to which one must open and raise to them and change by them both the subliminal and the surface being. ... But to begin by opening up the lower subconscious, risking to raise up all that is foul or obscure in it, is to go out of one's way to invite trouble. First, one should make the higher mind and vital strong and firm and full of light and peace from above; afterwards one can open subconscious with more safety and some chance of a rapid and successful change."[18]

As mentioned previously, Sri Aurobindo agrees with Freud that many of the obstinate psychopathological disturbances can be traced to the subconscious elements of the being but, while recognising the influence of the past, he nevertheless suggests that the seeker be cautious about reenergising painful processes from the past. The Freudian unconscious might be relatively cleared, but it can easily accumulate anew a large amount of conflictual material if the sadhak's mental habits and attitudes towards oneself and one's life are not changed. For Sri Aurobindo, the more the seeker is exclusively fixed on the darker areas the more one becomes subject to them; the innumerable rediscovered ego-desires only obscure the urge for spiritual realisation and turn the seeker away from the highest levels. "The superconscient, not the subconcient, is the true foundation of things. ... That is the promise of the greater psychology awaiting its hour before which these poor gropings will disappear and come to nothing."[19]

The seeker who practices sadhana may change profoundly in behaviour towards one's environment, without any systematic attempt by the seeker to modify it, and many psychological problems may disappear without the help of a psychoanalyst. Under the influence of some subtler Power or Consciousness-Force which permeates the whole being, these problems melt like ice in the sun. The sadhak tries to get in touch with this Divine Source and, in this journey, may even have to turn against the current in order to get closer to the Source. Freud would classify such a divine motive as a dream or selfish fantasy, far from one's real self.

According to Sri Aurobindo, the psychoanalyst takes up the darkest part of the lower vital and maintains that this lower vital part is responsible for all action in human life. In the exploration of this subconscious realm, Freud ignores the inner subliminal dimensions of consciousness, which are as much responsible for one's surface actions as one's subconscious processes. As mentioned before, these deeper, subliminal parts of the being are not at all incoherent but well organised, and Freud's lower vital subconscient is only a very inferior portion of the subliminal and psychic whole. For Sri Aurobindo it is certain "that when we go back into ourselves very deep away from the surface appearance, we find that the mind, heart and sensational being of man are moved by forces not under his own control and that he can become an instrument in the hands of Energies of a cosmic character without knowing the origin of his actions. It is by stepping into his subliminal consciousness that he becomes directly aware of them."[20] Sri Aurobindo describes the subliminal consciousness as: "The subliminal stands behind and supports the whole superficial man; it has in it a larger and more efficient mind behind the surface mind, a larger and more powerful vital behind the surface vital, a subtler and freer physical consciousness behind the surface bodily existence."[21] With the right attitude of opening to this subtle realm the sadhak can turn to the subconscious and purify its contents. Raising up the difficulties of the lower subconscient in the mass in order to observe, know and reject them may succeed in some cases, but it is not a safe or certain method. There is the danger of the old persistent habit of raising up and stressing the difficulties instead of rejecting them. The safest way is to remain in the higher part of the consciousness and, from there, put pressure onto the lower to change. That is why for Sri Aurobindo a guidance from a higher spiritual or inner subliminal consciousness is safer and more effective for a true and lasting change in dealing with repressed experiences of the past, instinctual energies or conventional social influences, than the guidance of a psychoanalytical therapist.

There are contemporary psychoanalysts who would challenge Sri Aurobindo's views on psychoanalysis. They would argue that "Freudians at least have their feet on the ground rather than their heads in the clouds, a good beginning if one wishes to travel reliably along the surface of the earth. Being concerned first and foremost with the development of ordinary competence in making a living, forming responsible relationships, enjoying sexuality and other natural appetites, raising a family and generally coping adequately with life, they help to establish a firm base from which an interest in deeper meaning can develop."[22]

Although he uses a different language, Ken Wilber would support such a view. He agrees with Sri Aurobindo that Freud's mistake lies in his description of the whole of a vast and complex reality in terms of a small part. They both emphasise that the seeker has to know more about the totality of one's being—the surface consciousness, the subconscient, the subliminal and the superconscient—before one can know the part. However, Ken Wilber, unlike Sri Aurobindo, aims at an equal and simultaneous development of the part as well as the whole. Each level/ stage has its own healthy and unhealthy manifestations, judged against the scale of the degree of integration. (Wilber 2002) Things can go wrong at each and any level which involves regression, arrest, repression, fixation and denial-defenses of self. He equates Freud's interpretation of the individual's depth with his upper left quadrant approach. Once one's interior depths are more adequately interpreted, one can more easily deal with one's pathological ego-defects. Merely focusing on high interior development, being too engaged in the upper quadrants, one creates a tendency to escape 'the messy flooded sewers of the lower quadrants'.

Ken Wilber agrees with Freud's assertion that, if the self represses various aspects of itself, then it will have less potential left for further self-development and might even stop developing entirely. As a process of clinging to lower levels, excessive defence mechanisms will use up a certain amount of energy in order to repress aspects of the self. By descending into the lower unconscious and becoming aware of those parts of the unconscious which are alienated by fear or anxiety, the individual is able to reintegrate that level. He or she thus releases that lower level of regressive tendencies and allows it to join the upward journey to a higher identity.

Ken Wilber, like Sri Aurobindo, is aware that Freud's depth psychology deals only with the lowest levels of the holarchy and that there are deeper or higher realms in the search for being which can be explored, rather than just pursuing a lifelong search into one's id. But, unlike Sri Aurobindo, Ken Wilber maintains that *"for just that reason* their narrow and narcissistic perspective can be so crippling ... with 'depth' psychology we can recontact these lower holons and expose them to consciousness, so that they can be released from their fixation and dissociation and rejoin the ongoing march of consciousness evolution. ... They can be reintegrated with your main self, so that your central self might now have 70 or 80 units of its potential available to it."[23] In order for a true integral orientation to emerge, 'One Taste' has to be complemented by the work done on the lower levels. For Ken Wilber, Freud's uncovering therapy aims at a relaxation of repressions and an understanding of the cause of repression. Relaxing repression against lower preconventional impulses creates simultaneously an opening to the descent of higher postconventional and spiritual impulses; the latter were not repressed in the past but are now able to emerge for the first time. In other words, relaxing the defences of repressed id impulses allows the descent of Spirit, because the early defences against a lower impulse tend to seal off the higher impulses. Undoing these early defences enables higher growth to proceed.

Ken Wilber gives full scope for regress to all those seekers who are struggling with pathological ego-defects. For them, it is better to recontact ego deformities first, before transcending the ego. According to Ken Wilber, "in psychoanalytic therapy, one engages in 'regression in service of ego' —that is, one descends back into a lower level that was alienated and split off by fear and anxiety, reintegrates that level by embracing it with love and acceptance, and thus releases that lower level from being a regressive pull, releases it from being in the grips of Thanatos (descent), and allows it to rejoin the ongoing march of a higher identity and a wider love of others (Eros)."[24]

Sri Aurobindo wants the ego to be dissolved in transcendence (a step forward into superconsciousness) and not to be dissolved in regressions (a step backwards into the chaotic, lowest region of the subconscious). He maintains that beyond defence mechanisms there are transformational processes, and the practitioner of integral yoga has the possibility of bringing down a higher power, which has its healing influence upon problems related to neurotic conflicts. But this view does not solve the problem, which is related to differential diagnosis; it needs a sound clinical judgment to distinguish the functioning of an automatic rigid defence mechanism from the process of genuine, transformation. Sri Aurobindo's integral Yoga does not explore the formative maturation process from early ego-childhood to ego-adulthood. Unlike Sri Aurobindo, Ken Wilber appreciates Freud's pioneering work and understanding of early infantile or prerational stages of human development and the types of pathology that are often rooted in complications at these early stages.

Nevertheless, although Ken Wilber admits that Freud's truths are important, they are also partial, as not all psychological anguish is due solely to repressing the *libido;* there may be other truths which, if repressed, would cause more psychic anguish. Ken Wilber agrees with Sri Aurobindo that in the deepest recesses of the psyche, one finds not repressed unconscious instincts but the superconscious Spirit. When he elaborates on the dynamics of repression, he refers to the illusionary repression of the universal consciousness or superconscious All. Freud's traditional theory of evolution lacks the notion of a meaningful purpose, i.e., to find fundamental Wholeness.

For Freud the meaning of the similarity between 'oceanic feeling' and psychopathology is unambiguous: these feelings usually involve something in disguise and are often related to a regression of the individual's earliest encounters, rather than the positive unfolding aspect of a creative experience. Much of religion and spiritual behaviour, according to Freud, is a projection of unconscious wishes. The transcendent state of consciousness has no validity on its own; it is only an infantile aberration intended to turn the adult away from reality. But it seems Freud mixed up the co-presence of different orders of experience, explaining one in terms of the other. Freud described the oceanic feeling as a sense of unbounded oneness with the universe that seeks "the resurrection of infantile helplessness." For

Sri Aurobindo, however, annihilation of the ego is not a return to the feelings of infancy but an emergence of the true spiritual person, who is no longer bound to ignorance and disharmony. But could it be that Sri Aurobindo (and also some of the transpersonal psychotherapist) may be mistaken about the utility of this 'oceanic feeling'? According to M. Epstein, "Freud's attempts to understand spiritual experiences are typical of psychologists both in and out of the transpersonal field. His recognition of the similarity between' certain mystical experiences and early infantile experiences of unconditional love cannot simply be dismissed as reductionistic. Because the two experiences are similar, such mystical states can be tremendously reassuring for those with deficits in their early experiences of intimacy ... transpersonal theorists have tended to ignore the ways in which mystical experiences of unity evoke primitive narcissistic cravings, focusing instead on the expansive or transcendent nature of those states. The expansive nature of the oceanic experience can clearly invigorate the self, but such states also provide the opportunity to work through early narcissistic issues in a new way. The spiritual path is ultimately about confronting one's own inherent narcissism, after all is said and done. Freud laid the foundation, however incomplete, for this understanding."[25]

Sri Aurobindo and Freud are both concerned with the removal of obstacles to increased awareness. But for Freud the removal of unconscious obstacles is related to the intensification of human happiness, whereas for Sri Aurobindo the removal of obstacles is related to the awakening of the Divine within. The transpersonal psychotherapist would say that when an individual does not attend to both the Divine and the narcissist in oneself, that person will move neither toward human happiness nor toward integral self-transformation. The language James Hillman uses for the issue of unconscious and superconscious explorations in the search for the soul is related to Maslow's peaks and valleys, and for Hillman valleys need more exposure. The psychological method analyses and reveals this valley world, whereas the spiritual method teaches the seeker to overcome the valleys and climb the peaks. "It is so much easier to transcend history [individual case history, our culture as history] by climbing the mountain and let come what may, than it is to work on history within us, our reactions, habits, moralities, opinions, symptoms that prevent true psychic change. Change in the valley requires ... a digging in the ruins, a re-collecting. ... spiritual teachings warn the initiate so often about introspective broodings about jealousy, spite and pettiness, about attachments to sensations and memories. These cautions present an accurate phenomenology of how the soul [the seeker] feels when the spirit bids farewell. ... If a person is concurrently in therapy and in a spiritual discipline, the spiritual teacher may well regard the analysis as a waste of time with trivia and illusions. The analyst may regard the spiritual exercises as a leak in the psychic vessel, or an escape into either physicality (somatizing a sort of sophisticated hysterical conversion) or into metaphysicality."[26]

According to Sri Aurobindo, "The significance of the lotus [the soul within] is not to be found by analysing the secrets of the mud from which it grows here; its secret is to be found in the heavenly archetype of the lotus that blooms forever in the Light above. The self-chosen field of these psychologists [psycho-analysts] is besides poor, dark and limited; you must know the highest before you can truly understand the lowest. That is the promise of the greater psychology awaiting its hour before which these poor gropings will disappear and come to nothing."27

Jeffrey Kripal meaningfully comments upon this quotation of Sri Aurobindo as follows: "Little better is Aurobindo's comment that psychoanalysis is 'inconsiderate, awkward and rudimentary, and that one cannot discover the meaning of the lotus by analysing the secrets of the mud in which it grows. The observations in these fields are of an initial character, they need to be supplemented by a direct inner psychological instrumentation, "which will drive large and wide roads into the psychologically Unknown". Although we can certainly appreciate Aurobindo's privileging of the final telos of the flower and understand his negative assessment of psychoanalysis as a reaction to the early grossly reductive stage of psychoanalytic thought, we must also, admit that such a statement virtually deconstructs itself for us ... we might also reasonably ask how anyone could hope to understand something as biological as a lotus without first beginning with the larger ecosystem, that is, with the secrets of the mud in which it grows. Put bluntly, there just is no such thing as a mudless lotus. We need not and should not *end* with the mud, but we certainly need to at least *begin* there. If psychoanalytically inclined thinkers, then, can be accused on concentrating too much on the mud of pathology, the body, and the libidinal drives, mystics such as Aurobindo can be accused of concentrating too much on solipsistic sexless lotuses growing out of nothing. Both perspectives are half perspectives, partial views that must be transcended by constant tacking back and forth 'in between'. It is pointless to deny the muddiness of the mud, but it is equally silly to deny the beautiful blooming nature of the blossom. *Both* are aspects of the flower. Only by accepting both, in dialogue and debate, will we be able to see a fuller picture (if never the full picture) of that iconic image and begin to understand its many truths."[28]

All in all, it would seem that the practice of integral Yoga requires as a prerequisite a stable, integrated and cohesive self, capable of exploring inner realms. To be more effective, it simultaneously needs aspiration, sincerity and a firm foundation of trust in the guidance of the Divine. Sri Aurobindo takes a reasonably developed ego as the starting point of his sadhana in which the sadhak is capable of being confronted by some pathological contents of the psyche. For Sri Aurobindo, psychopathological contents cannot be attributed merely to innate biological processes, early childhood experiences and social conditioning, the influence of hidden subconscious variables are also the pull and push of karma from previous incarnations. For the transpersonal psychotherapist it would be an oversimplification to refer the psychological problems, related to either character or inherited and environmental influences, to karmic principles and reincarnative processes. The transpersonal psychotherapist is not preoccupied with the early wounds of the seeker s personal history, but only helps in guidmg the seeker to approach painful blockages of the past in order to free the person from the psychological roots of his or her suffering. This is the reason why some of the transpersonal psychotherapists tend to explore various unconscious dispositions before moving to higher states of consciousness. For Sri Aurobindo, the process of healing subconscious traumatic experiences comes from the inner wellsprings of the psychic being or the higher universal Self, which will enable the seeker to outgrow such experiences. However, to depend only on the trust of the inner and higher guidance may stimulate the sadhak to avoid such threatening experiences. These traumatic experiences often need to be worked out with the help of psychological methods supported by the process of surrender to the inner or higher spiritual guidance. Mental analysis and scrutiny does give some insight into the working of the lower subconscious mechanisms and may be advisable in certain cases before the seeker moves on to the difficult path of Sri Aurobindo's integral Yoga.

Though Sri Aurobindo was very much aware of the general characteristics of those levels which were studied by psychoanalysts, could it be that he sometimes missed the precise details of Freud's psychology? It is clear that the attitude of Sri Aurobindo to psychoanalysis is more negative than positive, while that of the transpersonal psychotherapists is more positive than negative.

Could it be that the transpersonal psychotherapist is in a better position to blend the Freudian psychoanalytic approach with a transpersonal framework than Sri Aurobindo might have been, given his negative assessment of psychoanalysis? Maybe the unconscious is as important as the superconscious. To concentrate only on the inner and higher centres all the time, ignoring the difference between the ultimate and the proximate, may lead to obsessive and rigid patterns. There are different levels of our being and development, and maybe the seeker needs to work- on each of them at different times according to one's needs, rather than claiming one as the best. For some individuals in whom the lower forms of consciousness are blocking development, it is essential to know something about these lower unconscious processes in order to progress. But those seekers who are reasonably healthy may fully progress without excessively analysing past traumatic childhood experiences. These events do have an impact on the seeker, but with his or her determination, the seeker can move beyond them without reliving them.

One of the essential goals to be attained by the sadhak of integral Yoga is a certain change of consciousness, the spiritual change, and it is this change of the mind, heart and will which is obstinately resisted by the sadhak's ignorant nature. Sri Aurobindo advises the sadhak to look quietly at the resistance, detect its cause, acknowledge it, see its workings, reject it and call down the Power and Light from above for its removal. Sri Aurobindo is more or less aware of the problems described by Freud regarding the various defence mechanisms. He writes; "For the mind and vital will always find tricks and excuses for prolonging their own reign, imposing their likes and dislikes."[29] To get out of these imaginary obstacles, he continues; "It is why we [in integral yoga] always express depreciation of mental constructions and vital formulations—because they are the defence-works mind and vital throw up against their capture by the Divine ... The secret is to be firm in knocking it all down and making a *tabula rasa*, a foundation of calm, peace, happy openness for the true building."[30]

Sri Aurobindo is also aware of the frequent re-emergence of unconscious material into the conscious mind, but one of the preliminary goals of sadhana is to facilitate the development of the transcendence of the ego, and the eruption of unconscious material is only a secondary by-product of the practice. Sri Aurobindo prefers the surrender to the mysterious workings of the divine Grace in the individual, an action from above or from within, which decides its own movement. In the end, by a constant will and aspiration for change, the divine Grace can be brought down even into the body, where it can penetrate the subconscient also, and convert its resistance. But such a divine intervention seems psychologically vague, as the divine Grace is often working from behind and until the clouds vanish, making way for sunshine, the seeker is advised to insist quietly on the Light and wait in faith for it to come. According to Sri Aurobindo, "The state of grace is often prepared by a long tapasya [spiritual effort by concentrating the will to conquer the lower nature] or purification in which nothing decisive seems to happen... and it comes suddenly without a warning."[31] In integral Yoga, the first touches of the Divine Grace may rouse repressed appetites of the unregenerate nature which have to be eliminated. But the elimination of these repressed appetites is not the annihilation of the energy that impels it, but the egoistic force it takes. Once the egoistic moulds are dissolved, the force and the energy that feeds them can then be offered to the Divine, i.e., desires and hidden impulses are offered to the Divine for purification and transformation. Desires may continue to rise, but they need to be observed with equanimity, neither be neglected nor indulged, and offered to the transforming light of the Divine Grace.

An action from the Divine Grace is incalculable, it is

a power superior to any rule, even to the Cosmic Law, and its movement is not dependent on mental causes; it may sometimes bring apparently undeserved fruits, but the seeker cannot demand Grace as a right. For Sri Aurobindo, "Grace works in its own mysterious way, at first it works behind the veil, preparing things, not manifesting. Afterwards it may manifest but the sadhak does not understand very well what is happening; finally, when he is capable of it, he both feels and understands or at least begins to do so."[32] One cannot demand or compel Grace, "Grace is something spontaneous which wells out from the Divine Consciousness as a free flow of its being. The bhakta [the practitioner of the devotional path] looks for it, but he is ready to wait for it in perfect reliance—even if need be all his life— knowing that it will come, never varying in his love and surrender because it does not come now or soon... Length of time is no proof of an ultimate incapacity to arrive; it is only a sign that there is something in oneself which has to be overcome."[33] The miracle of Grace can come after years and years of flat failure and difficulty or terrible struggles, but it comes usually that way—as opposed to a slowly developing Grace—after much difficulty and not at once. Thus Grace comes of itself, intervening suddenly or with an increasing force, when all is ready.

Moreover, the descent of the Divine Grace has its own dangers. If the obscure mind or impure vital desire tries to use the descending Force for its own limited ideas or egoistic impulses, the sadhak can not escape suffering or other psychological obstacles. Could it be that, instead of waiting all one's life for the incalculable Grace which comes often as a response to a long and persistent course of sadhana *rightly* done, i.e., surrender to the Divine instead of surrender to one's egoistic attachments, that the transpersonal psychotherapist may be an expedient means of avoiding the danger of a preoccupation with an artificially created, enlarged ego-experience or with the bland euphoric enthusiasm of a self-induced state of pseudo-spirituality which counterbalances the inner call? After all, when the sadhak is in close contact with the divine Grace, all one's difficulties are not thrown aside. The Divine does not guaranty the sadhak against future misfortunes, and is the transpersonal psychotherapist not in a better position to establish a sufficiently stable foundation as a preparation for the development of a yogic consciousness, in which the divine Grace is allowed to work in the deeper roots of the individual's inner nature by removing obstructing unconscious resistances?

As mentioned before, it seems that the psychological aspects of Sri Aurobindo's metaphysical vision are based on his practice of integral Yoga only and are not always applicable to the present-day developments of clinical psychology or contemporary applied psychology.

PSYCHOPATHOLOGY AND THE ROLE OF CONSCIOUSNESS-FORCE

The increasing development of various scientific techniques and scientific achievements indicate that man lives in a completely different world as half a century ago. The data of psychological research go on changing in a rapid succession, and the question may be raised, where does Sri Aurobindo's metaphysical Yoga psychology stand in the face of the results of modern psychological development and research.

Sri Aurobindo's metaphysical views cannot always be placed on the same level as the present-day facts of actual experience and therefore call for some explanation. Though his metaphysical revelations are based on immediate perception and are not fully explicable in rational terms yet they must not contradict reason, as reason is aided by metaphysical revelations.

(I) Illness Due to Yoga

For Sri Aurobindo there exists a relation between health and the various planes of consciousness, and an illness of the body is always related to the expression of a break in equilibrium due to the disharmony, imbalance or wrong movement of the workings within or between the different parts of the being. As a result, there arises an incapacity to receive the descending Force. For Sri Aurobindo "all ill-health is due to some inertia or weakness or to some resistance or wrong movement there, only it has sometimes a more physical and sometimes a more psychological character."[34] In each case the cure of an illness requires finding its cause, either internal or external, and re-establishing the harmony through the light of the purifying spiritual Force. When the disturbance is the result of a movement in Yoga, then it is related to an inner difficulty in the sadhak's spiritual life. The outer phenomena may be similar to those who don't practice Yoga, but for those who practice sadhana the causes of disequilibrium are of a different nature. One of the main causes is related to the descending Force which acts upon many different lines and its results depend on the nature that receives it. According to Sri Aurobindo, "All illnesses are obviously due to the imperfect nature of the body and the physical nature. The body can be immune only when it is open to the higher consciousness and the latter can descend into it."[35] Rapid progress in one part of the being which is not accompanied by the same progress in other parts produces disharmony which manifests itself as illness. However, the sources of an illness are manifold, each can have a multitude of causes but it always indicates where the weak part of the being is.

There are two ways of curing an illness spiritually; one consists in dynamic faith in the Divine Force and, in other cases, if the body lacks receptivity, the seeker analyses the inner psychological state which has brought about the illness and acts on that. Nevertheless, removal of the psychological roots of ill health can be done only by a total enlightenment of the different parts of the being from the unifying Divine Force.

Ken Wilber relates physical illness to his four quadrant model; every physical event has at least four dimensions. The individual's interior states (subjective factors) are intimately related to the cause and cure of physical illness, but individual consciousness is also inextricably embedded in shared cultural values and worldviews, i.e., illnesses cannot be defined without reference to a shared cultural background. Ken Wilber's medical model attempts to understand the multi-level nature of disease and its cure by adding the emotional, mental and spiritual levels of the medical model.

(II) Psychological Health in Integral Yoga

Disturbances in the upward, inward and downward movements along the hierarchies of consciousness may create certain forms of disease. Illness, as a disharmony at any plane of consciousness, manifests itself ultimately in the physical plane and healing, to be effective, has to act on this level. Sri Aurobindo describes how illness manifests at three levels, as follows:

(a) The physical level of consciousness also has, besides its gross material part—the inert and subconscient earthly and bodily-physical as experienced by the outward senses—a subtle physical part with a subtler luminous consciousness called body consciousness, a consciousness which can act independently of the mental will. According to Sri Aurobindo, "in matters of health and illness for instance ... the body acts on its own and is not a servant of the mind ... there is a body-consciousness which can do things at the mind's order, but has to be awakened, trained, made a good and conscious instrument. It can even be so trained that a mental will or suggestion can cure the illness of the body."[36]

(b) The vital level, as the seat of desire, is the source of conflicting emotions such as anger, fear, depression and anxiety. Forceful repression or overindulgence of these vital desires may be the cause of disharmony. The vital plane of consciousness is characterised by the life-energy, a source of energy that supplements the material energy of the physical plane. The vital energy itself has a creative impulse and a lack of this life energy is another cause of ill-health. However, a gradually controlled, purified and transformed vital, through the synthetic integrative principle of the psychic being, functions as an effective will for inner progress, which ultimately leads to the Bliss aspect of Sachchidananda.

(c) The mental level is able to creatively master the world, but is also the source of man's greater maladies. Through mental discipline and self-reflection the mind can improve its thought-power, which furthers the possibility of thought-control, through which the mind can separate itself from its thought- patterns to take the witness attitude. In integral Yoga the mind itself cannot wholly resolve all kinds of mental conflicts; it is the supra-rational faculties of knowledge such as intuition, revelation, and inspiration which are able to resolve mental conflicts through the process of sublimation and transformation. "Illness has come as something that has to be past through ... for illness is a deformation of the physical nature just as lust, anger, jealousy, etc., are deformations of the vital nature and error and prejudice and indulgence of falsehood are deformations of the mental nature. All these things have to be eliminated and rejection is

> the first condition of their disappearance while acceptance has a contrary effect altogether."[37]

If 'all life is yoga', then, can practising sadhana also lead to psychopathological conditions? Sri Aurobindo does not elaborate extensively on the psychopathological disturbances which occur in the lower realms, as he is more concerned with the development of the higher and inner realms. While doing so he does describe, in detail, various forms of psychospiritual pathologies which may come up during the process of sadhana, but these psycho-spiritual pathologies are only related to spiritual development. Could it be that Sri Aurobindo overlooked the fact that problematic behaviour is also determined by the social conditioning of the environment, inherited parental conditions and the enormous influence of genetics, which play an important role in the individual's development?

The Western psychotherapeutic approach considers a breakdown of ego-functions due to inner conflicts or environmental factors as one of the main causes of psychopathology. For Sri Aurobindo, psychopathology is often related to a withdrawal from the world of external reality which is mostly facilitated by too intense a concentration upon oneself and, as a consequence, the individual sinks into the vital part of one's being. The vital world is full of conflicting emotions, greed, anger, etc.

For Sri Aurobindo, the physical mind is responsible for compulsive neurosis, as it is connected with repetitive thoughts and customary old movements. However, obsessivive neuroses can also be traced to the blind and chaotic action of the subconscient elements of our being. All kinds of lust, greed, fear which stem from the subconscious need not be suppressed but faced with an attitude of detachment and perfect equanimity. An active life presents every oppertunity for all the lower energies of nature to come up to the surface. All hidden impulses and desires which invade the being have to be faced and conquered by a mental control when the seeker is not in touch with the highjer spiritual forces

Depression occurs generally in the vital and is often a sign of acute egoism, which lacks receptivity to the divine forces. Sri Aurobindo is aware that it is impossible to escape from depression, almost all sadhaks go through these attacks. It is not easy to overcome depression because it is ingrained in the human vital and difficult to throw out. "The rule in yoga is not to let the depression depress you, to stand back from it, observe its cause and remove the cause; for the cause is always in oneself, perhaps a vital defect somewhere, a wrong movement indulged or a petty desire causing a recoil, sometimes by its satisfaction, sometimes by its disappointment."[38]

Depression is like an illness to which the body consents from habit and from belief in the illness even though it suffers from it. If the vital mind withdraws its consent and refuses to be dominated by the habitual suggestions, then the recurrences of depression may ease. The seeker should react against fits of depression and not allow them by any kind of mental encouragement to persist or grow chronic.

Depression cuts the sadhak off from the light of the divine Power and prevents the Force from flowing through. According to Sri Aurobindo "If there are always forces around which are concerned to depress and discourage, there are always forces, above and around us which we can draw upon,—draw into ourselves to restore, to fill up again with strength and faith and joy and the power that perseveres and conquers. It is really a habit that one has to get of opening to these helpful forces and either passively receiving them or actively drawing upon them—for one can do either."[39]

By choosing for the Divine, the seeker receives an inner confidence and certitude in which one has the courage to stand face to face against any obstacle. So in order to control depression, the sadhak is advised to get out of the vital and enter into a deeper consciousness which has the power to drive away the depression. By the discipline of sadhana and a total confidence in the divine Grace the sadhak can overcome and lose the habit of depression.

(III) Psychopathology and the role of Consciouness Force

It seems clear by now that for Sri Aurobindo the cure for psychopathological symptoms requires a shift of consciousness. Those whose consciousness is turned inwards and upwards need less external support and respond more easily to inner means. In the awakening of the inner and higher realms of being, there is a more subtle energy which is able to change the whole meaning of the healing process. This subtle spiritual Consciousness-Force, beyond the outer instrumental personality, supports the whole of man's psychological complexity, and in integral Yoga the seeker aims at becoming aware of this secret spiritual Force, to bring it to the foreground and activate its healing powers, as it is the source of health.

For Sri Aurobindo this world is nothing but a play of force, or energy, a mind-energy, life-energy and energy in matter, but there is also a spiritual force behind all other forces from which they originate, a Divine Force above, which can be used as a force for purification, illumination and transformation. Nature, as the outer or executive side of the Consciousness-Force, forms and moves the world. This outer side appears to be a play of gross forces, but behind it is the living consciousness and the Force of the Divine, i.e., the Divine *Shakti.* By a spiritual evolution man becomes less subject to the lower Nature and gradually establishes a contact with the higher Nature. By an ascent into it, it can activate its descent into the seeker and this double process is able to transform the lower nature.

The action of the Force does not exclude the need for

sadhana, its action comes rather as an answer or help to sadhana. This does not mean that it sometimes acts without sadhana, it may give a response in those who do not seem to be ready. However, usually it does not act like that, as it is not a physical force that acts in the same way on everybody, but a spiritual Force whose action cannot be reduced to mechanical rules.

This Divine Force is the original source and other forces are derived from it, i.e., the Divine Force uses them as instruments. In this way the invisible Divine Force can produce mental, vital and physical results, it can "alter the mind, develop its powers, add new ones, bring in new ranges of knowledge, master the vital movements, change the character, influence men and things, control the conditions and functioning of the body, work as a concrete dynamic Force on other forces, modify events, etc., etc... However, it is not a Power that acts without conditions and limits. The conditions and limits under which yoga and sadhana has to be worked out are not arbitrary or capricious."[40]

The Yogic or Divine Force works according to a certain law and under certain conditions, and in man this Force acts according to the nature of one's instrument. Man is a complex living instrument and if the seeker has the capacity and develops responsiveness, then the Force can work perfectly. It is for this reason that Sri Aurobindo insists on the perfection of the instrument so that its lack of receptivity need not block the Force. The powers of mind, life and body have their limitations and cannot rise above their natural ultimate limits. However, the lower instrumentation can open itself to what is beyond and call down a supramental Power to work in the seeker. Thus Sri Aurobindo observes that, "If the supramental Power is allowed by man's discerning assent and vigilant surrender to act according to its own profound and subtle insight and flexible potency, it will bring about slowly or swiftly a divine transformation of our fallen and imperfect nature."[41]

Integral Yoga can succeed only if there is a complete willingness to let the Divine Power, as it descends, do with the seeker whatever is needed for the work that has to be done. For Sri Aurobindo it is due to Yogic consciousness that, "illness can be repelled from one's own body or cured, even chronic or deep-seated illnesses and long-established constitutional defects remedied or expelled."[42]

As pharmacological therapeutic agents are used at the energy level of the outermost physical consciousness, so can more subtle treatments like acupuncture and homeopathy be applied to life-energy of the vital plane. On the mental plane of consciousness various forms of psychotherapy combined with some simple meditation techniques can be effective to awaken hidden forces veiled behind the mind. However, in integral Yoga these therapeutic techniques when applied to the surface level of consciousness need to be supplemented by the extension of the seeker's inner and higher yogic consciousness to effectuate a complete healing process. It is this greater inner individual and Universal Divine pranic force which supplies and sustains all one's physical, vital and mental activities. According to Sri Aurobindo, "This pranic force we can use for any of the activities of life, body or mind with a far greater and effective power than any that we command in our present operations, limited as they are by the physical formula. The use of this pranic power liberates us from that limitation to the extent of our ability to use it in place of the body-bound energy. It can be used so to direct the Prana as to manage more powerfully or to rectify any bodily state or action, as to heal illness and to liberate an enormous amount of mental exertion and play of will or knowledge. The exercises of Pranayama are the familiar mechanical means of freeing and getting control of the pranic energy."[43]

The greatest obstacle to the action of the Divine Force is the ego-sense and in order to overcome the limitations of the ego, Sri Aurobindo emphasises the replacement of the ego by the psychic being; the latter is able to free the action of the pranic force from the ego. Once the psychic being comes to the foreground and when simultaneously the knowledge of the workings of the force is developed, it not only heals all sorts of illnesses but also functions as an opportunity for psychological growth. For Sri Aurobindo, it is only the psychic or spiritual Force that is able to recreate a perfect harmony and proper functioning of the entire being.

If "Yoga is nothing but practical psychology"44, then it must also deal with psychological disturbances, which are the subject-matter of clinical psychology. When referring to the state of psychological health Sri Aurobindo relates this state to the development of the psychic inmost part of the being, which supports and purifies the outer nature. However, when viewed in the context of psychotherapeutic language of psychological health, could it be that Sri Aurobindo's integral Yoga lacks a detailed analysis and understanding of clinical psychopathology and may, therefore, not be effective for reducing psychopathological symptoms?

The discovery of the psychic being is considered of utmost importance as it is the psychic being, the psychological center of truth, love and beauty that controls and guides the individual's destiny. For Sri Aurobindo, the psychic being , as the true integrating principle, is free from psychological disturbances and the centrality of the psychic being is, therefore, the basis of psychological health and growth. The means for its attainment are not based on the fulfilment of cravings—external or internal— and the avoidance of aversions, but on the control, rejection and, finally, transformation of them. But for the clinical psychologist the question arises that, if a person lacks contact with or development of the psychic being, does this mean that the same person is psychologically immature?

Sri Aurobindo elaborates extensively on the psychological problems related to the various parts of the being, but all these psychological disturbances are signs or different forms of an exacerbated egoistic state. He could not have been aware of today's development in neuro-physiological psychology, including brain-research and neuropharmacology. Psychopathology may be a physiological dysfunction, and certain classes of depression, thought disorders, uncontrolled anger, etc., are partially curable by pharmacological agents. The underlying root-idea is based on the assumption that each specific psychopathology has a specific physiological correlate and can, therefore, be modified with the treatment of a pharmacological agent.

Certain aspects of human behaviour can very well be understood in neurological terms even though a sufficient explanation for consciousness cannot be given in neurophysiological terms. For Sri Aurobindo, there must be non-material, psychospiritual principles to satisfactorily explain the fact of direct intuitive experience of the individual's self-awareness and one's capacity for making conscious decisions. Consciousness has the capacity to function as a witness of all various processes that take place in the individual's psychophysical system, i.e., the witnessing function of consciousness is able to establish the individual's freedom from psychophysical determinism. Sri Aurobindo maintains that freedom from psychological disturbances can be attained only by developing a higher state of consciousness beyond the physical, vital and mental consciousness.

But is it only the lack of or increase in Consciousness-Force which determines psychological changes or are there other forces which determine behaviour? Did Sri Aurobindo fully integrate biochemical predispositions and genetic neurophysiological factors as mediators of mental change? The use of tranquillisers often reduces disorderly thought processes and behaviour, which proves that these symptoms are biochemically related. Neuroscientific research in brain-related disorders, both neurological diseases and mental illnesses, has shifted from the mind to the brain, and the biological basis of mental disorders has been firmly established.

Could physiology possibly develop in such a way that along with chemistry it can explain *some* of the psychological laws which determine behaviour and thus become capable of explaining in physical terms *some* of the events of psychospiritual processes?

Sri Aurobindo's detailed map of consciousness often denigrates important physical aspects of mental disorders, but his spiritual vision should not contradict physical facts. The medical model has proved that the physical body does not only respond to metaphysical forces which can be manipulated by the practice of integral Yoga. A mental disorder may be due to the influence of inherited predispositions, genetic components, traumatic arrests, biological drives, or a distorted complexity of the brain. Modern clinical and biotechnological research has proved that genetic, anatomic and metabolic processes are related to altered states of consciousness. Genetic predispositions, brain disorders and stresses in adulthood are the three main causes that render the individual vulnerable to psychotic states of consciousness. They cannot always be explained away by karmic principles and reincarnation.

Norepinephrine, dopamine, serotonin and other complex molecules (neurotransmitters) are engaged in chemical reactions that affect moods, thoughts and emotions. Physically altering the brain changes subjective experiences, but simultaneously life experiences, mental events and spiritual practices also have their impact on the brain which, in turn, affects the neurotransmitters. Molecular biology has learned us much about our origination. At the moment scientists have much more detailed knowledge about genes and are able to determine the genome sequention. Through gentechnology scientists have discovered the causes of many heredity diseases.

Though healing takes place through the medium of consciousness—consciousness as a primary force that interacts with the brain and mind—there are also anatomical and chemical strata which influence the healing processes of the human mind. Neurophysiology and neurochemistry are significant matters and cannot be treated as unimportant manifestations in the transcendent reality. It seems clear that the transcendental experience of divine Bliss is not an experience of the Spirit alone, but also involves the body, the nervous system and influences the cerebral matter of the brain of the sadhak: they are all inextricably interwoven. Did Sri Aurobindo underestimate the correlation (but not its reduction) of transcendental Divine Consciousness with the organic biomaterial brain and the empirical organism?

If the mystical experience is only an encounter of Spirit with incorporeal Divinity, then it leaves aside the state of physical health, mental disposition and the environment of the sadhak, which do colour the mystical experience. Patanjali's yoga, for example, assumes that the spiritual realm can be controlled by the material, i.e., bodily mastery can be used for spiritual attainment. In *Hatha* **and** *Raja Yoga* sadhana is done through the body and the mind, and the psychodynamic therapists, like Patanjali, discovered the impact of the physical on the non-physical; changes in physical and mental attitudes can bring about a change in spiritual values. For the transpersonal psychotherapist the lower physical aspects are understood as contributing to the realisation of the seeker's higher aspirations. Self-analysis and individual effort are some of the important means of healing psychological disorders.

Sri Aurobindo is not so much concerned with the

clinical presentation of spiritually based phenomena, but for the transpersonal therapist a clinical presentation of such phenomena seems essential to avoid misdiagnosing of the suffering seeker. For Sri Aurobindo, a psycho-spiritual framework within a clinical setting leaves out a fully developmental metaphysical grounding, i.e., the Divine within, in its individual, universal and transcendental aspects. He assumes that spiritual experiences such as the cosmic or supramental realisations leave their influence on the physical as well as the mental level and, more than that, these experiences have some degree of power over these levels. Sri Aurobindo does not deny the biological and physiological factors in psychopathology, but affirms that these factors need to be transformed by the inner and higher spiritual realm. However, in doing so, he appears to subtly denigrate these factors as if they were lower, less significant aspects in the transcendent reality.

Although not denying the reality of psychopathology but giving it only a subordinate status, could it be that Sri Aurobindo, unlike the transpersonal psychotherapist, failed to turn various forms of psychopathology into inner teachings, as John A. Nelson did in *Healing the Split?* It may therefore be questioned whether or not Sri Aurobindo fully succeeded in establishing the all-comprehensive and integral character of his yoga psychology.

Did Sri Aurobindo bypass the meaning, purpose and richness of psychopathology to the soul in the inward and upward spiritual journey of the sadhak? Why are psychopathological phenomena not instrumental to the development of a divine life? For Sri Aurobindo human dissatisfaction is necessary to the evolution of a divine life. Could untoward psychopathological phenomena, therefore, not serve as one of the stepping-stones toward the divine life? Sri Aurobindo assumes that psychopathological phenomena are in the end only apparent and transitional, but could it be that such a view overlooks the instrumental value of these phenomena? Psychopathology can function as a motivator for and initiating force in the discovery of new frontiers of growth.

Psychopathological distress, therefore, need not always be classified as undesirable or treated as a curse, these critical life experiences have the potential for behavioural change and may be used in the service of spiritual development. But Sri Aurobindo does not want the sadhak to dwell on these psychopathological events, as analysis of them may lead to fragmentation rather than integration into the higher. Ultimately, the Divine is in the centre of the lotus, not in the mud of psychopathological symptoms. However, no theory of Integral Psychology can be complete without taking into account the entire spectrum of human behaviour. Does Sri Aurobindo's metaphysical Yoga psychology overemphasise the importance of mystical experiences? If we are to arrive at a better understanding of human nature, then psychopathological phenomena should not be underestimated. These phenomena are as real and valuable as spiritual processes, they are both ways of finding the soul and part of the divine manifestation. The Spirit cannot be pathogenic, this is confined only to the psyche, but is denying or underestimating the role of psychopathology in the process of transcendence, without a recognition of the psychopathological tendencies that reside in the psyche, not in itself pathological.

KEN WILBER ON PSYCHOPATHOLOGY

For Ken Wilber, consciousness is pluridimensional and pathology can and does occur at any level. Each of the different schools of Western psychotherapy primarily addresses a different level of the spectrum of consciousness. In his spectrum model of psychology, the self is faced with the task of differentiation and then integration (fulcrum of self-development), at each major stage of development. If anything goes wrong at a given fulcrum (failure of differentiation), then it shows itself in the form of a specific corresponding type of pathology. In other words, a developmental "lesion" at a particular stage manifests itself as a particular type of psychopathology. Development may also proceed too fast, which may end up in dissociation (the contact with the preceding stages is lost); sometimes the succeeding levels do not include but repress or deny the lower stages, or the higher stages may get into the grip of the preceding lower stages. Pathological hierarchies may replace communication by domination or rationality may be used in irrational ways.

Each developmental fulcrum from the prepersonal to the personal to the transpersonal has its own characteristic pathology. Ken Wilber elaborates extensively on all the stages of human development, specifically on the infantile prepersonal stages and the psychopathologies that often result from complications at these early stages. He does not deny the importance of brain neurochemistry and developmental neurobiology in the genesis of psychopathology, but he also includes Freud's theory of previously repressed feelings which reappear in disguised forms as painful neurotic symptoms.

He asserts that psychological conflicts from earlier stages of growth can influence spiritual development, and contemplative practices may be used as a defence against neurotic tendencies. Western psychodynamic approaches have collected sufficient evidence to show that pathologies at these prepersonal stages are more related to the regression or resurgence of the prepersonal 'id' (preconscious harmony of paradise) than the intuitive realisation of the transpersonal God. Ken Wilber meaningfully differentiates psychopathological problems at the various levels of being and treats them as "different phenomena with very different treatment modalities."[45]

In *Integral Psychology,* he relates pathological development to his four quadrant model. All the quadrants mutually interact and an understanding of individual psychopathology needs to include all the levels of all the quadrants. In the words of Ken Wilber, "We are fast approaching an understanding that sees individual pathologies as but the tip of an enormous iceberg that includes self-stages, cultural worldviews, social structures, and spiritual access to depth.[46] Developmental psychopathology should not only focus on dysfunctional parenting or child abuse, but should also integrate biologically influenced models such as neuroscientific processes or genetic factors and psychosocial currents.

Sri Aurobindo's integral model of development does not pay much attention to differential diagnosis (i.e., the difference between spiritual emergency and psychose on the lower realms of being), as he is more concerned with the realms of the inner and higher being. His integral Yoga is a way of life for spiritual growth, whereas Ken Wilber's psycho-spiritual developmental model is also based on clinical concepts. But are concepts which pertain to the medical model appropriate when applied to the contemplative model of higher levels of consciousness? For Sri Aurobindo clinical concepts and spiritual development are two different orders and levels of development, and should not be confused with each other.

HEREDITY

In the Eastern views of life, karma implies a sort of metaphysical or psychic theory of heredity based on the hypothesis of rebirth. Psychic heredity, such as predispositions to disease, character traits, etc., need not always be reduced to physical aspects as maintained by natural science. Within certain limits the individual is free to choose; even heredity and environment are only elements that are provided by an All-seeing Intelligence to the free choice of the soul at every graded step of its evolution. It is the soul that initially chooses its own destiny in the future by means of karma. Sri Aurobindo relates heredity to samskaras— impressions of past habits which are stored up in the subconscious—and most of our predispositions and tendencies of reaction are from past lives.

He admits the utility of the scientific theory, which claims that genes and chromosomes are the cause of hereditary transmissions of physical and psychological variations, "but we do not discover how psychological characteristics can be contained and transmitted in this inconscient material vehicle. We do not see or know that a play of electrons, of atoms and their resultant molecules, of cells, chemical'secretions and physiological processes manages by their activity on the nerves and brain of a Shakespeare to produce a Hamlet.... These formulae of Science may be pragmatically correct and infallible, they may govern the practical how of Nature's processes, but they do not disclose the intrinsic how or why."[47] Sri Aurobindo contends that his metaphysical theory of Matter is necessary to understand how inconscient vehicles can perform such a function. As he observes, "There would be no difficulty either in understanding on this principle how infinitesimals of a material character like the gene and the chromosome can carry in them psychological elements to be transmitted to the physical form that has to emerge from the human seed ... for we see that the subconscient physical carries in it a mental psychological content, impressions of past events, habits, fixed mental and vital formations, fixed forms of character, and sends them up by an occult process to the waking consciousness, thus originating or influencing many activities of our nature."[48]

For Sri Aurobindo, the terrestrial evolution of Nature has a double process: (1) the scientific visible physical evolution with birth as its machinery, in which each body is maintained through its heredity, and (2) the invisible spiritual soul evolution with rebirth into ascending grades of forms and consciousness as its machinery. He agrees with the scientific theory of heredity as a life-evolution process for keeping a type of species in unchanged being, but he questions if it is also an instrument for progressive variation. It is one thing that a type can vary within its own specification, but it is quite another thing that a type can go beyond it. There must be other forces than variations in physical heredity at work in bringing about new characteristics, and for Sri Aurobindo there are invisible life forces and psychological forces at work, responsible for variations in Nature.

Sri Aurobindo accepts the principle of hereditary variation, but for him the existence of different grades or types of Being are all due to the Force of consciousness in the material universe rather than the different results of the cumulative influence of hereditary variations. The creation of various types cannot be framed *exclusively* in terms of heredity. The process of evolution need not be mere mechanical, and typal variation is successfully brought about by the Force of Consciousness. The course of evolution cannot be explained without teleology and Sri Aurobindo interpretes the evolution of man with the idea of purposeful evolution.

He regards the process of evolution as fundamentally a revelation of higher powers of consciousness, and only secondarily as a development of more complex biological forms. Sri Aurobindo agrees that Western science has done quite a lot to explain the facts of material evolution but it has neglected the evolution of consciousness. According to him, "A theory of spiritual evolution is not identical with a scientific theory of form-evolution and physical life-evolution; it may accept the scientific account of physical evolution as a support or an element, but the support is not indispensable. The scientific theory is concerned only with the outward and visible machinery and process, with the physical development of things in Matter and the law of development of Life and Mind in Matter; its account of the process may have to be considerably changed or may be dropped altogether in the light of new discovery, but that will not affect the self-evident fact of a spiritual evolution, an evolution of Consciousness, a progression of the soul's manifestation in material existence."[49]

Sri Aurobindo maintains that consciousness is the centre of the entire evolutionary process expressing itself in material form. When the organisation of matter comes to a point of sufficient complexity, life emerges and begins to dominate matter, after which mind emerges and dominates life and matter. According to Sri Aurobindo, "If evolution is a truth and is not only a physical evolution of species, but an evolution of consciousness, it must be a spiritual and not only a physical fact. In that case, it is the individual who evolves and grows into a more and more developed and perfect consciousness and obviously that cannot be done in the course of a brief single human life. If there is the evolution of a conscious individual, then there must be rebirth. Rebirth is a logical necessity and a spiritual fact of which we can have the experience."[50]

For Sri Aurobindo, the scientific claims of heredity may account for our physical make-up, our temperament and vital peculiarities, but it fails to account for psychological phenomena of a higher kind such as genius or inborn faculty. Science will not be able to explain supraphysical phenomena by some physical fact or heredity; it extends a physical truth into the psychological field, i.e., science's theory of heredity forces its extended application of the physical truth into a basis for explaining the subtle complex phenomena of our psychological being.

In the inner reality of things, evolution has always had a spiritual significance and the physical change was only instrumental. According to Sri Aurobindo, "In the old Indian version of this theory, evolution, heredity and rebirth are three companion processes of the universal unfolding;

evolution the processional aim, rebirth the main method, heredity one of the physical conditions. That is a theory which provides at least the framework for a harmonious explanation of all the complex elements of the problem. The scientific idea starts from physical being and makes the psychical a result and circumstance of body; this other evolutionary idea starts from soul and sees in the physical being an instrumentation for the awakening to itself of a spirit absorbed in the universe of Matter."[51] This means that the body or the physical part of our life action is not only the result of biological heredity, there is also an assisting psychical cause (the law of karma), an evolutionary heredity which shapes the individual's temperament, character and predispositions.

Our present personality is bound by many things, by one's physical and vital heredity, environmental forces and ignorance. However, the soul, which is beyond our present personality, is not the result of our heredity, but has prepared by its own actions and affinities this heredity. According to Sri Aurobindo, "What is supremely important is what I make of all this surrounding and invading present and not what it makes of me ... I have created by my past Karma my own conditions and my relations with the life of others and the general Karma. That shapes my heredity, mv environment, my affinities, my connections, my material, my opportunities and obstacles ... and on this groundwork I build new Karma, enlarge experience, go on with my soul evolution."[52]

So, Sri Aurobindo acknowledges that there are many things in the body, and some in the mind and vital which are inherited from the parents, but there are other things that are peculiar to one's own nature or developed by the happenings of this life and not genetically inherited.

A CRITICAL ESTIMATE OF SRI AUROBINDO'S INTEGRALISM

As a special contribution to the present-day humanity, Sri Aurobindo's spiritual synthesis does not aim merely at uniting all the great spiritual disciplines and blending them into a vast harmony, it envisages much more and takes the whole being and nature of man as its field.

According to Arabinda Basu, "Sri Aurobindo's synthetic spirituality is two-fold; it is an integration within his own consciousness of the different elements of his being and nature and outside of himself, the establishing of a new pattern of relationship with his fellows based on an immediate and intimate knowledge of their being and nature which are equally manifestations of the integral Truth- Consciousness of which his own being and nature are formulations. Such a comprehensive conception of life can be easily seen to include all types of activity which man undertakes now. Economics and politics, commerce and industry, education and culture, art and craft of all kinds, physical perfection, purified vital expansion and enjoyment, intellectual development and enrichment; nothing need be excluded, indeed will certainly be included in a new integral life. However, it must be pointed out that these will not be conducted as now, that is, on the basis of Ignorance of the essential and active truth of things. It will not be mental but supermental."[53]

Sri Aurobindo found out that the solution of all human problems lay in the divinity latent in man and that the purpose of humanity is to discover this divinity and create a divine humanity. His integral Yoga aims at a radical change of consciousness and the transmutation of the whole earthly existence into something Divine. This idea behind Sri Aurobindo's philosophy of transformation and a divine life on earth is based on a metaphysical position. He assumes the positive presence of the Divine at every grade of our existence—physical, vital, mental. They all have the inherent potentiality of being transformed into divine elements, and it is not only the indwelling soul which aspires to be in touch with the Divine. The root of the philosophy of the Life Divine seems to be the search for the meaning and perfection of life. Sri Aurobindo's concept of a divine life is a metaphysical vision with a spiritual programme which makes it more than a mere theory. Each individual is urged to find one's own line of inner development within the broad framework of integral Yoga.

Sri Aurobindo's metaphysical vision gives the reader insight into his integralism, which refers to the acceptance and sublimation of the opposition between Matter and Spirit. However, after explaining Sri Aurobindo's contribution, some of his insights are challenged by various critics, but always in a meaningful perspective or a constructive way, giving a sympathetic overview of Sri Aurobindo's exceptional metaphysical vision.

If Sri Aurobindo's philosophical vision can be considered a *darshan,* a point of view, and be understood as *sadhana,* he would admit in the ultimate integration the validity of other points of view without combating them. This integration does not seek mere logical harmony or non-contradiction, but it also seeks accommodation for every opposing concept in the great system of ideas, i.e., it does not eliminate or exclude all that has significance in a wider sphere than its immediate context.

Does his metaphysical system admit certain limits of his own perspectives and the possibility of other viewpoints? Which place does postmodern understanding take in Sri Aurobindo's integral vision, i.e., does his integral synthesis allows for a radical plurality of perspectives? Sri Aurobindo has described human beings as complex creatures operating on many levels, but can a single vision of a future way of being encompass all that?

His theoretical and experiential views on a better understanding of the evolution of consciousness attempts to find an answer for a question for which there may never be a final answer. Evolution need not take place only through an inevitable sequence of unidimensional development. There may be also a multidimensional developmental course to different goals, for example described by R. Coan as, "there is more than one possible goal and no clear reason to contend that all of us as individuals must develop toward the same common psychic end.... We can distinguish a number of possible goals in the evolutionary process and that we probably need to recognize a still larger number of pathways leading to them."[54] He classifies five models of developmental goals—efficiency, creativity, inner harmony, relatedness and transcendence—and he uses these modes to explain the evolution of consciousness.

The thousands of souls who are thirsting for self-knowledge through Herculean labour may not all be aware of the confusion about the real nature of their thirst on account of a confused or disintegrated personality structure. Could it be that such seekers fall victim to deception due to improper guidance on the path? Could it be that without the living presence of a proper guide, their integral sadhana ends up in some form of hypocrisy when beliefs that were of value more than seventy five years ago are not transformed by the seeker into a lived experience? Could it be that out of the many who enter the path of integral Yoga only a few determined sadhaks may come out at its sunlit exit, whereas others might lose their way to their spiritual destiny in a chaotic labyrinth? May the seeker on the inward journey get lost when unconscious forces are unchained, or may one get engulfed during the process of sadhana by spiritual energies which the self is unable to integrate and as a consequence may cause psychological disturbances in the form of confusion and fear? Could it be that during the practice of sadhana the seeker avoids unconscious and defensive processes of the self, which may create later on some form of psychopathology or puffed-up egos? Did Sri Aurobindo overlooked the practitioner's unique psycho-spiritual dispositions? The practice of his integral discipline may not always conform his spiritual pathway and may not be suited for each follower. How to deal with this question when related to the present-day disciples where his guidance is merely based on a matter of faith?

Sadhana is very helpful in purifying and transforming the psychological dimension of the sadhak, but is spiritual practice alone sufficient to deal with and solve various deep-rooted psychological obstacles which, sooner or later bog down many sadhaks? No doubt, the practice of sadhana brings the seeker into greater union with the healing Divine Force, but does full connection with the Divine Force guarantee perfect mental health? The privileging of the divine Grace may be utilized to avoid direct encounters with repressive barriers, which as a consequence, limits the sadhak's ability to work through and integrate unresolved psychological conflicts. It is obvious that man differ in their capacities for spiritual development, and the discipline the sadhak has to undergo needs to be adjusted to this level of progress. Who is there to guide and check the sadhak in one's individual development besides the divine force of Grace?

Can transpersonal psychotherapy be helpful in skilfully navigating through these problematic inner psychological areas during the sadhak's search for one's soul within? Although transpersonal psychotherapy is probably helpful to the sadhak when the seeker is encountering psychological hang-ups during one's spiritual journey, this does not mean that transpersonal psychotherapy is absolutely necessary.

For Sri Aurobindo, a spiritual transformation includes a psychological transformation, but it is difficult to translate his metaphysical vision into contemporary transpersonal language. His metaphysical vision includes the practice of sadhana, and the resolution of various psychological difficulties occurs only when the seeker him or herself opens to the Divine Grace.

It is not always clear whether the crucial questions regarding Sri Aurobindo's psychological insights, which are raised by the transpersonal psychotherapist, are merely an apparent disagreement or whether the two visionaries are locked into different dynamics.

Sri Aurobindo's vision was originally transmitted only to those seekers who were seriously committed to the demanding discipline of sadhana at the Sri Aurobindo Ashram. To prevent easy access, the Mother (of the Ashram) had to be sure that an applicant was ready and inwardly prepared before admitting him or her into the Ashram.

.

In elaborating the spiritual changes in the divine life that he expects to occur in the future, Sri Aurobindo maintains that the worth of the emergence of such a divine life can be determined by the actual occurrence, though this future fulfilment may take millennia. Only time can tell. The spiritual changes which he predicts will occur through the seeker's effort, by the practice of sadhana, together with the descent of the Divine Grace. Each sadhak, by consciously participating in the spiritual evolution has some power to accelerate the realisation of the changes in humanity necessary for a divine life. The non-occurrence of these changes in the near future, either within the individual or in the collective humanity, may imply that the individual has failed in his or her yogic efforts. However, Sri Aurobindo emphasises the primary importance of the divine Grace which is almost exclusively responsible for the future spiritual evolution. Grace will act and bring results in its own time, provided the seeker rejects everything that stands in the way of the action of its transforming Force. But how long can an individual seeker rely and be dependent on Grace, without any pragmatic result in one's life? In encountering all the various difficulties while attempting to achieve some progress in sadhana, when the fruits of the sadhak's labour are denied, it seems unreasonable to rely on the divine Grace indiscriminately when this does not produce some pragmatic effects in the sadhak's life.

In Patanjali's Yoga or some form of Buddhist practices, liberation is achieved through one's own efforts with the help of intensive introspection and practice of discipline, without the mediation of the divine Grace. Mystical experiences in Patanjali's yoga system, for example, can be brought about through conscious human effort, discipline and training, asceticism and meditation, and need not be inspired by a divine Power.

Do Aurobindonians allow a high degree of critical thinking and analytical judgement in their spiritual life? In other words, does their sadhana involve critical reflection? Does it bring sound scholarship into the spiritual domain?

In Sri Aurobindo's integral Yoga the sadhak needs faith as a condition for one's sadhana and he warns the practitioners against doubt, insecurity, etc. But does this mean that he wants the sadhak to accept blindly, without being critical, his psycho-spiritual interpretations and evaluations? Indeed *initially,* the beginner needs to be receptive, give up one's intellectual attitude, and accept and surrender to his vision without questioning the grounds of his prescribed methods. Too many doubts in the initial stages will hinder the sadhak's ability to enter pathways. But what happens if the sadhak omits a critical judgment in the later stages of the sadhana? Can the same sadhak enter the new path as a sleep-walker, without gaining knowledge or insight? Sri Aurobindo's brilliant vision is often taken for granted as an explanation of the whole reality; his followers, with a lack of critical attitude and analysis, and without deeper knowledge, may fall back to copying and parroting his words, which finally may deteriorate Sri Aurobindo's vision into a rigid system of formulas. In such cases, sadhana becomes mechanical; the sadhak may not be ready to face the extreme difficulties in integral sadhana and the seeker is not able to apply Sri Aurobindo's spiritual practices and insights into one's day- to-day life.

Sri Aurobindo's metaphysical concepts and claims are a mental translation of his own powerful mystical experiences, and in his theoretical speculative intelligence he is mainly influenced by Indian spiritual traditions and English Romantic poets. In his positive conception of the destiny of the individual, he provides us a theory which explains in general how such a divine life might become possible in the future.

However, Sri Aurobindo does not always make a clear distinction between a metaphysical theory and a psychological fact in his metaphysical claims. Reason is not strong enough to provide the true metaphysical view unless it is supported by supramental Knowledge. Sri Aurobindo claims to possess significant extraordinary powers, and the facts of these supramental powers prove the evidence and reveal the essential nature of the Divine. He tries to incorporate scientific findings, but they get only pragmatic value, whereas he gives a special emphasis to the data of his mystic experiences.

Sri Aurobindo's creative achievement, integral Yoga, including the psychological aspects of his metaphysical vision, is mainly attributed to the practice of his yoga and scarcely to analytical study, empirical research and the force of logical argument.

For D.P. Chattopadhyaya, Sri Aurobindo's attempt "to develop a comprehensive philosophical theory of Reality and Society highlighting the integral character of the parts and the whole—individuals and society—and of everything with the rest of the world does not by itself establish the practical credibility of the theory. I am aware of the position taken by some followers of Sri Aurobindo claiming that Sri Aurobindo's views on related matters are truths of fact and should not be regarded as theories. Personally speaking I do not see how a particular view can claim immunity against rational criticism on the ground that it is based on the truth of facts."[55]

Though reason gets its due by playing an important role in man's quest for truth and justice, yet Sri Aurobindo often exposes the limitations as well as the hollowness of its lofty claims; the integral truth of things is truth not of reason but of spirit. Analytical and logical reason do not provide the inmost truth within us, they do not enable the human mind to get in direct touch with reality, which can be done only by the faculty of intuition. The pragmatic constructions of analytic reason play an important role in presenting us a clear picture for understanding external reality, but it does not make available the deepest truth of our life; for the purpose of finding out and realising the complex truth analytic reason seems inadequate. Nevertheless, philosophical articulation of the immediacy of yogic experience is needed for the communication of spiritual insights to others, and for scientific investigation with the facts of spiritual experience.

D.P. Chattopadhyaya is aware of Sri Aurobindo's objection to 'normal' reason due to its alleged association with sense perception and emotion, but he fears that "too much emphasis on supranormal reason or spiritual vision demands of man to believe in something for which he has neither good reason nor necessary experience at his disposal. Consequently, he feels obliged to fall back on faith, unsupportable belief, or some sort of authority."[56] He further observes that "One's commitment to an ideal and the difficulties involved in realising it should not lead one to pin one's faith in some metaphysical principle, 'ensuring' the practical success of the ideal within an undefined time-frame. For this metaphysical faith, although the expression of a noble sentiment, is hardly of any practical consequence."[57]

Could it be that questionable assumptions may be rationally preferable to unquestionable faith? D.P. Chattopadhyaya concludes that, "For scientific theory construction, bold and creative imagination is extremely important. An exclusive reliance on facts or what I have called fact-fetish is inconsistent with the very aim of science and other forms of rational inquiry ... both of them [K. Marx and Sri Aurobindo] have been accused of grand-theory construction and not of fact-fetish. One might even go a step further and say against Sri Aurobindo, in particular, that he refers to facts only in order to illustrate his theories and laws and not to establish them. One cannot fail to note that he is not a sterile inductivist. Certainly he cannot be accused of excessive reliance on empirical data ... when the critic says that his theory [any grand-theory or highly general laws] is purely speculative and not fair to facts, he *is* under a rational obligation to show the connection between his abstract theories and concrete facts. This exercise of relating the former to the latter at times turns out to be very difficult and delicate. For facts may refuse to confirm the theories and conform to the concepts used in these theories. In other words, some facts may really prove very 'awkward' and uncompromising."[58]

Ken Wilber's Integral psychology, with a metaphysical commitment is open to contemporary scientific inquiries which have factual content and is open to empirical verification. Ken Wilber's works contain extensive data collected through continuing research, and it is one of the reasons why he has been critisised; some of his empirical data are challenged by the different data and results from case material of other transpersonal researchers.

Is Sri Aurobindo's metaphysical vision able to

withstand the latest present-day discoveries in various fields of research? Are the followers of his vision able to take in certain contemporary ideas, and deal with them in a constructive manner without deconstructing the deeper content of his suggestions?

In his emphasis on unity, did he overlook empirical facts and logical consistency? Did he pay sufficient attention to the possibility of realising some of the Western views by means of Eastern techniques? Can mystical experiences in the spiritual realm only be interpreted with the help of supramental knowledge or can they also be partially interpreted with the help of the rational psychological analysis of processes such as conditioning, association, projection, cognitive development, learning, education and other environmental processes? The followers of Sri Aurobindo claim that they do not need the acknowledgement of the academic world, but does this mean that Sri Aurobindo's metaphysical psychology can omit an objective analysis which needs some empirical proofs for his claims? Could the disciples, in the initial stages, be more open to some of the scientific discoveries without being dependent on these discoveries, knowing that the spiritual dimension reveals itself, in the ultimate stages, in the inner realm of being? As a matter of fact, the dogmatism of many of Sri Aurobindo's devotees does not offer any new insight. A dogmatic approach to Sri Aurobindo's integral vision often implies that his integral practice is relatively impervious to debate. Such an attitude often prevents the freedom of the academic researcher to explore or investigate questions which are related to the relevance of Sri Aurobindo's vision to contemporary research. Sri Aurobindo did not want a cult, religion or system of belief. It is impossible to avoid entirely Sri Aurobindo's metaphysical assumptions, but should they be kept to a minimum? For those Aurobindonians who would like to remain faithful to the terminology of Sri Aurobindo's psychological insights and his metaphysical assumptions, they should be able to integrate the developments in other contemporary new fields of psychology.

According to this author, not much research work has been undertaken to inquire into the relevance of Sri Aurobindo's ideas in our present time, and the kindled and faith-frosted attitudes of the devotees of Sri Aurobindo are not making sufficient moves to rationally assess his ideas, as this may cause a fear that offends the divinity of Sri Aurobindo and his ideas. The devotees are grateful to Sri Aurobindo for giving them a faith in human unity, and one does not turn to the Guru to provide an adequate empirical substantiation for his metaphysical vision of spiritual transformation. Such attitude leaves hardly any scope to re-evaluate Sri Aurobindo's vision even while human understanding advances.

Sri Aurobindo's emphasis on yogic research through contemplative methods does not mean that his devotees can bypass the development of empirical scientific research. Sri Aurobindo nowhere denies the practical validity of such research, though he points out its limitations and its inadequacy in providing the seeker with spiritual oneness. However, before arriving at a new science with supraphysical certitudes, the sadhaks are advised to adhere to the rigorous methods of science (like Ken Wilber's three strands of actual practice, direct experience of data, and confirmation/rejection), but not to its purely physical instrumentation and external standards.

THE ASHRAM

The ashram was founded as "a centre and a field of practice for the evolution of another kind and form of life, which would be sustained by a higher consciousness and embody a full life of the Spirit."[59]

It was created to provide a place where individual seekers could work out a complete change of their nature.

The ashram was "to provide a secure atmosphere, a place and life apart, in which the consciousness of the individual might concentrate on its evolution in surroundings where all was turned and centred towards the one endeavour and, next, when things were ready, to formulate and develop the new life in those surroundings and in this prepared spiritual atmosphere. It might be that, in such a concentration of effort all the difficulties of the change would present themselves with a concentrated force; for each seeker carring in himself the possibilities but also the imperfections that has to be transformed, would bring in not only his capacities but his difficulties and the oppositions of the old nature and, mixed together in the restricted cycle of a small and close common life, these might assume a considerably enhanced force of obstruction which would tend to counterbalance the enhanced power and concentration of the forces making for the evolution. This is a difficulty that has broken in the past all the efforts of mental man to evolve something better and more true and harmonious than the ordinary mental and vital life. But if Nature is ready and has taken her evolutionary decision or if the power of the Spirit descending from the higher planes is sufficiently strong, the difficulty would be overcome and a first evolutionary formation or formations would be possible."[60]

The seekers in the ashram have opted to dedicate their lives completely to the practice of sadhana through integral Yoga, a synthesis of karma (action), bhakti (devotion), and jnana (knowledge) Yoga. There are general laws of discipline, but each individual is given the freedom to pursue one's sadhana according to that which is congenial to his or her temperament. The problem of transformation deals with all sorts of favourable and unfavourable elements and the sadhaks in the ashram, the laboratory of supramental yoga, are therefore representative of all quarters of life.

It is not easy to verify objectively Sri Aurobindo's claims of a divine life. It seems that the Ashram is still in the initial formative stages, where any kind of assessment is mainly based on faith. In the course of integral Yoga each plane of being has to be dealt with and people in the Ashram are not yet free in their outer selves from ego and wrong movements. The character of life in the ashram is different from the ordinary environment of life. When the sadhak enters this place, it often takes quite some time to be aligned with the main stream. During this period, the recalcitrant elements—egoism, revolt, etc.—come into reactionary play and they can persist for quite a long time. Other seekers may hand over the responsibility for their life to the Divine, in the supposition that the Divine will do all the work for them, without their needing to examine their own inner world. This is one of the main reasons why all sorts of difficulties arise and which explains much in the Ashram (and also in Auroville) that people do not expect there. Difficulties do not cease by coming here, but have to be faced and overcome. However, it is extremely difficult to overcome the forces which have controlled mankind for centuries. The old forces are not to be avoided but, on the contrary, have to come to the surface first, before they can be rejected, purified and transformed.

The Ashram sometimes faced difficult periods in its survival after the Mother left her body. Recently, on the 125th year of Sri Aurobindo's birth anniversary, an insider's personal view on Sri Aurobindo's ashram was published, after some negative publications appeared in the press regarding some serious conflicts within the ashram. For the author, Jugal Kishore Mukherjee, these problems are only transitionary and should not unduly discourage the sadhaks. He gives a forthright overview of the development of the ashram from the past up to the present, and its future prospects and destiny. In this essay, Mukherjee endeavours to answer various critical questions from students of the Sri Aurobindo International Centre of Education. Some of the questions were: "Is there any specific goal towards which the Ashram is moving, are the ashramites not slowly veering round the status of a religio-cultural community, and has the ashram outlived its value as a spiritual institution?"[61]

Mukherjee notices that "the real worth and importance of the ashram is not in its opulent eye-catching facade but in its common spiritual character.[62] He assumes that the ashram's constant growth is under the silent guidance of the divine conscious Force and the sadhak has to make sincere efforts to receive this Grace and collaborate in the work of each one's spiritual transformation- "A collective spiritual life--the goal of the ashram—is meant to express the spiritual and not merely the physical, vital or even the mental being of man; it has therefore to found and maintain itself on greater *values* than the mental, vital, physical values of ordinary human groupings." 63

He concludes that the main concern of the ashramites is related to their development of a spiritual consciousness, but in this process he warns the sadhak "not to be complacent in our attitude and allow things to drift on. On the one side we have to remember that the Ashram is an epitome of the human nature that has to be changed. On the other side we should not lapse into the indolent attitude, we need not bother; the Mother will do everything for us."[64]

The seekers in the Ashram are still on a path of preparation. The great adventure of transforming human consciousness and establishing this transformed consciousness in collective humanity is a great work which is still going on.

AUROVILLE, THE CITY OF HUMAN UNITY

The Ashram is the first step towards the acconiplishment of the creation of a new being and a new consciousness. Auroville is the next step, more exterior, where Aurovilians attempt to make a collective experiment for the progress of humanity; the experiment puts emphasis on the creation of a new type of society, which is based on human unity. Auroville is envisioned as consciously evolutionary and as the city of the twenty-first century for the twenty-first century man. Its citizens seek a new culture that is universal and integral through an experiment with the evolution of consciousness and its powers. This transcendental humanism involves full human development through the inner psychic and higher spiritual being. In its proper context, Auroville, like the Ashram, has to be seen in its spiritual character, i.e., the transformation of earth life through the descent of the supramental consciousness in matter and the beginning of a new spiritualised collectivity based thereon.

It is difficult, sometimes even impossible, to understand the meaning of the global experiment called Auroville. To give an objective view of what is happening in Auroville raises a serious problem, as it tries to achieve something that has never existed before. The description of the state of the community at present can only be an outward gaze, a half-light, sometimes even a false light, yet an attempt can be made at the evaluation of the present state of the community even though opinions about this state differ widely amongst Aurovilians themselves. It is obvious that the ideas about the multi-faceted character of Auroville, as expressed by this author, do not represent the views of the entire community. Auroville, as a growing international township, attempts to find an answer to the global pressure for change. The Aurovilians represent one conscious section of humanity which is ready to offer its energy for the realisation of a 'city the Earth needs'. Their work towards the growth of a new life and the acceleration of the process of evolution is a continuous research work which is not effected by merely mystical means, as it is by life itself that the Divine has to be discovered. Auroville has nothing to do with religion, dogma or ideology. It is a place where Aurovilians aim at an integral change of consciousness and a change of institutional, social, educational, economic and organisational patterns. The Mother—who, in 1926 took up the full charge of the Ashram when Sri Aurobindo retired into seclusion —launched the project of Auroville in 1968, and described the universal township as "a place where man can live away from all national rivalries, social conventions, self-contradictory moralities and contending religions; a place where human beings, freed from all slavery to the past, can devote themselves wholly to the discovery and practice of the Divine Consciousness that is seeking to manifest. Auroville wants to be this place and offers itself to all who aspire to live the Truth of tomorrow."[65]

The town is being developed around four fundamental aspects of man's activities, i.e., the residential, industrial, cultural and international zones. These zones are separated more in theory than in practice. At the centre stands the Matrimandir, the Soul of Auroville, that "wants to be the svmbol of the Divine's answer to man's aspiration for perfection, union with the Divine manifesting in a progressive human unity." The various functions of life are all integrated in the unique purpose of the city. All sorts of activities are represented or aimed at in Auroville and include environmental regeneration, industrial growth, organic agriculture, educational research, including body awareness, physical training and sports, alternative healing, village development, economic self-sufficiency, artistic creativity of all kinds, architectural designing, appropriate building technology, alternative energy sources and business enterprises. But the products of the outward manifestations do not offer clear and polished results, and do not change Auroville's unsettled nature.

The basic structure of Auroville is based on a synthesis of spiritual and material life. As a spiritual community, Auroville attempts to combine spirituality with modern technology and science; in their synthesis, inner spiritual and outer scientific knowledge serve each other. This town as a model of integral living intends to actualise a new man who forms the basis of a new society; all the problems of human unity find their solution in the levels of consciousness beyond the mind. A unity of mankind can therefore not be long lasting, if it is based on the compulsions of economic, social, technological or political needs. The solution of contemporary problems requires a sounder foundation in the deeper psychological needs of man, i.e., a new knowledge and deeper exploration of consciousness not undertaken by mankind so far. However, all the external means should not be abandoned, but transformed and made to serve the Divine Consciousness. A genuine human unity becomes possible only if the citizens of Auroville move towards the realisation of the divine Reality that we are all One. It is this secret Spirit and not the ego which will become the centre of all life through the emergence of a new consciousness. This new consciousness is able to transform humanity and its life on earth. Auroville, as a laboratory for the materialisation of this new consciousness, has been created for those seekers who want to surrender their ego and who want to develop their inner and higher spiritual being. Aurovilians are not in Auroville to fall back into their old habits, desires, and an easy life; life in Auroville means an almost superhuman effort, aspiration, sincerity and surrender for the divinisation of man.

Auroville gets a lot of publicity about its external developments, but not much is known about the inner spiritual development that its citizens are seeking through these externalities. The external development need not always reflect a new consciousness and forces of the old world, from egoism to spiritual dogmatism, are still rampant in Auroville like anywhere else in the world. These old manifesting forces have to be encountered and dealt with fully in the initial stages, before they can be transformed.

A brochure on Auroville describes this situation as follows: "it's not easy to live in Auroville, in spite of its comparative lushness during the winter months. It's not just the climate, nor the sensory and emotional overload, nor the galloping entropy that causes almost everything to fall apart very quickly. Nor is it merely that Auroville reflects so many of the negative trends—politics, money, power, manipulation, small-town gossip, etc.—that exist everywhere else. It's more to do with the fact that everybody who comes to live here seems to be confronted, sooner or later, with difficulties on a scale and of an intensity rarely experienced before. ... What's going on? At first sight it appears inexplicable. Here is a place dedicated to the highest ideals which appears to magnify individual and community problems rather than to solve them. But if one sees that the purpose of Auroville is individual and collective progress, and if one understands that such progress is impossible unless all personal and collective problems are confronted and dealt with fully, then one begins to understand why Auroville is the way it is."[66]

It is for this reason that progress in the process of integral transformation is rather slow. Though some Aurovilians talk about their inner centre, what to do with those citizens who bv self-deception take their ego for the psychic? Can they be prevented from such regressive tendencies in their endeavour for spiritual development? Who will guide those those Aurovilians who lack a transparent sincenty and aspiration for a higher life, the greatest safeguards on the slippery road?

Do Aurovilians have the courage to see that there is a certain lack of coherence in the collective organisation within the community? The Charter of Auroville indicates that 'the City of Dawn' is a place of continual research in human unity. Is the core of Aurovilians strong enough to keep this experiment on the right track in its contribution to the ideal of human unity? Are they willing to learn some useful tools what has been achieved elsewhere, and are they capable of accepting diverse approaches to a shared common goal, without the fear that different new pathways dilute the experiment of their collective yoga?

The citizens of Auroville do not claim to know all the answers to the present global problems; they are nevertheless determined to succeed in their efforts in the spiritual adventure which is based on the integral vision of Sri Aurobindo and the Mother. In this adventure, Auroville stands at the beginning of the beginning and still has a long way to go on the road to genuine human unity. Through the development of the citizen's inner and higher levels of consciousness, the divisive forces occasioned by differences in culture, race, religion, language and lifestyle could be overcome. Despite all its innumerable practical difficulties and all its failures, it is in the diversity of experimentation that Auroville hopes to establish its own identity and that this project can be realised. As a collective experiment for the progress of humanity, Auroville seems to develop gradually with all the perplexities of the complicated human laboratory. Each Aurovilian represents and works out something for humanity, and in order to avoid a gradual collapse of the experiment itself, Aurovilians try to draw ceaselessly on the source of the Divine Force. All the activities in Auroville are opportunities to establish contact with that Divine Consciousness Force, the ultimate supporting principle of Auroville.

NOTES

1. Sri Aurobindo, *The Hour of God,* p 23.
2. Ibid., p.21.
3. Ibid., p.22 Sri. Aurobindo, *The synthesis of Yoga,* p. 23.
4. Sri Aurobindo, *The Synthesis of Yoga,* p.39.
5. Sri Aurobindo, *Letters on Yoga,* p.1281.
6. Sri Aurobindo, *Essays Human and Divine,* p. 340.
7. Sri Aurobindo, *The Foundation of Indian Culture,* p. 59.
8. Sri Aurobindo, *Essays Human and Divine,* p. 322.
9. Sri Aurobindo, *The Life Divine,* p. 828.
10. Sri Aurobindo, *The Human Cycle,* p.l.
11. Sri Aurobindo, *The Synthesis of Yoga,* p.597-598.

12. Ibid., p.593-594.
13. Sri Aurobindo, *Letters on Yoga, p.* 898.
14. Sri Aurobindo, *The Life Divine,* p. 735.
15. Sri Aurobindo, *Letters on Yoga,* p.354.
16. Ibid., p.354-363.
17. Ibid., p. 1607-1608.
18. Ibid., p. 1606.
19. Ibid., p. 1609.
20. Sri Aurobindo, *The Life Divine,* p. 604.
21. Sri Aurobindo, *Letters on Yoga,* p.1606.
22. J. Needleman & D. Lewis, *On the way to self-knowledge,* p 219.
23. Ken Wilber, *A Brief History of Everything,* p. 155.
24. Ken Wilber, *Sex, Ecology, Spirituality,* p.636.
25. B. Scotton, B. Chinen and J. Battista, *Textbook of Transpersonal Psychiatry,* p.33.
26. J. Needleman & D. Lewis, *On the way to self-knowledge,* p. 125-126.
27. Sri Aurobindo, *Letters on Yoga,* p. 1609.
28. J. Kripal, *Vishnu on Freud's desk,* p. 449.
29. Sri Aurobindo, *Letters on Yoga,* p. 619.
30. Ibid., p. 613.
31. Ibid., p. 621.
32. Ibid., p. 610.
33. Ibid., p. 792.
34. Ibid., p. 1567.
35. Ibid., p. 1563.
36. Ibid., p. 324.
37. Ibid., p. 1566.
38. Ibid., p. 1347.

39. Ibid., p. 1506.
40. Ibid., p. 218.
41. Sri Aurobindo, *The Hour of God p. 72.*
42. Sri Aurobindo, *On Hintself,* p. 209
43. Sri Aurobindo, *The Synthesis of Yoga.,* p. 727.
44. Ibid., p 39'
45. Ken Wilber, Transformation of Consciousness, p 146.
46. Ken Wilber, *Integral Psychology,* p. 113.
47. Sri Aurobindo, *The Life Divine,* p. 299.
48. Ibid., p. 835.
49. Ibid., p. 835.
50. Sri Aurobindo, *Letters on Yoga,* p. 47.
51. Sri Aurobindo, *The Problem of Rebirth,* p. 24-25.
52. Ibid., p. 104-105.
53. A. Basu, *The relevance of Sri Aurobindo today,* p. 25-26.
54. R. Coan, *Human Consciousness and its Evolution,* p. 21.
55. D.P. Chattopadhyaya, *Sri Aurobindo and K. Marx,* p. 216.
56. Ibid., p. 218.
57. Ibid., p. 250.
58. Ibid., p. 197-198.
59. *Mother India;* Volume XX, No.10-11, 1968, p. 4.
60. Sri Aurobindo, *The Life Divine,* p. 1062.
61. J.K. Mukherjee, *Sri Aurobindo Ashram,* p. XXIII
62. Ibid., p. 18.
63. Ibid., p. 51.
64. Ibid., p. 66.
65. *Mother's Agenda,* 20.09.1969.
66. Auroville, Auroville Publication Group, p.6.

Epilogue

Psychology has become a 'dusty discipline'. It is being eaten alive by the scientific approaches of the Right-Hand quadrants (such as cognitive science) and it is being dissolved and deconstructed by the mean green meme in the Left-Hand quadrants. It [psychology] seems to be on its last legs.[1]

A direct experiential and experimental psychology seems to be demanded if psychology is to be a science and not merely a mass of elementary and superficial generalisations with all the rest guesswork or uncertain conclusion or inference. We must see, feel, know directly what we observe; our interpretations must be capable of being sure and indubitable; we must be able to work surely on a ground of sure knowledge.[2]

In a recent interview with Shambhala Publications, Ken Wilber officially announced his resignation from the transpersonal psychology movement and his withdrawal from his work as a consulting editor of *The Journal of Transpersonal Psychology*. He resigned because of differences with the major role players of the transpersonal movement, which have led to an impasse in which none of the factions has much to offer the others and where they will likely never to be able to agree with each other. These divisions within the ranks are related to their idea of the nature, scope and role of transpersonal psychology. There is also a great deal of disagreement as to what constitutes transpersonal psychology. Ken Wilber categorizes the four major factions of transpersonal psychology as:

1. the magic-mythic group, which tends to confuse

prerational mythic forms with transrational formless Spirit (New Age);

2. the altered states group, which looks at temporary non-ordinary states, avoids development, stages and sustained practices (retro-Romantics);
3. the postmodernists, with their pluralistic relativism, criticise universalism and the perennial philosophy, which finally leads to boomeritus;
4. the integral school incorporates the essentials of all the other schools "but that is exactly what is sharply disputed by all of them".

Ken Wilber set forth the theory that integral psychology will no longer be affiliated with the transpersonal movement and will be referred to, from now on, as an integral approach wider than any particular approach to psychology. The many positive and brilliant insights and contributions of these four approaches have to be included in a more integral approach but taken by themselves, they lead to difficulties because each of them ignores other equally important aspects of the psyche.

Differentiating the first-tier and second-tier approaches within his integral model, Ken Wilber felt a need to establish the Integral Institute, in an attempt to bring together second-tier thinkers who will use Integral solutions to today's problems in education, medicine, politics, business, ecology, spirituality, and art. In an announcement of the formation of the Integral Institute, he describes it in this way: "Integral Institute is a non-profit organization dedicated to the integration of body, mind, soul and spirit in self, culture and nature. This integral vision attempts to honor and integrate the largest amount of research from the greatest number of disciplines—including the natural sciences (physics, chemistry, biology, neurology, ecology), art, ethics, religion, psychology, politics, business, sociology, and spirituality. Integral Institute is dedicated to the proposition that piecemeal approaches to the world's problems—war, hunger, disease, famine, over-population, housing, technology, education—not only no longer help but often compound the problem, and they need to be replaced by approaches that are more comprehensive, systematic, encompassing—and integral."[3]

The members of the Integral Institute, using integral approaches to all the above-mentioned fields, "are trying to position themselves as surfing the front crest of that rising incoming wave of second-tier consciousness." The younger generation will receive training in all aspects of integral thinking and integral practice and carry on the integral vision in the future. The gathering of second-tier researchers and integral theorists creates, some sort of sanctuary where integral second-tier research and writing can occur and where they can come together to share their ideas and experiments.

The general vision that guides the Integral Institute is mainly based on the all-quadrant, all-level model, a union of subjective (I), intersubjective (we) and objective (it) dimensions of reality. This four quadrant model is able to examine parallel developments in each quadrant, i.e., developmental stages in each quadrant correspond with developments in the others. At the moment there are four hundred members and various branches (psychology, business, politics, medicine, education, art, spirituality and media) and each of them has its "core teams", gifted and influential integral theorists and researchers in a specific area. Each of the branches is giving and receiving research from all the others, as the findings of one field will have direct relevance to other fields.

At times Ken Wilber's all-quadrant, all-level model, which attempts to integrate the scientific system approach and metaphysical system speculation, has the tendency to be immune to criticism. In two published interviews of Ken Wilber with Shambhala Publications, entitled *On Critics, Integral Institute, My Recent Writing and Other Matters of Little Consequence and Do Critics Misrepresent My Position?* as well as the Introductions of *The Collective Works,* he gives the reader detailed explanation regarding the various criticism he has received and the motives for the discriminative and argumentative attitude found in his later works. For Ken Wilber, a healthy scepticism rather than blind faith or a critical and sometimes even polemical attitude is a proper guide for him on the road to truth. An integral vision can never flourish in the domain of deconstructive postmodernism or of pluralistic relativism infected with emotional narcissism of the baby boom generation. He claims his occasional polemical and sarcastic tone in *Sex, Ecology, Spirituality; A Brief History of Everything* and *The Eye of Spirit* was necessary in order to remove the major barriers to a universal integralism. Ken Wilber assumes that most of the critical reactions to his works largely reflect a green-meme (first- tier) attack on his second-tier thinking. In the introduction to Volume 8 of *The'Collective Works,* he defends himself, as follows, in a rather emotional tone: "In today's climate of postmodern pluralism, since there is no such thing as *objective* truth, then arguments are conducted almost entirely by attacking the *subject* who holds the beliefs. ... the easiest way to fight this integral view is not to engage the ideas and evidence head on, but simply to try to discredit me as a person (the two most common forms: I don't fit their version of spiritual, and I am apparently slightly more authoritarian than Mussolini). Those charges are made exclusively by people who have never met me, which I think speaks volumes. ... Moreover, my work is such an imposing structure, many theorists feel that in order to make their own contributions, they have to differentiate themselves from me by attacking me—the only way they can make a name for themselves is by tearing me down. ...

I have one major rule: *Everybody* is right. More specifically, everybody—including me—has some important pieces of truth, and all of those pieces need to be honored, cherished, and included in a more gracious, spacious, and compassionate embrace.... My critical writings have never attacked the central beliefs of any discipline, only the claims that the particular discipline has the only truth—and on those grounds I have often been harsh. But every approach, I honestly believe, is essentially true but partial. And on my own tombstone, I dearly hope that someday they will write: He was true but partial" 4

Most of Ken Wilber's criticism in these three books is directed towards the green-meme approach, and is an attempt to get green to examine their own views more extensively. Ken Wilber expresses his anger at the deconstructive postmodernists through his second-tier criticism of the first-tier green wave. Most of the hostile criticism he received came from the greens, who look at his second-tier views but see nothing except their first-tier stage. Ken Wilber assumes that these green critics simply project their own shadows onto him.

In an Online dialogue between Ken Wilber and Allen Combs, on their differences regarding states and structures of consciousness Allen-describes such an attack on Ken Wilber as follows: "it is no honor to original thinkers of the caliber of Plotinus, Sri Aurobindo or Jean Gebser to lump them into a kind of jargon-laden transpersonal soup with *Great Chain of Being* as the stock, as if their original writings could really be geometrically compounded in some uncompromised fashion. *Syncretism* (the idea that all great religions and philosophies are at the same core) was popular in the late days of antiquity, and is again popular today. Perhaps it contains a serving of truth, but boiling everyone down into the same pot does not do justice to their all- important individual flavors. It gets worse ... Wilber's efforts to glue a stack of subtle planes of being on top of integral consciousness in order to make it more spiritual is like pouring sugar into spring water to make it more clear."[5]

In a reply to this attack Ken Wilber writes; "Actually, in my 'whole model' there are the temporary states, the levels of consciousness, and the various developmental lines that move through these levels. Combs is here completely confusing them, and thus once again claims that I don't differentiate them. What Combs is doing, I believe, is using he phase-2 model presented in *Up from Eden,* as most of his attacks do. I accept those attacks, belatedly, as accurate criticism of a view I held 15 years ago…he [Allen] is not very good at interpreting even the major themes of my work beyond the Up from Eden period."[6]

Ken Wilber does admit that much of the misrepresented reviews of his work are related to the huge amount of his written material which makes it hard for anyone to grasp it accurately. In his multiple perspectives on different issues, Ken Wilber outlines several different meanings of the topic and he includes all of them in his integral theory. Merely focusing on one of his simplified or popularised statements often creates misleading accounts of his real position. To get a whole picture one has to read at least six or seven of his books, including the endnotes as they present his technically correct but often obscure views. Fortunately, he has also received negative but accurate and constructive criticism from second-tier readers. Those criticisms that he found valid were incorporated into subsequent writings. All the criticism related to misrepresentations of his work has spurred him to start teaching his materials and disclosing his views personally to the outside world.

Ken Wilber's style of argument and his harsh critique of those who offer thoughtful and critical reflections and who disagree with parts of his integral model are not always appreciated by his opponents within the transpersonal movement. It is often difficult for them to relate Ken

Wilber's engagement in critical discourse on the vision-logic level with his dismissive commentaries and sometimes combative attitudes that are contrary to transpersonal values and discriminating wisdom. Polemical language could be counterproductive to the effort to reach a deeper insight if it lacks cooperation and sympathy for the critical views of his opponents.

This author has attempted not to distort or misrepresent Ken Wilber's views in order to establish his own views or to highlight his own position and concerns. To present Ken Wilber's integral views faithfully and to avoid misrepresentations of his insights it was necessary to use his own words to a great extent, often even without using quotation marks.

When Ken Wilber incorporates Sri Aurobindo's ideas in his comprehensive theory, he does not always quote Sri Aurobindo's writings directly, and it is often not clear which aspects of Ken Wilber's ideas are originally his own and which one's he borrowed from Sri Aurobindo and other integral thinkers. In his attempt 'to transcend and include' in order to differentiate his own from narrower or less inclusive approaches, is Ken Wilber paying sufficient attention to the overall aim of that which he differentiates? He frequently attempts to find parallels with Sri Aurobindo's integral approach but, while doing so, he often leaves out the profound differences between the two approaches.

The aim of Ken Wilber's integral approach is One Taste, where the individual merges with the unified consciousness of the non-dual Spirit. In One Taste, "subject [as the unmanifest world of 'empty' consciousness] and object [the manifest world] are *both* distinct realities *and* aspects of the same thing: a true unity-in-diversity."[7] In the realisation of One Taste, having completely transcended the world of Form, consciousness awakens to a radical embrace of all Form, i.e., there is a perfect union of the manifest and unmanifest, and the finite world is included in the infinite Spirit. Ken Wilber, like Shankara's Advait Vedanta puts this ultimate 'transcend and include' as follows:

> This world is illusory
> Brahman alone is real
> Brahman is the world."[8]

The absolute Self, as pure radiant Emptiness, is the goal and ground of the entire manifest world. But this view does not solve the problem between the ultimate Reality as emptiness and the illusion of object/subject in the other three quadrants. When he relates consciousness to depth, Ken Wilber does not mean depth which is qualifiable, such as sensation, perception or intention, as these particular levels of depth are all forms of consciousness. According to Ken Wilber, "Consciousness is not a thing or a process—we can just as well, with William James, deny that it even exists, because it is ultimately Emptiness, the opening or clearing in which *the form* of beings *manifests* themselves and not any *particular* manifestation itself.... The Being of beings is depth, which, being unqualifiable as such, is finally Emptiness as such (consciousness as such)."[9] Consciousness is, therefore, not an emergent quality but it allows qualities to emerge.

For Ken Wilber, consciousness as depth increases with the complexity of forms in the ascending scale of development until it experiences itself at the level of One Taste, where it is liberated and has no further need of forms. As mentioned above, Ken Wilber relates the realisation of the ultimate Reality with emptiness, however, such a realisation does not seem to bridge the status of the forms in the other three quadrants. In the realm of manifestation, we are never without these quadrants, but in the formless there are no quadrants. If these quadrants are absorbed into emptiness, does this mean that they are ultimately illusory?

Ken Wilber's integral approach does not only focus on the relative or manifest planes in order to arrive at relative solutions, as this would leave out the infinite Spirit as the ground of all four quadrants. He is aware that ultimate solutions are not found in relative mental constructions, but in the development of the nondual pure awareness of One Taste that persists through waking, dream and deep sleep states. A full understanding of any solution involves therefore the development of consciousness that discloses the supramental states of nondual awareness. In Ken Wilber's integral Kosmic framework the four quadrants, as the forms of the manifest phenomenal world on the relative plane, ultimately arise from nondual Spirit. Only by going beyond the forms into the formless realms are contradictions dissolved and only then is the seeker able to realise Oneness with the entire Kosmos.

Sri Aurobindo acknowledges the existence of the transcendent non-dual Spirit, but it seems that Ken Wilber overlooks Sri Aurobindo's idea of the Supermind as a creative Consciousness-Force. In the metaphor of vertical height or the ascent of consciousness into the superconscious, Ken Wilber does mention Sri Aurobindo's supermind, but he uses it in a different context. He points out that "the metaphor of vertical height also works well because in many spiritual experiences, we sense that Spirit is *descending* from above into us (a factor emphasised in many spiritual practices, from Aurobindo's descent of supermind to the Gnostics' descent of the holy spirit). We reach up to Spirit with Eros; Spirit reaches down to us with Agape."[10] In describing the descent as the Agape of the supermind, he relates this descent to goodness, compassion and universal love of the Kosmos reaching down to us. According to Ken Wilber, "Many Tantric and yogic schools--Aurobindo's for example — put prime emphasis on 'the descent of the supermind', the agape of the supermind that 'comes down' in order to pull us up to an identity with it, so that we then express that agape or compassion for all beings now 'in' us."[11]

For Sri Aurobindo, the supreme Reality is basically Consciousness and it contains within itself a Consciousness Force which, when manifested, becomes an active, dynamic Creative-Force. The creative Consciousness- Force of Brahman is responsible for the process of evolution. This Force, as the Becoming, is the action of the Conscious Being and its results are forms of that Conscious Being, i.e., matter, life, mind, soul and spirit. Consciousness-Force, as an expression of the universal force of life, manifests as physical energy in matter and emotional energy in all living beings. This Consciousness-Force, as an expression of evolved consciousness is able to interact with any form up to sub-atomic levels, though it is not dependent on forms. For Sri Aurobindo, "the supramental Consciousness-Force from above and the evolving Consciousness-Force from behind the veil acting on the awakened awareness and will of the mental human being would accomplish by their united power the momentous transition."[12] Only the supramental consciousness can bring about an integral transformation and transform the human life into a divine life. Such transformation cannot be reached merely through a process of spiritual ascent of consciousness but needs the descent of this higher spiritual consciousness into life and matter in order to transform each and every aspect of existence. In Sri Aurobindo's integral Yoga, this supramentai Consciousness-Force is the real force for the transformation of the postmodern stages of development, unlike Ken Wilber's psycho-spiritual development, which culminates in the liberation of a nondual pure consciousness. In integral sadhana, once "One Taste" is realized after a prolonged preparatory stage the seeker must bring down this realisation to the exterior world and change the conditions of life upon earth until an integral transformation is accomplished. In Sri Aurobindo's sadhana, the Brahman experience is not excluded from his Yoga, it is a necessary stage which can be achieved only after a prolonged period of self-discipline. Sadhana in integral Yoga is a means to expedite the descent of the supramental Consciousness-Force. As the Consciousness-Force descends in matter and radiates, it seeks fit instruments to express and manifest itself. The more the instrument is open, the better are the results. The aim of integral Yoga is therefore not merely liberation *from* life, but a total transformation *of* human life and action on earth. In other words, his goal is the evolution of the human race living a life divine.

Sri Aurobindo did not want to establish a school of philosophy, an integral institute or any isms, but "to create a ground of spiritual growth and experience and a way which will bring down a greater Truth beyond mind but not inaccessible to the human soul and consciousness."[13] In integral Yoga the sadhak aims at bringing down a new consciousness into life, and a change in the physical, vital and nervous being, so that they become fit instruments of the truth. The Ashram is a centre of spiritual life which serves as a means to bring down the higher consciousness and make it a power for a divine life on earth. The practice of his yoga needs not only individual effort, but also the influence of the Divine Grace or the direct guidance of a Guru, who represents to the disciple the divine wisdom and conveys to the seeker something of the divine ideal.

Ken Wilber admits that he is not a Guru but a pandit. A Guru accepts devotees and when the compassion of the Guru meets the devotion of the disciple then the Guru absorbs the karma of the devotee. The intense bond between the Guru and devotee is an important part of the devotee's awakening and transformation. Ken Wilber does not take people as devotees or disciples and work with them personally because he does not want to be a Guru and enter into a therapist/client relationship with people. He admits that he is not qualified "to wrestle with people over their spiritual destinies". He tries instead to legitimise spiritual practice within Western secularised culture and to find an academic basis for it. As a writer he may reach thousands of people, and his intellectual approach (at the integral visionlogic level) to spirituality, combined with his integral transformative practice makes him an ideal Western pandit.

Ken Wilber's integral psychotherapy aims not at a mere development and integration of the surface empirical self, but also at the discovery of the central being (Atman). His integral transformative practice includes exercises on all the major levels of the human bodymind—physical, emotional, mental, social, cultural and spiritual. However, this leaves out Sri Aurobindo's complementary, interdependent intrapsychic processes of aspiration and surrender to the Divine, which depend on faith in the existence of the soul that is conscious of God. Along with this foundation, Sri Aurobindo emphasises an uncompromising movement of rejection of all egoistic habits and insistences, which can be achieved by the realisation and control of the psychic being. When sadhaks are in touch with their psychic being, it becomes possible to open and uplift their whole "lower nature" to the Divine and it becomes possible to purify the external nature. After its purification, the surface nature is able to function as an instrument fit for the manifestation of the divine in one's life, which then becomes a 'life divine'. Once one's psychic being has come to the fore, a group of sadhaks must simultaneously try to transform the external world by bringing down collectively the divine into it. This means that various transformed sadhaks together must have the corresponding effect in stimulating cultural, social and educational transformation.

By moving from Wilber-II to Wilber-III and Wilber-IV and adopting his all-quadrant, all-level model, Ken Wilber was not denying Sri Aurobindo's integral vision but enriching it. While discussing with Ken Wilber (via a series of e-mail exchanges) the attitude of the Whiteheadian defenders who are not able to extend Whitehead's enterprise in order to fill in the blanks, Keith Thompson sees a similarly constrained attitude in the Aurobindonians. He has "never understood the impulse of 'Aurobindonians' who say that Aurobindo's system is 'complete'. (It is not; Wilber has identified weak areas and fleshed them out impressively)."[14] This lack of completeness may be interpreted as an omission on the part of Sri Aurobindo but, in fact, he did not overlook the social, cultural and scientific context in the process of transformation to the divine life. His metaphysics include a socio-cultural orientation and in his writings these issues are definitely one of his major concerns, although they were not his *central* or ultimate concern. In *The Human Cycle* and *Foundations of Indian Culture,* Sri Aurobindo deals systematically and comprehensively with the social and cultural life of man, indicating the effects of the individual's spiritual development upon the evolution of man's socio-cultural life. Sri Aurobindo elaborated extensively on the interaction between the. evolution of the Upper Left quadrant and the transformation of the Upper Right, Lower Right and Lower Left quadrants. No doubt, Sri Aurobindo did emphasise the individual "subjective quadrant" as this determines and is an expression of the "objective quadrant". Ken Wilber's all-quadrant, all-level approach aims at a multi-causal analysis without reducing one to the other. Could it be that the weak areas that Ken Wilber identified are more closely related to Sri Aurobindo's disciples than to his vision?

Ken Wilber claims that his integral model is a refinement of Sri Aurobindo's integral view as it provides an opening to the contributions of Western psychology and psychotherapy, and is set in the context of the all-quadrant all-level model. Ken Wilber maintains that without integrating these contributions Sri Aurobindo's integral yoga remains limited and partial. As long as Aurobindonians remain enclosed in Sri Aurobindo's revealed teachings, treating them as final truths, and refuse to link Sri Aurobindo's integral Yoga with contemporary scientific and spiritual research and its practical concerns, it becomes difficult to for them to gain insight into Ken Wilber's critical questioning and his assumed improvement of Sri Aurobindo's vision. Without integrating the developments and insights from other systems of contemporary Eastern spiritual disciplines and modern Western psychology, merely preserving and repeating the original psychological insights of Sri Aurobindo limits the scope of his yoga psychology and makes his vision exclusive.

The author, while critically examining the core assumptions and claims of each, tried to overcome this barrier by giving equal importance to the integrative perspectives of both Sri Aurobindo and Ken Wilber, and by sympathetically exploring the points of convergence as well as points of divergence in the two views.

Ken Wilber outlines "a dozen different fields of consciousness studies, all of which need to be brought together in an integral view: cognitive science, introspectionism, neuropsychology, individual psychotherapy, developmental psychology, psychosomatic medicine, non-ordinary states of consciousness, Eastern and contemplative traditions, quantum consciousness approaches, and subtle energy research. ... each of them has something extremely important and valuable to say. And that means, inescapably, that we will measure our progress towards a truly integral orientation based precisely on our capacity to include, synthesize, and integrate all twelve of those important approaches ... anything less than that simply cannot claim the adjective integral."[15] In his attempt to unify all the various aspects of human knowledge, Ken Wilber honours the scientific and spiritual dimensions of man. If the disciples of Sri Aurobindo omit a dialogue about the insights gained through these twelve approaches and maintain that such components are merely palliatives which leave the ordinary consciousness fundamentally the same, and that a radical change from the ordinary consciousness to the divine consciousness is only possible through the of descent of Grace and the practice of integral Yoga, then it becomes difficult to bridge the gulf between Sri Aurobindo's metaphysical Yoga psychology and Ken Wilber's endeavor to unify all the various aspects of modern human and spiritual knowledge. In his integral approach, Sri Aurobindo never overlooked historical contributions in other fields of knowledge, and it is up to his followers to integrate the benefits and contributions of modern contemporary Eastern and Western psychology. The true scientist according to Sri Aurobindo is "always ready to reconsider old conclusions in the light of new facts, to give a candid consideration to every new idea or old idea revived if it deserves a hearing, no matter how contradictory it may be of previously ascertained experience or previously formed conclusion, is the sceptical temper, the temper of the inquirer, the true scientist."[16]

It may be necessary that the integral views Sri Aurobindo once held have to be partially modified by his followers in the field of present-day knowledge. Ken Wilber's current integral views may likewise soon be seen as naive. That's why further revision of both integral approaches is necessary for future application to each seeker's unique life and circumstances.

Before arriving at giving Ken Wilber credit for his integral reconstruction of science, based on the quadrant model, it may be useful to refer once more to his integral approach to science, consciousness, and spirituality.

In order to arrive at a spiritual science of the transcendental realm, Ken Wilber meaningfully distinguishes 'narrow' science, which uses sensorimotor experiences tied to a rational analysis, from 'broad' science, which uses empiricism in a wider fashion, including direct mental and spiritual experiences as presented to consciousness. Each science is based on the investigation of its specific objects or phenomena. In their truth claims, both types of science share the three common tests for knowledge: injunction, experience and confirmation, though each has its own domain and its own degree of certainty. Besides this distinction between 'narrow' and 'broad' science, Ken Wilber also classifies various levels of science which he relates to the various levels of consciousness: sensory or gross science refers to narrow science, whereas mental or subtle science and spiritual or causal science refer to interpretative and spiritual phenomena respectively. For Ken Wilber, different stages of consciousness development require different spiritual approaches. On its pre-rational level, spirituality can best be approached through image, metaphor and faith in myths. At the rational stage, spirituality involves a rational scientific approach through faith in reason. At the transrational level, spirituality shifts from the contents of the mind to the contents of the spirit and can best be approached through direct practice. This transpersonal spirituality is akin to Ken Wilber's postmetaphysical science; its conclusions are not based on dogmatic theories but on the evidence of those individuals who have demonstrated developmental competence confirmed by reconstructive science.

This postmetaphysical view is meaningfully described by Ken Wilber as follows: "although all of the contemplative traditions aim at going within and beyond reason, they all *start* with reason, start with the notion that truth is to be established by *evidence*, that truth is the result of *experimental* methods, that truth is to be tested in the laboratory of personal experience, that these truths are open to all those who wish to *try the experiment* and thus disclose *for themselves* the truth or falsity of the spiritual claims—and that dogmas or given beliefs are precisely what hinder the emergence of the deeper truths and wider visions.... the claims about these higher domains are a *conclusion* based on hundreds of years of experimental introspection and communal verification. ... These spiritual endeavors, in other words, are purely scientific in any meaningful sense of the word, and the systematic presentations of these endeavors follow precisely those of any *reconstructive science.*"[17]

For Ken Wilber, each higher level of complexity is not a predetermined or fixed set of levels through which each and every individual must pass on one's own realisation, but an open field of developmental potentials for higher functioning. Only when the higher or subtle levels of consciousness emerge or unfold in various people does it become something of a fixed level and a cosmic pattern with universal features for future development. Ken Wilber maintains that before a particular level of higher consciousness emerges in evolution, that higher stage can unfold in an infinite number of ways; it is determined and formed by the four quadrants, which are constantly changing. This pattern can be investigated by reconstructive science on the basis of extensive empirical phenomenological and experiential research on stages of development.

For Sri Aurobindo, the objective ultimate truth of science is not able to explain all subjective domains of our being which lie behind the obvious surface levels. Nevertheless, subjectivity and objectivity are interdependent realities, as the Being offers itself to its own consciousness as object to the subject and looks at itself as subject on the object. We know the objective universe through our subjective consciousness whose instruments are the physical senses.

There is no difference in the essential laws of the objective physical and the subjective psychical, they only differ in their energies, instrumentation and exact processes. The subjective phenomena must be pursued by a subjective method of inquiry, observation and verification. Research into subjective yogic experiences which belong to an inner domain requires exact observation and scrupulous experimentation but it must evolve, accept and test other means and methods which are used in the examination of the objective external realm. It needs the capacity of spiritual experience and the inner methods by which that experience and verification are made possible. In Sri Aurobindo's yoga psychology we deal with subtle, flexible materials that exceed common physical science. Its field is wider than modern psychology, as it includes experiences beyond sense perception and beyond rationality; i.e., it uses subtler inner senses and intuitive perception to evaluate those experiences pertaining to higher states of consciousness. Through this direct psychological instrumentation, the seeker can arrive at certain data and results that can be verified by "sure data" and by the results of other sadhaks, like Ken Wilber's reconstructive science.

To test the validity of spiritual experience, Sri Aurobindo's yoga psychology uses a method that is similar to Ken Wilber's research methodology in the higher levels of consciousness. It requires a genuine knowledge through the accumulation of direct experience or apprehension of data (direct apprehension), an all-round actual practice (instrumental injunction), and an intuitive discrimination for its verification (communal confirmation or rejection). *Any sadhak who is not prepared to go through the vast field of spiritual phenomena has to accept the guidance of the Guru until the seeker has accumulated sufficient experience and knowledge of the inner and higher subtle forces.*

From what is described above, it should be clear that

in his integral approach to science and spirituality, Ken Wilber does not only correlate the various *types* of science with his four quadrant model, but he also correlates major *levels* of science with the various levels of human existence: sensory, mental and spiritual. He does not reduce the higher realms to mere science. Science (it) is only one third of the gross subtle and causal realm. These levels include art (I), and morals (We). Each level follows its own different methodology and validity claims. By incorporating the higher spiritual realm in his model, he creates an academic basis for a spiritual worldview. This does not mean that he reduces spirituality to rationality, on the contrary, his postmetaphysical approach offers a scientifically reliable understanding of spirituality. Ken Wilber does not want to mystify plain facts and he uses his quadrant model in order to explain his theory of everything without merely using a transcendental hypothesis. His comprehensive theory construction tries to unite all kinds of disparate facts together and his postmetaphysical approach has a necessary relation with the present facts of life. In the practice of spiritual discipline, the results of academic research go side by side with the results of the search for one's inner being. However, ultimately, only Spirit (the depths of one's inner being without objects, thoughts, space and time) is the evidence for Spirit.

Sri Aurobindo, like Ken Wilber, is not denying scientific development and the pragmatic truth which science offers to humanity. He preserves the truths of material science and its real usefulness in the final harmony, although many of its existing forms have to be broken or left aside. Sri Aurobindo, unlike Ken Wilber, attributed his spiritual achievements mainly to the practice of his integral Yoga, and not with the help of academic empirical research. His metaphysical vision is hardly based on the objective approach which is related to observable facts and sense experience. On the contrary, his subjective approach is more related to intuition, insight and introspection, which makes his concept of man highly metaphysical and speculative for those people who are not able to move beyond the rational realm.

Should the followers of Sri Aurobindo include in their integral model the rational and academic approach with a view to determine its degree of authenticity (vertical transformation; permanent and ultimate) and legitimacy (horizontal translation; temporary and relative)? A translative spirituality focuses on autonomous individuals who consciously choose communities of other autonomous individuals, whereas transformative spirituality relates to the transformative opening of spirituality in terms of true authenticity.

It is the external and experimental verification that confers its potentially believable status to us and, even within broad limits, allows us to judge the relative degree of maturity or authenticity of the transrational or spiritual development of a particular person. What happens if the upward movement to self-realisation and self-transcendence begins to go sour when the followers demand allegiance to the Guru's worldview without their own rational and logical inquiry and postconventional needs?

Reason has certainly a legitimate part to play in relation to the higher fields of one's spiritual experience and divine knowledge, even though that part is quite subordinate. Describing the utility of the intellect in the context of yogic development, Sri Aurobindo insists that, although "the intellect cannot be a sufficient guide in the search for spiritual truth and realisation, yet it has to be utilised in the integral movement of our nature. ... The seeking intelligence has to be trained to admit a certain large questioning, an intellectual rectitude not satisfied with half-truths, mixtures of error or approximations and, most positive and helpful, a perfect readiness always to move forward from truths already held and accepted to the greater correction, completing or transcending truths which at first it was unable or, it may be, disinclined to envisage. A working faith of the intellect is indispensable, not a superstitious, dogmatic or limiting credence attached to every temporary support or formula, but a large assent to the successive suggestions and steps of the Shakti, a faith fixed on realities, moving from the lesser to the completer realities and ready to throw down all scaffolding and keep only the large and growing structure."[18]

Aided by his overall spectrum model of human development, Ken Wilber's approach is able to demonstrate the nature of a *bona fide* authentic spiritual movement. In his all-level all-quadrant model, all waves and streams of development, and states and types of consciousness, can be disclosed by reputable non-reductionistic researchers who are working with second and third-tier conceptions.

What is the present state of Sri Aurobindo's disciples? Are those who have moved to second-tier consciousness (yellow and turquoise) ready to open up to the conclusions from researchers working with second or third-tier conceptions, using premodern, modern and postmodern sources?

. Researchers working with these conceptions may be able to investigate certain developmental events which may turn 'pathological' in the process of realisation of the Aurobindonians' ideals, when 'the higher' do not transcend and include 'the lower' but deny and abuse the lower in the service of the emergence of the higher. Such events are not only related to individual processes but can also be applied to socio-cultural aspects of development, where progress comes at the cost of the exploitation of the lower members of the community. The effect of such pathological events on new levels needs to be critically reviewed.

Sri Aurobindo did not care to have his name in any blessed place—for serious work, advertisement or propaganda is a poison, "as it means either a stunt or a boom—and stunts and booms exhaust the things they carry on their crest and leave it lifeless and broken high and dry on the shores of nowhere—or it means a movement. A movement in the case of a work like mine means the founding of a school or a sect or some other damned nonsense. It means that hundreds or thousands of useless people join in and corrupt the work or reduce it to a pompous farce from which the Truth that was coming down recedes into a secrecy and silence. It is that what has happened to the 'religions' and is the reason of their failure."[19]

Sri Aurobindo had no intention of becoming a 'traditional Guru'. As a phase-specific authority, he guided the devotees during the awakening of their true self and as such Sri Aurobindo as a teacher is a virtual necessity on the road. But at some point in the journey when this centre of the Self gradually awakes, Sri Aurobindo's authority as a guru gradually diminishes. He did not encourage dependency on his legacy. On the contrary, he emphasised the disciples using their own spiritual resources to find the true guidance within.

Sri Aurobindo describes the Teacher of integral yoga as follows: "The wise Teacher will not seek to impose himself or his opinions on the passive acceptance of the receptive mind. ... He will give a method as an aid, as a utilisable device, not as an imperative formula or a fixed routine. ... His whole business is to awaken the divine light and set working the divine force of which he himself is only a means and an aid, a body or a channel ... what will most stimulate aspiration in others is the central fact of the divine realisation within him governing his whole life and inner state and all his activities.... It is this dynamic realisation that the Sadhaka must feel and reproduce in himself according to his own nature. ... He is a man helping his brothers, a child leading children, a Light kindling other lights, an awakened Soul awakening souls." [20]

Aurobindonians must be aware that the contexts of any system are constantly shifting. Sri Aurobindo's integral vision, like Ken Wilber's integral theory, is an open-ended system and how it evolves does not depend on Sri Aurobindo's views, but on the attitude of his followers in the Ashram and in Auroville. Those Aurobindonians who like to remain faithful to his tradition should nevertheless be able to readjust or partially refine Sri Aurobindo's open-ended system in order to integrate the discoveries and the demands of contemporary psychological, social, cultural and scientific development that had been hitherto unknown. Do the followers of Sri Aurobindo unjustifiable assume that Sri Aurobindo's spiritual insights are based on an unchanging identity which may be threatened by foreign invaders?

The followers of Sri Aurobindo may have faith and find refuge solely in Sri Aurobindo's metaphysical views, which may comfort them, but through methodical contemplative experiential investigation and research—collecting data from those followers who are already advanced in their sadhana and who are able to compare their spiritual experiment with other seekers (researchers) in the community—the Aurobindonians themselves may be able to explore and verify the authenticity of the spiritual truth with respect to Sri Aurobindo's supramental claims and place them in the context of the mainstream disciplines of psychology, philosophy, sociology, ecology, physics, etc. In other words, through a process of re-experiencing and mastery of the various phenomena at play within the subtle dimensions of the human psyche, using Sri Aurobindo's experiential methodology to reproduce in consciousness his spiritual insights, the sadhak is able to know and verify the experiential foundation of integral Yoga rather than merely depending on the faith in Sri Aurobindo's claims. Are Aurobindonians reducing Sri Aurobindo's integral vision to mere dogmatic theories and thereby becoming counterproductive? And are they not opening their approach to outside research and evidence because it does not fit their prevailing convictions and belief system, or are some genuine aspirants able to experiment with and integrate the results of the scientific, technological and information revolution with the overall insights as expounded by Sri Aurobindo?

It is the spirit of free inquiry that is able to unsettle dogmatism and comfortable beliefs. This spirit of free inquiry finds its expression, not only in the fields of physical science and technology, but also in fields beyond its narrow departments. Those Aurobindonians who do not easily accept the spirit of critical inquiry into Sri Aurobindo's vision may easily produce a mood in which they omit any rational scrutiny. However, Sri Aurobindo does not present his integral vision as a finished creed or dogma to be accepted without questioning, but as a subject of experiment and research. This yoga proceeds from the initial belief to the investigation of it, so that each sadhak knows Sri Aurobindo's claims to be true for him or herself.

Recently the Sri Aurobindo Centre of Reseach for Human Unity was inaugurated in Auroville (C.I.R.H.U). This all-encompassing university-like centre functions for interaction between Auroville and the world. It provides a platform for research on the world's quest for human unity, and welcomes research scholars from all over the world to take part in the Auroville experiment while Aurovilians can benefit from their knowledge and expertise. Despite the various differences between the two approaches, it seems that there are also striking similarities between the experimental project of Auroville and Ken Wilber's Integral Institute: both projects aim at bringing together the ancient spiritual wisdom of the East with the material achievements of the West, in order to create new integral solutions to the global problems of life. The members of Ken Wilber's Integral Institute and the citizens of Auroville aim in their research activities to change their present human consciousness, i.e., an exploration of psychological ranges of man's inner and higher consciousness. Could Auroville offer a contribution in bringing forth some fresh perspectives to the noble endeavour of the all-quadrant, all-level approach where the physical, emotional, mental and spiritual levels of being are exercised simultaneously in the I, we, and it domains? At the same time, could the establishment of the Integral Institute offer some methods to those Aurobindonians who are in the process of re-evaluating Sri Aurobindo's vision in the context of contemporary scientific development without deconstructing the deeper contents of Sri Aurobindo's integral insights?

NOTES

1. Ken Wilber Online, *A Shambhala Interview,* p. 6.
2. Sri Aurobindo, *Essays Divine and Human,* pp. 335-336.
3. Ken Wilber Online, *Announcing the Formation of Integral Institute,* p. 1.
4. Ken Wilber, *The Collective Works,* Introduction, pp. 41-42.
5. Ken Wilber Online, *Allen Comb's Open Reply to Ken Wilber.*
6. Ken Wilber Online, *Ken Wilber's Second Response to Allen Combs.*
7. Ken Wilber, *Integral Psychology,* p.181.

8. Ibid., p. 155.
9. Ken Wilber, *Sex, Ecology, Spirituality,* p.539.
10. Ken Wilber, *Integral Psychology,* p.lll.
11. Ken Wilber, *Sex, Ecology, Spirituality,* p.339.
12. Sri Aurobindo, *The Life Divine,* p.922.
13. Sri Aurobindo, *Letters on Yoga,* p.559.
14. Ken Wilber Online, *Do Critics Misrepresent my Position?* p.14.
15. Ken Wilber, *One Taste,* p.104.
16. Sri Aurobindo, *Essays Divine and Human p.23.*
17. Ken Wilber, *Sex, Ecology, Spirituality,* p.265.
18. Sri Aurobindo, *The Synthesis of Yoga,* p.749.
19. Sri Aurobindo, *On Himself,* p.375.
20. Sri Aurobindo, *The Synthesis of Yoga,* p.60-61.

Bibliography

1. Ajaya, Swami; *Psychotherapy East and West: A Unifying Paradigm,* The Himalayan International Institute, Honesdale, 1985.
2. Aurobindo, Sri; *The Life Divine,* Sri Aurobindo Ashram Publication, Pondicherry; 10th impression, 1993.
3. Aurobindo, Sri; *Essays Divine and Human,* Sri Aurobindo Ashram Publication, Pondicherry, 1994.
4. Aurobindo, Sri; *The Foundations of Indian Culture,* Sri Aurobindo Ashram Publication, Pondicherry. 8th impr., 1995.
5. Aurobindo; Sri/' On *Himself,* Sri Aurobindo Ashram Publication, Pondicherry, 5th impr., 1989.
6. Aurobindo, Sri; *The Hour of God,* Sri Aurobindo Ashram Publication, Pondicherry, 1972.
7. Aurobindb,'Sri; *The Human Cycle,* Sri Aurobindo Ashram Publication, Pondicherry, 6th impr., 1992.
8. Aurobindo, Sri; *Letters on Yoga,* I. II, III, Sri Aurobindo Ashram Publication, Pondicherry, 5th impr., 1988.
9. Aurobindo, Sri; *More Lights on Yoga,* Sri Aurobindo Ashram Publication, Pondicherry, 3rd impr., 1995.
10. Aurobindo, Sri; *The Supramental Manifestation.* Sri Aurobindo Ashram Publication, Pondicherry, 2nd edition, 1989.
11. Aurobindo, Sri; *The Synthesis of Yoga,* Sri Aurobindo Ashram Publication, Pondicherry, 9th impr., 1992.

12. Aurobindo, Sri; *Bases of Yoga,* Sri Aurobindo Ashram Publication, Pondicherry, 5th impr., 1998.

13. Basu, Arabinda; *The Relevance of Sri Aurobindo Today,* Publ. by Manik Mitra, Calcutta, 1975.

14. Basu, Soumitra; *Integral Health,* Sri Aurobindo's Int. Institute for Integral Health and Research, Pondicherry, 2000.

15. Beidler, William; *The Vision of Self in Early Vedanta,* Motilal Banarsidass, New Delhi, 1975.

16. Boorstein, Seymour, Ed; *Transpersonal Psychotherapy,* Science and Behavior Books, Stanford, 1991.

17. Boorstein, Seymour; *Clinical Studies in Transpersonal Psychotherapy,* State University of New York Press, Albany, 1997.

18. Boss, Medard; *A Psychiatrist Discovers India,* Oswald Wolf, London, 1965.

19. Brahma, N. Kanta; *Philosophy of Hindu Sadhana,* Motilal Banarsidas, New Delhi, 1993.

20. Brown, D.J. Peddar; *Introduction to Psychotherapy,* Tavistock Publications Ltd., London, 1979.

21. Chakravorti, Satya Jyoti; *The Philosophy of Sri Aurobindo,* Sterling Publishers, New Delhi, 1991.

22. Chattopadhyaya, D.P; *Sri Aurobindo and Karl Marx:* Integral Sociology and Dialectical Sociology, Motilal Banarsidass, New Delhi, 1991.

23. Chaudhuri, H; *Sri Aurobindo; the Prophet of Life Divine,* Sri Aurobindo Ashram Publication, Pondicherry, 1973.

24. Coan, R. W; *Human Consciousness and Its Evolution,* Greenwood Press Inc., Connecticut, 1987.

25. Corsini, R. J. and Wedding D, editors; *Current Psychotherapies,* F.E. Peacock Publication, Illinois, 1989.

26. Cortright, Brant; *Psychotherapy and Spirit,* State University of New York Press, Albany, 1997.

27. Coxhead, Nanda; *Beyond Psychology: The Potential of Conscious Thinking,* Mandala Press, London, 1991.

28. Dalal, A.S; *Psychology, Mental Health and Yoga,* Sri Aurobindo Ashram Publication, Pondicherry, 1992.

29. Dasgupta, S.N; *History of Indian Philosophy,* Vol. I - V, Motilal Banarsidass, New Delhi, 1975.

30. Deikman, Arthur; *The Observing Self: Mysticism and Psychotherapy,* Beacon Press, Boston, 1982.

31. Deutsch, Eliot; *Humanity and Divinity,* University of Hawaii Press, Honolulu, 1970.

32. Ellis, A; *Why Some Therapies Don't Work; The Dangers of Transpersonal Psychotherapy,* Prometheus Books, Buffalo, 1989.

33. Evans-Wentz, W. Y, Ed; *The Tibetan Book of the Dead,* Oxford University Press, Oxford, reprinted, 1988.

34. Fort, Andrew. O; *The Self and its States,* Motilal Banarsidass, New Delhi, 1990.

35. Gandhi, Kishore; *Social Philosophy of Sri Aurobindo and The New Age,* Sri Aurobindo Ashram, Publication, Pondicherry, 1991.

36. Gay, Peter, Ed; *The Freud Reader,* Vintage, London, 1995.

37. Grof, S; *Beyond the Brain: Birth, Death and Transcendence in Psychotherapy,* State University of New York Press, New York, 1988.

38. Grof S; *The Adventure of Self-Discovery,* Sunny Press, Albany 1988.

39. Grof, C and Grof, S. *The Stormy Search for the Self,* Jeremy. P. Tharcher/ Puntam Book, New York, 1990.

40. Hendricks, G and B. Weinhold; *Transpersonal Approaches to Counseling and Psychotherapy,* Love Publishing Company, Denver, 1982.

41. Hillman, James; *Re-visioning Psychology,* Harper Perennial, New York, 1992.

42. Hiriyanna, M; *Outlines of Indian Philosophy,* Motilal Banarsidass, New Delhi, 1994.

43. Hiriyanna, M; *The Essentials of Indian Philosophy,* George Allen and Urwin Ltd, Bombay, 1973.

44. Iyengar, Srinivasa K.R; *Sri Aurobindo, a Biography and a History,* Sri Aurobindo Integral Centre of Education, Pondicherry, 1985.

45. J acobs, Hans; *Western Psychotherapy and Hindu Sadhana,* George Allen and Urwin, London, 1961.

46. Kakar, Sudhir; *The Analyst and the Mystic,* Viking, New Delhi, 1991.

47. Kripal, Jeffrey and T.G. Vaidyananathan; *Vishnu on Freud's Desk; A Reader in Psychoanalysis and Hinduism,* Oxford University Press, New Delhi, 1999.

48. Kovel, Joel; *A Complete Guide to Therapy,* Penguin Books, London, 1991.

49. Maitra, S.K.; *The Philosophy of Sri Aurobindo,* Sri Aurobindo Ashram Publication, Pondicherry 5th impr., 1993.

50. Maitra, S.K; *The Meeting of the East and the West in Sri Aurobindo's Philosophy,* Sri Aurobindo Ashram Publication, Pondicherry, reprinted, 1988.

51. Mann, Richard; *The Light of Consciousness,* Sunny Press, Albany, 1984.

52. Maslow, A; *The Farther Reaches of Human Nature,* The Viking Press, New York 2nd edition, 1968.

53. Maslow, A; *Eupsychian Management,* Irwin Press, Illinois, 1971.

54. Maslow, A; *Psychology of Science,* Regnery, Chicago, 1969.

55. Maslow, A; *Religions, Values, and Peak-Experiences,* The Viking Press, New York, 1970.

56. Maslow, A; *Towards a Psychology of Being,* Van Nostrand Reinhold Comp, 2nd edition, New York, 1968.

57. Misra R.S; *Integral Advaitism of Sri Aurobindo,* Motilal Banarsidass, New Delhi, 1998.

58. Mukherjee, Jugal Kishore; *Sri Aurobindo's Ashram: Its Role, Responsibility and Future Destiny,* Sri Aurobindo International Centre of Education, Pondicherry, 1997.

59. Needleman, J. and D. Lewis, editors; *On the Way to Self-Knowledge,* Alfred A. Knopf Inc, New York, 1976...

60. Nelson, John. E; *Healing the Split: Integrating Spirit Into Our Understanding of the Mentally Ill,* State University of New York Press, Albany, 1993. Okun B. F; *Seeking ConnectionsJn Psychotherapy,* Jossey-Bass Publishers, „ San Francisco, 1990.

61. Organ, Troy Wilson; *The Hindu Quest for the Perfection of Man,* Munshiram Manoharlal Publishers, New Delhi, 1994.

62. Raju, P.T; *The Philosophical Traditions of India,* Motilal Banarsidass, New Delhi, 1992.

63. Raju, P.T; *Spirit, Being and Self,* Motilal Benarsidas , New-Delhi

64. Rama, Swami; *Yoga and Psychotherapy: The Evolution of Consciousness,* The Himalayan Intern. Institute, Honesdale, 1981.

65. Reddy Madhusudan; *Integral Yoga Psychology,* Institute of Human Study, Hyderabad, 1990.

66. Rischabhchand; *The Integral Yoga of Sri Aurobindo,* Sri Aurobindo Memorial Fund Society, Pondicherry, 1974.

67. Rowan, John; *The Transpersonal: Psychotherapy and Counselling,* Routledge, London, 1993.

68. Roy, D.K., *Sri Aurobindo Came to Me,* Sri Aurobindo Ashram Publication, Pondicherry, 1952.

69. Rothberg, D., and Sean Kelly, *Ken Wilber in Dialogue,* Theosophical Publishing House, Wheaton, 1998.

70. Radhakrishnan, S; *Indian Philosophy* Vol I and II, Oxford University Press, New Delhi, 5th impr., 1999.

71. Sachdeva, I.P. *Yoga and Depth Psychology,* Munshiram Manoharlal, New Delhi, 1978.

72. Safaya, Raghunath; *Indian Psychology,* Munshiram Manoharlal, New Delhi, 1976.

73. Saksena, S.K.; *Nature of Consciousness in Hindu Philosophy,* Motilal Banarsidass, 2nd edition, New Delhi, 1971.

74. Satprem, *Sri Aurobindo or the Adventure of Consciousness,* Sri Aurobindo Ashram Publication, Pondicherry reprinted, 1987.

75. Schaef, Wilson; *Beyond Therapy, Beyond Science,* Harper Collins Publishers, New York, 1992.

76. Scotton, Bruce, Allan B. Chinen and John, R. Battista; *Textbook of Transpersonal Psychiatry and Psychology,* Harper Collins Publishers, New York, 1996.

77. Sen Indra; *Integral Psychology: The Psychological System of Sri Aurobindo,* Sri Aurobindo Institute Centre of Education, Pondicherry, 1986.

78. Sharma H.L; *Yoga Technique of Psychotherapy,* G.D.K. Publications, New Delhi, 1979.

79. Sharma, S.L; *The Therapeutic Dialogue: A Theoretical and Practical Guide to Psychotherapy,* University of New Mexico Press, Albuquerque, 1986.

80. Srivastava, G.M.L; *The Yoga of Patanjali and the Integral Yoga of Sri Aurobindo,* Vishwa-kala Prakashan, New Delhi, 1987.

81. Staal, F; *Exploring Mysticism,* Penguin Books Ltd, Middlesex, 1975.

82. Tart, Charles; *Transpersonal Psychologies,* Harper and Row Publishers, New York, 1975.

83. Vaughan, F; *The Inward Arc: Healing and Wholeness in Psychotherapy and Spirituality,* Shambhala Publication, Boston, 1985.

84. Vrinte, Joseph; *The Concept of Personality in Sri Aurobindo's Integral Yoga Psychology and A. Maslow's Humanistic/Transpersonal Psychology,* Munshiram Manoharlal, New Delhi, 1995.

85. Vrinte, Joseph; *The Quest for the Inner* Man, Motilal Banarsidass, New Delhi, 1996.

86. Walsh R, and F. Vaughan; *Beyond Ego: Transcendental Dimensions in Psychology,* Jeremy Thatcher Inc, Los Angeles, 1980.

87. Walsh R, and F. Vaughan, Ed; *Paths Beyond Ego,* Jeremy Thatcher, Los Angeles, 1993.

88. Watts, A; *Psychotherapy East and West,* Penguin Books, Middlesex, 1973. Warrier, E, I; *Sri Aurobindo's Integral Yoga and Shankara's Advaita,* Vohra Publishers, Allahabad, 1990.

89. Weiner, Irwin; *Principles of Psychotherapy,* John Wiley and Sons, N-York, 1975.

90. Wei wood, John, Ed; *Explorations in East/West Psychology: The Meeting of the Ways,* Stocken Books, New York, 1979.

91. Wilber, Ken; *The Atman Project,* Quest Book, Illinois, 1980.

92. Wilber, Ken; *The Spectrum of Consciousness,* A Transpersonal view of Human development. Theosophical Publishing House, Illinois, 1982.

93. Wilber Ken; No *Boundary: Eastern and Western Approaches to Personal Growth,* Shambhala, Boston, 1985.

94. Wilber, Ken; *Up From Eden: A Transpersonal View of Human Evolution,* Routledge and Kegan Paul, London, 1983.

95. Wilber, Ken; *Eye to Eye: The Quest for the New Paradigm,* Shambhala, Boston, 1990.

96. Wilber, Ken and J. Engler, D.P. Brown; *Transformations of Consciousness,* Shambhala, Boston, 1986.

97. Wilber, Ken; *Sex, Ecology, Spirituality, The Spirit of Evolution,* Shambhala, Boston, 1995.

98. Wilber, Ken; *The Eye of Spirit,* Shambhala, Boston, 1997.

99. Wilber, Ken; *The Marriage of Sense and Soul: Integrating Science and Religion,* Random House, New York, 1998.

100. Wilber, Ken; *One Taste: The Journals of Ken Wilber,* Shambhala, Boston, 1999.

101. Wilber, Ken; *Integral Psychology: Consciousness, Spirit, Psychology, Therapy,* Shambhala, Boston, 2000.

102. Wilber Ken, *A Theory of Everything,* An Integral vision for business, politics, science and spirituality. Shambhala, Boston, 2001.

103. Zerg, J.K. and M. Munion Ed; *What is Psychotherapy? Contemporary Perspectives,* Jossey-Bass Publishers, San Francisco, 1990.

Index

D

E

M

N

O

P

Y

JOSEPH VRINTE was born in the Netherlands, graduated from Lucknow University and afterwards joined Rohilkhand University, Bareilly, where he obtained his M.A. psychology/philosophy and his Ph.D.

For the last twenty years he has been working intermittently as a mental health worker in various mental health institutions in the Netherlands.

During the present research work he actively participated in various activities in Auroville, where he lives. Dr. Vrinte, an established researcher in the field of Sri Aurobindo's integral Yoga and the transpersonal psychology movement, is the author of *The Concept of Personality in Sri Aurobindo's Integral Yoga Psychology and A. Maslow's Humanistic/ Transpersonal Psychology*, and *The Quest for the Inner Man.*